I0044330

A Clinical Guide to Maternity and Women's Health Care

A Clinical Guide to Maternity and Women's Health Care

Editor: Tim Grayson

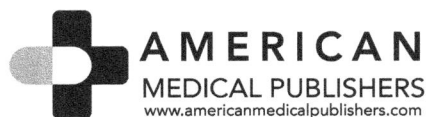

AMERICAN
MEDICAL PUBLISHERS
www.americanmedicalpublishers.com

AMERICAN
MEDICAL PUBLISHERS
www.americanmedicalpublishers.com

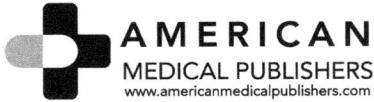

Cataloging-in-Publication Data

A clinical guide to maternity and women's health care / edited by Tim Grayson.
   p. cm.
Includes bibliographical references and index.
ISBN 978-1-63927-444-4
1. Maternal health services. 2. Women's health services. 3. Maternal and infant welfare. I. Grayson, Tim.
RG940 .E87 2022
618.24--dc23

© American Medical Publishers, 2022

American Medical Publishers,
41 Flatbush Avenue,
1st Floor, New York,
NY 11217, USA

ISBN 978-1-63927-444-4 (Hardback)

This book contains information obtained from authentic and highly regarded sources. Copyright for all individual chapters remain with the respective authors as indicated. All chapters are published with permission under the Creative Commons Attribution License or equivalent. A wide variety of references are listed. Permission and sources are indicated; for detailed attributions, please refer to the permissions page and list of contributors. Reasonable efforts have been made to publish reliable data and information, but the authors, editors and publisher cannot assume any responsibility for the validity of all materials or the consequences of their use.

Trademark Notice: Registered trademark of products or corporate names are used only for explanation and identification without intent to infringe.

Contents

Preface

This book has been a concerted effort by a group of academicians, researchers and scientists, who have contributed their research works for the realization of the book. This book has materialized in the wake of emerging advancements and innovations in this field. Therefore, the need of the hour was to compile all the required researches and disseminate the knowledge to a broad spectrum of people comprising of students, researchers and specialists of the field.

Maternity refers to the time period during pregnancy and soon after childbirth. It presents various health risks to a woman. It comes with major changes and challenges in the physical, emotional and social health of a woman. It is necessary to provide appropriate health care to the woman going through the maternity period. The conditions such as hemorrhage, eclampsia, sepsis and obstructed labor often lead to maternal death. Maternal health is affected by several factors such as early marriage, home birth and various cultural attitudes towards sexuality. The woman going through pregnancy often deals with various non-fatal health problems such as ectopic pregnancy, preterm labor, gestational diabetes, hyperemesis gravidarum, obstetrical fistulae, and anemia. This book contains some path-breaking studies in the field of maternity and women's health care. It will also provide interesting topics for research which interested readers can take up. Those in search of information to further their knowledge will be greatly assisted by this book.

At the end of the preface, I would like to thank the authors for their brilliant chapters and the publisher for guiding us all-through the making of the book till its final stage. Also, I would like to thank my family for providing the support and encouragement throughout my academic career and research projects.

Editor

Spatial variation in the use of reproductive health services over time: a decomposition analysis

Gordon Abekah-Nkrumah

Abstract

Background: The paper argues that several Sub-Saharan African countries have recorded marked improvements in the use of reproductive health services. However, the literature has hardly highlighted such progress and the factors responsible for them. The current study uses Ghana as a case to examine progress in the consumption of reproductive health services over the last two decades and the factors responsible for such progress.

Methods: The study uses two rounds (1998 and 2014) of Demographic and Health Survey data from Ghana. Standard frequencies, a logit model and decomposition of the coefficients of the logit model (i.e. Oaxaca-type decomposition) was employed to examine changes in the use of reproductive health services (4+ antenatal visits and skilled attendance at birth) at national and sub-national levels (i.e the four ecological zones of Ghana) between 1998 and 2014 as well as factors explaining observed spatial changes between the two periods.

Results: Descriptive results suggest that the highest level of improvement occurred in resource-poor zones (i.e. northern belt followed by the southern belt) compared to the middle belt and Greater Accra, where access to resources and infrastructure is relatively better. Results from Oaxaca-type decomposition also suggest that women and partner's education, household wealth and availability and accessibility to health facilities are the key factors explaining spatial variation in reproductive health service consumption over the two periods. Most importantly, the marginal efficiency of investment in women and partner's education and access to health services were highest in the two resource poor zones.

Conclusion: There is the need to target resource poor settings with existing or new pro-poor reproductive health interventions. Specifically, the northern and southern zones where the key drivers of education and availability of health facilities are the lowest, will be key to further improvements in the consumption of reproductive health services in Ghana.

Keywords: Spatial variation, Reproductive health, Decomposition

Background

Africa's unfavourable mother and child health outcomes is often the subject of policy and academic discourse. Mortality and morbidity episodes related to women and children constitute a major challenge on the continent. For example, out of 289,000 maternal deaths in 2013, 286,000 occurred in developing countries with 179,000 of these deaths occurring in Sub-Saharan Africa (SSA) alone [1]. In addition, SSA accounted for 49% of global under-five deaths (6,914,300) in 2011, with low birthweight and stunting prevalence being 12% and 40% respectively from 2007 to 2011, [2, 3].

Notwithstanding the above, it is important to emphasise that some SSA counties (e.g. Ghana, Rwnada, Kenya, Tanzania etc) have over the last two decades made tremendous progress in improving mother and child health outcomes through improved access to reproductive and child health services. In Ghana for example, the Maternal Mortality Rate (MMR) reduced by 49% in 2013 [1]. Besides maternal health, child health outcomes have also improved, with infant and under-five mortality declining by 28% and

Correspondence: gabekah-nkrumah@ug.edu.gh
Department of Public Administration and Health Services Management, University of Ghana Business School, P. O. Box 78, Legon, Accra, Ghana

44% respectively for the period 1998 to 2014 [4]. Also, the percentage of children under-five, who are stunted, wasted or underweight dropped by 16%, 3% and 7% respectively from 2003 to 2014 [4]. Most importantly, these outcome improvements are taking place at a time of increased use of reproductive health services (e.g. antenatal and delivery care), which is considered a key strategy for improving mother and child health outcomes in Ghana [5]. Estimates from the 2014 Ghana Demographic and Health Survey (GDHS) suggest that the percentage of women receiving antenatal care from a skilled provider increased from 82% in 1988 to 97% in 2014, with 4+ antenatal visits (78% in 2008 to 87% in 2014) and health facility deliveries (42% in 1988 to 73% in 2014) improving tremendously [4].

The existing reproductive and child health literature abounds in several studies [6–10] that explain generally, factors that influence the use of reproductive health services such as antenatal and delivery care. Majority of these studies have concluded that individual, household and community level factors influence the use of reproductive health services. What is however not clear in the existing literature is the extent to which these determinants explain changes that have occurred over time. The few studies (i.e. from Ghana, Rwanda and Uganda) [11–13] that have tried to address this issue, have focused their analysis at the national level. This limit one's ability to understand spatial nuances that may be taking place especially at sub-national levels such the different regions or a group of regions with similar characteristics (ecological zones). In the case of the Ugandan paper [13], the authors mainly computed and compared the probability of using health services conditioned on selected determinants across two periods. Although useful, this approach makes it difficult to know the contributions of the determinants to period changes in the use of such health services.

Thus, the current study uses the Ghana Demographic and Health Survey (GDHS) data to highlight changes in the use of reproductive health services (RHS) (antenatal and delivery care) at the national and ecological zone level between 1998 and 2014 and factors responsible for such changes. Specifically, the study:

1. Examines trends in the use of RHS at the national and ecological zone level between 1998 and 2014.
2. Examine the determinants of use of RHS at the national and ecological zone level using a pooled cross-section of 1998 and 2014.
3. Examine factors contributing to or explaining changes in the use of RHS between 1998 and 2004 at the national and ecological zone level.

The importance of this study is seen in its added value to the existing literature. First, highlighting changes in the use of RHS over the last two decades could constitute a good source of information to guide policy formulation. Secondly, identifying specific factors responsible for any identified changes can be crucial not only for policy formulation, but also appropriate targeting. Finally, the current paper extend the analysis beyond the national level to include the four ecological zones in Ghana. Thus, the study does not only identify factors contributing to changes in the utilisation of RHS over time, but also capture spatial (ecological zone) variation in the contributions of determinants to changes in the use of RHS over time.

Methods
Data source
The study used two rounds (1988 and 2014) of GDHS datasets collected by the Ghana Statistical Service and supported by OR/IFC Macro and IFC International Company. The GDHS is nationally representative and based on a two-stage probability sampling strategy. In the first stage, the country was divided into regions and each region into urban and rural areas. Based on the latest available population census sampling frame, primary sampling units (PSU's) known as clusters were selected from each region in a manner that reflect the rural/urban divide and proportional to the size of the regions. This is done using systematic sampling with probability proportional to size. In the second stage, households are selected from the clusters using systematic sampling with equal probability. Females of reproductive age (15–49) who were either usual members or visitors in the selected households were interviewed. In addition, men aged 15–59 years from a sub-sample of a second or third of total households selected were also interviewed. The survey also collected information on children aged between 0 and 59 months. Information from the survey relevant to this study includes: background characteristics of women and their husbands/partners, reproductive histories, current use of contraceptives, antenatal visits and delivery assistance. The main reason for using the two rounds of the GDHS is to make it possible to examine changes in the use of both antenatal and delivery care as well as examine factors that have contributed to such changes.

Variable definition and measurement
Given that antenatal and delivery care constitute a major strategy adopted by policy makers in Ghana to improve RHS, we have for the purpose of this study used antenatal and delivery care to capture use of RHS. Antenatal care is captured by a single indicator; whether a pregnant woman had four or more antenatal visits (4+ antenatal visits). Delivery care is also captured by a single indicator; whether a pregnant woman had skilled attendants at birth (doctor, nurse or midwife) when delivering her baby (skilled attendants at birth).

The use of 4+ antenatal visits is based on the WHO recommendation that a pregnant woman needs at least four antenatal visits to be deemed protected from pregnancy-related risk and complications [14, 15]. Thus, we assume that all antenatal visits fewer than four constitute a risk to the pregnant woman. Hence the variable was coded as 1 if a woman had 4+ antenatal visits, else 0 (i.e. a binary choice variable). The strategic value of delivery taking place in a health facility and assisted by skilled birth attendants is that it gives women in labour, access to various delivery services and most importantly, emergency obstetric care (EOC), the absence of which can increase the risk of complicated deliveries. It is therefore assumed that childbirth with the assistance of skilled birth attendants reduces the risk exposure of expecting mothers. Thus, we code any birth assisted by skilled birth attendants as 1 else 0.

Independent variables used in the study are standard determinants of use of reproductive health services also used by several other authors [7–9, 16]. The variables include individual level factors (i.e., woman's age and age squared, birth order, woman's level of education and that of her partner, religion and ethnicity), household factors (i.e., household wealth and number of elderly women in the household) and Community factors (i.e., place of residence and availability and accessibility to health services). Bivariate correlation coefficients between the determinants and the outcome variables (results not shown) were calculated to ensure that the determinants where not redundant in the estimated models. Besides, the determinants in the estimated model were introduced into the model in a stepwise fashion to ensure that redundant variables were not included.

Within the RHS literature, availability and accessibility of health services has often been captured using variables such as distance to health facility, category of health personnel and health infrastructure [7, 17, 18]. However, the GDHS data does not have these variables. Thus, we follow existing authors [19–21] by calculating the non-self cluster proportion of households with access to good water (NSCPHGW) and non-self cluster proportion of households with flush toilets (NSCPHGT) as proxies to capture availability and accessibility of health facilities. In principle, the two variables capture and accessibility to and availability of social services such as healthcare within the neighbourhood. For ease of interpretation of the two proxies, determining thresholds (i.e. specific cut-off values) that indicate lower or higher levels of access will be appropriate. However, such cut-off values may be arbitrary and therefore less relevant for purposes of policy. Thus, we follow prior authors [10, 20, 21] by rescaling the two variables to lie between 0 and 1, where values closer to 0 suggest lower levels of access

or availability of health services and vice versa. The definition and measurement of all other variables used in the study are contained in Table 1.

Four ecological zones (i.e. southern zone, middle zone, northern zone and Greater Accra), based on Ghana's ten administrative regions are used for the analysis. The southern zone is made up of three regions along Ghana's coastline; Western, Central and the Volta regions. It is important to emphasise that although Greater Accra region is part of Ghana's coastline, it has not been added to the southern zone on the basis that it hosts the national capital in addition to having different geographical and climatic conditions from the other regions along the coastline. Hence, Greater Accra is used in the analysis as a separate ecological zone. The middle belt is made up of another three regions located at the middle part of the country; Ashanti, Eastern and Brong-Ahafo regions. The northern belt is equally made up of three regions in the northern part of the country; Northern, Upper East and Upper West regions (see both Figs. 1 and 2 for the ecological zone demarcation).

Econometric model
Estimating determinants of reproductive healthcare use
As indicated in Section 1, a key objective of the paper is examining the determinants of a woman's decision to use or not to use any of the two reproductive health services. Framing the objective in this manner reduces the utilization decision of a woman into a binary choice set, making it possible to estimate the determinants of use of reproductive health services with a logit model. Thus, if the binary choice set (i.e. having or not having 4+ antenatal visits or skilled birth attendants) is generalized as J, and an indirect utility derived from choosing any of the two alternatives as V, then the log odds of a woman using any of the two reproductive health services can be expressed as in Eq. 1

$$Ln\left(\frac{P(V_j)}{1-P(V_j)}\right) = X_j\beta + \varepsilon_j \qquad (1)$$

Where, for instance, $V_j = 1$ if reproductive healthcare is used based on the definition of the variables in Table 1, and $V_j = 0$ if otherwise. X represents a vector of determinants at the individual, household and community level, with β being coefficients to be estimated and ε, the error term. It is important however to emphasise that the β's reported in Tables 3 and 4 are marginal effects and not log odds. The use of the marginal effects makes it possible to interpret the β's as change in the outcome variable as a result of a unit change in the determinants.

Table 1 Summary statistics for dependent and independent variables – pooled data for 1998 and 2014

Variables	Obs.	Mean	SD	Variables	Obs.	Mean	SD
4+ Antenatal Visits				Ethnicity			
No	6386	0.214	0.410	Akan (Ref)	6386	0.399	0.490
Yes	6386	0.786	0.410	Ga/Dangme	6386	0.052	0.222
Woman's Age	6386	30.493	7.229	Ewe and Guans	6386	0.136	0.343
Woman's Age Sq.	6386	982.076	460.205	North ethnicities	6386	0.393	0.488
Birth order				Others	6386	0.020	0.140
One child (Ref)	6386	0.214	0.410	Number of elderly	6386	1.340	0.665
Two children	6386	0.193	0.395	Household wealth			
Three children	6386	0.161	0.368	Poorest (Ref)	6386	0.315	0.465
Four and above	6386	0.431	0.495	Poorer	6386	0.214	0.410
Woman's education				Middle	6386	0.183	0.387
No educ (Ref)	6386	0.374	0.484	Richer	6386	0.157	0.364
Primary	6386	0.193	0.395	Richest	6386	0.130	0.336
Secondary	6386	0.404	0.491	Ecological zones			
Tertiary	6386	0.029	0.168	Southern belt (Ref)	6386	0.283	0.451
Partner education				Greater Accra	6386	0.085	0.279
No educ (Ref)	6386	0.296	0.457	Middle belt	6386	0.308	0.462
Primary	6386	0.100	0.300	Northern belt	6386	0.323	0.468
Secondary	6386	0.459	0.498	Rural dummy	6386	0.651	0.477
Tertiary	6386	0.074	0.261	NSCPHGW	6386	0.663	0.340
Missing Partners	6386	0.071	0.256	NSCPHFT	6386	0.100	0.209
Muslim	6386	0.298	0.458	Sample Dummy			
Year Dummy				Skilled Attendance at Birth	6665		
Year 1998	2242						
Year 2014	4144						

Source: Authors' calculations. Calculations take account of sample weights. Note that the models on skilled attendants at birth is based on slightly different sample per the sample dummy. NSCPHGW and NSCPHFT are the non-self-cluster proportion of households with good water and non-self-cluster proportion of households with flush toilets respectively. Note, partner's education includes a 5th category (missing partners). This was added to cater for women who do not have partners and would otherwise have been dropped from the regressions. The age variable has also been categorized with number of observations and percentages as follows: 15–19 (2645: 18.6%), 20–24 (2958: 17.3%), 25–29 (2421: 17%), 30–34 (2004: 14.1%), 35–39 (1887: 13.3%), 40–44 (1516: 10.7%) and 45–49 (1308: 9.2%)

This notwithstanding, the log odds results have also been reported in Additional file 1: Table S1and Table S2.

Decomposition of changes in the use of reproductive health services

To decompose period (1998–2014) changes in 4+ antenatal visits and skilled attendants at birth over their determinants both at the national and ecological zone level, we used the binary analog of the standadard Blinder [22] and Oaxaca [23] decomposition technique developed by Fairlie [24–26]. The use of the Fairlie approach is due to the fact that the standard Blinder-Oaxaca decomposition is not suitable for decomposing changes in a binary variable such as 4+ antenatal visits, and skilled attendants at birth.

Following from Fairlie [24], the decomposition of a nonlinear equation $Y = F(X\hat{\beta})$, can be expressed as:

$$\overline{Y}^R - \overline{Y}^B = \left[\sum_{i=1}^{N^R} \frac{F\left(X_i^R \hat{\beta}^R\right)}{N^R} - \sum_{i=1}^{N^B} \frac{F\left(X_i^B \hat{\beta}^R\right)}{N^B} \right] + \left[\sum_{i=1}^{N^B} \frac{F\left(X_i^B \hat{\beta}^R\right)}{N^B} - \sum_{i=1}^{N^B} \frac{F\left(X_i^B \hat{\beta}^R\right)}{N^B} \right]$$

(2)

Where $\overline{Y}^j$ is the average probability of the outcome of interest for group j, N_j is the sample size for group j, R is reference group (i.e. 2014), B is the base group (1998), and $\hat{\beta}$ a vector of coefficient estimates for group j, and F,

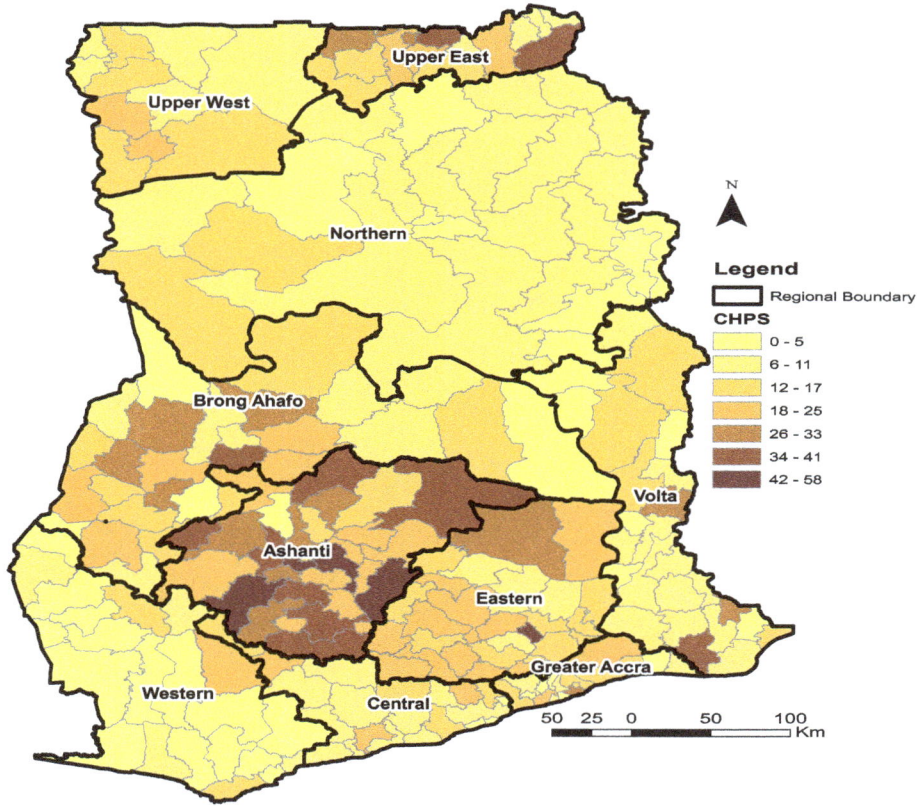

Fig. 1 Distribution of CHPS Facilities in Ghana as at 2016. Source: Fig. 1 is constructed by the author using health facility data from GHS. Fig. 1 covers four ecological zones; Northern zone (Upper West, Upper East and Northern Region), Middle zone (Ashanti, Eastern and Brong Ahafo), Southern zone (Western, Central and Volta) and Greater Accra. Note also that CHPS is an acronym for Community Planning and Services; a lower level health facility in Ghana

a cummilative distribution function from a logistic distribution. The first term in the bracket represents that part of the gap in the dependent variable that is due to group differences in the distribution of Xs. The second bracket represent the gap arising from differences in group processes that determines the level of Y as well as the proportion of the group difference captured by unobserved endowments [26]. Thus, Eq. 2 is used to estimate the contribution of period (1988 to 2014) differences in the entire set of determinants to the gap in the dependent variables.

To estimate the independent contributions of individual determinants to the period gap in the dependent variables, coefficients $\hat{\beta}^*$ from the logit regression for a pooled sample of the two periods are used as in Eq. 3 below, to estimates the contributions of $X_1 \ldots\ldots X_n$.

$$\frac{1}{N^B} \sum_{j=1}^{N^B} F\left(\hat{a}^* + X_{1j}^R \hat{\beta}_1^* + X_{2j}^R \hat{\beta}_2^*\right) - F\left(\hat{a}^* + X_{1j}^B \hat{\beta}_1^* + X_{2j}^R \hat{\beta}_2^*\right) \quad (3)$$

As has been the case in many studies, we donot focus on the decomposition of the error term and so not reported in the results.

Additionally, standard errors can be calculated for the decomposition and thereby make it possible to test the significance of the estimated contributions of the covariates. As shown by Fairlie [26], Eq. 3 can be rewritten as Eq. 4 using the delta method to approximate the standard errors.

$$\hat{D}_i = \frac{1}{N^B} \sum_{i=1}^{N^B} F\left(X_i^{RR} \hat{\beta}^*\right) - F\left(X_i^{BR} \hat{\beta}^*\right) \quad (4)$$

From Eq. 4, the variance of $\hat{D}_i$ can be approximated as Eq. 5 below:

$$Var\left(\hat{D}_1\right) = \left(\frac{\delta \hat{D}_1}{\delta \hat{\beta}^*}\right) Var\left(\hat{\beta}^*\right) = \left(\frac{\delta \hat{D}_1}{\delta \hat{\beta}^*}\right) \quad (5)$$

Where $\frac{\delta \hat{D}_1}{\delta \hat{\beta}^*} = \frac{1}{N^B} \sum_{i=1}^{N^B} f(X_i^{RR} \hat{\beta}^*) X_i^{RR} - f(X_i^{BR} \hat{\beta}^*) X_i^{BR}$ and f is the logistic probability density function.

To estimate Eqs. 3 and 5, one will need a 1 to 1 matching of the observations of the 1998 and 2014

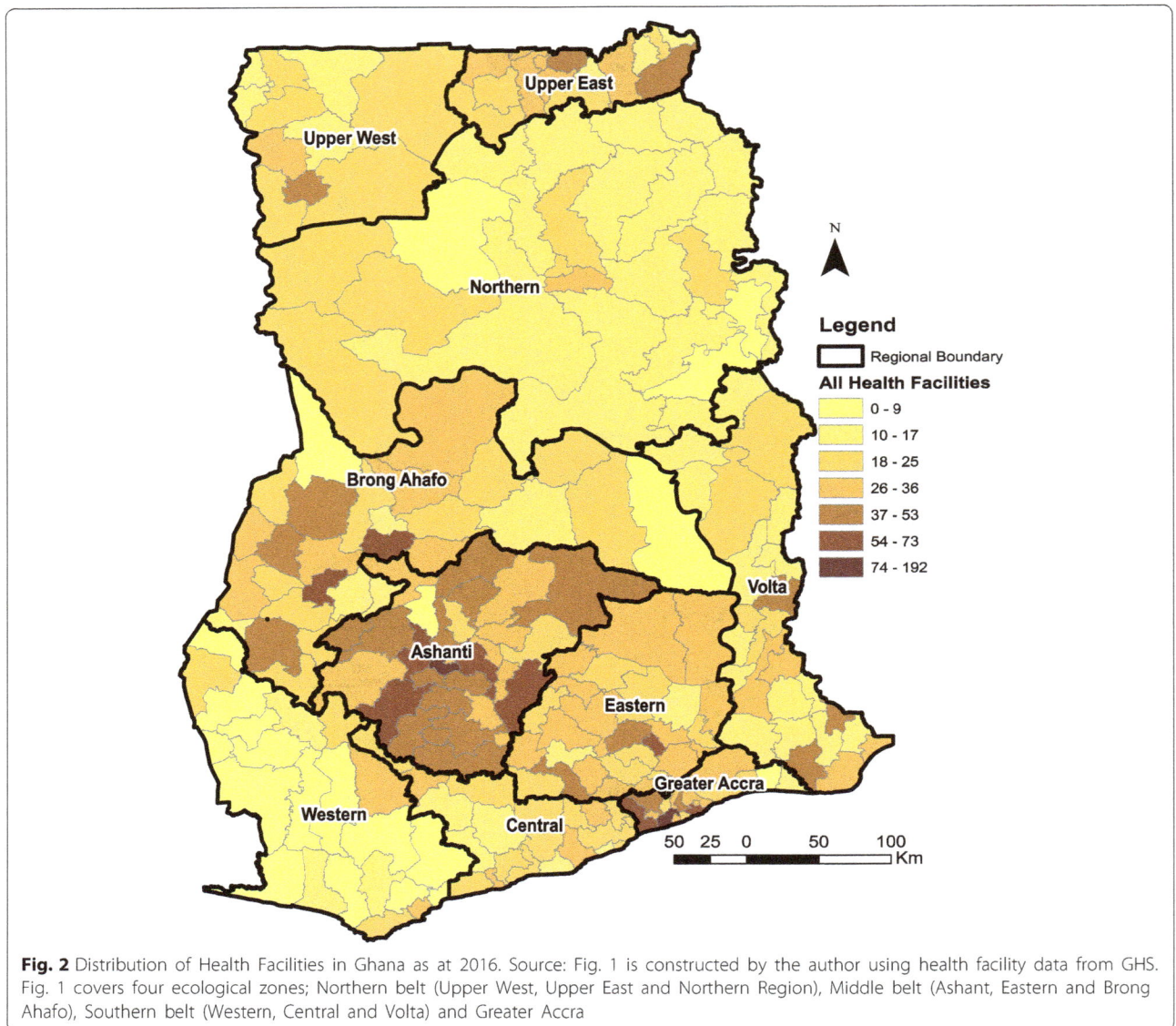

Fig. 2 Distribution of Health Facilities in Ghana as at 2016. Source: Fig. 1 is constructed by the author using health facility data from GHS. Fig. 1 covers four ecological zones; Northern belt (Upper West, Upper East and Northern Region), Middle belt (Ashant, Eastern and Brong Ahafo), Southern belt (Western, Central and Volta) and Greater Accra

samples. However, it is the case that the 2014 sample is larger than the 1998 sample (see Table 1). To overcome this challenge, we follow Fairlie [26] and draw a large number of random samples (5000) from the 2014 sample and match each of the random samples to the 1998 sample to calculate the decomposition. The reported result is therefore the mean of the repeated calculations.

Results

Descriptive results

In this section, we present results on the use of the two reproductive health inputs (4+ antenatal visits and skilled birth attendance) using a pooled sample for two periods (1998 and 2014) at the national level and across the four ecological zones. The results in Table 2 suggest that at the national level, women making 4+ antenatal

visits increased by 22.9%, with birth attended by skilled personnel also increasing by 29.8%. The improvement in utilization at the national level is also reflected in utilization at the ecological zone level. The southern zone recorded the highest level of improvement in 4+ antenatal visit (25.2%), followed by the middle zone (23.6%), the northern zone (21.2%) and finally the Greater Accra region (15.5%). In the case of skilled birth attendants, the northern zone recorded the highest increase (36.8%), followed by the southern zone (31.9%), the middle zone (27.4%) and Greater Accra (17.2%).

Table 2 also shows trends in key policy variables such as education, household wealth and availability and accessibility of health services. The northern zone witnessed the greatest level of improvement in women's education at all levels except for the tertiary level.

Table 2 Trends in 4+ antenatal visits and skilled birth attendance and selected independent variables

Variables	National		Southern Belt		Capital		Middle Belt		Northern Belt	
	1998	2014	1998	2014	1998	2014	1998	2014	1998	2014
4+ Antenatal	64.86	87.71	62.78	87.95	76.11	91.59	65.77	89.36	59.53	80.7
Skilled Birth Attendants	46.22	75.99	42.12	74.03	75.96	93.18	53.67	81.07	17.2	54.02
Woman's Education										
No education	29.12	19.07	25.94	15.82	14.76	8.33	21.09	12.86	76.88	56.26
Primary	18.05	17.79	21.29	19.81	15.63	14.21	19.53	18.60	8.66	16.77
Secondary	50.58	56.80	50.74	59.63	63.84	63.78	58.29	63.42	12.95	24.64
Tertiary	2.25	6.34	2.03	4.74	5.78	13.69	1.08	5.13	1.51	2.34
Partner's Education										
No education	22.77	20.11	14.30	12.65	8.87	6.57	13.86	12.98	77.26	65.76
Primary	7.84	8.85	9.54	10.13	4.56	4.76	8.24	9.19	6.05	10.65
Secondary	60.66	58.87	65.44	66.04	73.67	68.28	71.19	66.91	11.24	16.66
Tertiary	8.73	12.17	10.72	11.18	12.90	20.38	6.71	10.92	5.45	6.93
Household Wealth										
Poorest	20.26	16.09	18.63	7.96	2.33	1.82	16.30	9.59	57.61	68.60
Poorer	17.22	17.41	20.53	24.73	3.78	2.51	19.53	20.90	19.28	14.89
Middle	18.20	20.62	26.52	31.20	4.06	10.30	20.79	22.84	7.32	8.42
Richer	20.12	22.53	20.87	22.94	22.55	29.06	22.40	25.48	8.99	5.13
Richest	24.21	23.35	13.45	13.16	67.28	56.31	20.98	21.20	6.81	2.95
NSCPHGW (Mean)	.5659	.7961	.5066	.7457	.8425	.9384	.5249	.7746	.4822	.7498
NSCPHGT (Mean)	.0874	.2381	.0372	.1425	.3084	.5709	.0564	.2113	.0242	.1083

Source: Calculated by author using data from the 1998 and 2014 Ghana DHS. Note estimates uses sample weights

Women with no education reduced by 20.6%, whiles those with primary and secondary education increased by 8.1% and 11.7% respectively. The southern zone also witnessed appreciable improvements in women's education with a 10.1% drop in women with no education and an 8.9% increase in women with secondary education. At all levels of women's education, Greater Accra had the least improvement except that it had the highest increase in women with tertiary education (7.9%). The performance of the northern zone with respect to partner's education is even more pronounce compared to the other ecological zones. Partners with no education reduced by 11.5%, whiles those with primary and secondary education increased by 4.6% and 5.4% respectively.

In addition, the southern zone showed the strongest improvement in household wealth, with a 10.7% drop in women in the poorest wealth quintile, but a 4.9% and 2.1% increase in the middle and richer quintiles respectively. Whereas the middle zone witnessed some improvement in household wealth, the northern zone exhibited the least progress, recording an increase of 11% in women categorized as the poorest as well as a 3.8% drop in the number of women categorized as richer or richest. On availability and accessibility of health services, the northern zone recorded the biggest increase

(0.268) in the mean proportion of women who have access to good water in the neighbourhood compared to the lowest increase (0.096) recorded by the Greater Accra region. On the contrary, Greater Accra recorded the highest increase in the proportion of women in the neighbourhood with access to flush toilets, followed by the middle and southern belts.

Determinants of use of reproductive health services

In this section, we present the results of the determinants of 4+ antenatal visits and skilled attendants at birth. Although results on log odds are reported in Additional file 1: Table S1 and Table S2, the discussion in this section is based on marginal effects as reported in Table 3 to Table 4. Given that the results are not different from what is known in the existing reproductive health literature, we summarise the results, but highlight key findings, especially at the ecological zone level. The results in Tables 3 and 4 shows that whiles women's age has a quadratic effect on the two RHS, birth order, being a Muslim woman, number of elderly women in the household and living in a rural area are all significantly negatively correlated with both 4+ antenatal visits and skilled birth attendants. On the contrary, women and partners education, household wealth and access to and availability

Table 3 Determinants of 4+ antenatal visits in Ghana – marginal effect estimates

Variables	Ecological Zones				
	National	Southern	Gt Accra	Middle	Northern
Woman's_Age	0.0223***	0.0261**	0.0216**	0.0246***	0.0061
	(0.0054)	(0.0114)	(0.0099)	(0.0089)	(0.0102)
Woman's age Square	−0.0003***	−0.0003*	−0.0003**	−0.0003**	−0.0001
	(0.0001)	(0.0002)	(0.0002)	(0.0001)	(0.0001)
Birth Order: 2nd Birth	−0.0422**	−0.0533	−0.0810*	−0.0638*	0.0210
	(0.0190)	(0.0357)	(0.0435)	(0.0357)	(0.0355)
Birth Order: 3rd Birth	−0.0572**	−0.0642	−0.0699	−0.0971**	0.0078
	(0.0228)	(0.0453)	(0.0454)	(0.0472)	(0.0384)
Birth Order: 4th Birth	−0.0944***	−0.1145**	−0.0622	−0.1193***	−0.0237
	(0.0214)	(0.0447)	(0.0476)	(0.0396)	(0.0417)
Woman's Education: Primary	0.0310***	0.0388*	0.0142	−0.0133	0.0764***
	(0.0119)	(0.0212)	(0.0185)	(0.0221)	(0.0254)
Woman's Education: Secondary	0.0808***	0.1096***	0.1094***	0.0276	0.0702**
	(0.0141)	(0.0252)	(0.0322)	(0.0241)	(0.0335)
Woman's Education: Tetiary	0.1148***		0.0595***		0.1320**
	(0.0326)		(0.0226)		(0.0670)
Partner Education: Primary	0.0336**	0.0274	−0.0133	0.0202	0.0698***
	(0.0136)	(0.0261)	(0.0353)	(0.0256)	(0.0247)
Partner Education: Secondary	0.0437***	0.0704**	0.0011	0.0251	0.0607*
	(0.0138)	(0.0287)	(0.0286)	(0.0247)	(0.0335)
Partner Education: Tetiary	0.1089***	0.1347***	0.0471*	0.1273***	0.0368
	(0.0166)	(0.0238)	(0.0280)	(0.0238)	(0.0516)
Muslim Dummy	−0.0216	0.0133	0.0078	−0.0649***	−0.0282
	(0.0159)	(0.0277)	(0.0204)	(0.0249)	(0.0280)
Ethnicity: Ga/Dangme	−0.0727**	−0.0029	0.0228	−0.1891***	
	(0.0327)	(0.0586)	(0.0262)	(0.0510)	
Ethnicity: Ewe and Guan	−0.0383**	−0.0496**	−0.0239	−0.0707**	−0.3705
	(0.0178)	(0.0243)	(0.0372)	(0.0318)	(0.3045)
Ethnicity: Northern Groups	0.0344*	−0.0098	0.0422**	0.0275	−0.1515**
	(0.0207)	(0.0416)	(0.0200)	(0.0239)	(0.0628)
Ethnicity: Others	−0.0184	−0.0014	0.0279	−0.0146	−0.5808**
	(0.0374)	(0.0608)	(0.0323)	(0.0633)	(0.2370)
Number of Elderly Women in HH	−0.0208***	−0.0089	−0.0174	−0.0082	−0.0288**
	(0.0074)	(0.0128)	(0.0125)	(0.0136)	(0.0131)
Wealth Quintile: Poorer	0.0483***	0.0544**	0.0280	0.0355**	0.0637***
	(0.0117)	(0.0211)	(0.0225)	(0.0181)	(0.0233)
Wealth Quintile: Middle	0.0493***	0.0712***	0.0321	0.0474**	0.0599
	(0.0133)	(0.0243)	(0.0279)	(0.0212)	(0.0389)
Wealth Quintile: Richer	0.1020***	0.1398***	0.0603	0.0884***	0.1322***

Table 3 Determinants of 4+ antenatal visits in Ghana – marginal effect estimates *(Continued)*

Variables	Ecological Zones				
	National	Southern	Gt Accra	Middle	Northern
	(0.0131)	(0.0218)	(0.0384)	(0.0199)	(0.0322)
Wealth Quintile: Richest	0.1379***	0.1397***	0.1846*	0.1359***	0.0105
	(0.0142)	(0.0217)	(0.0953)	(0.0204)	(0.0769)
Eco_Zone: Greater Accra	−0.0466				
	(0.0331)				
Eco_Zone: Middle	0.0006				
	(0.0139)				
Eco_Zone: Northern	0.0475**				
	(0.0230)				
Rural Dummy	−0.0097	0.0147	−0.0224	0.0028	−0.0548
	(0.0155)	(0.0254)	(0.0519)	(0.0251)	(0.0366)
NSCPHGW	0.0718***	−0.0269	−0.0040	0.0334	0.1898***
	(0.0254)	(0.0380)	(0.0556)	(0.0268)	(0.0617)
NSCPHFT	0.0811*	0.2519*	−0.0254	0.1763**	0.0999
	(0.0486)	(0.1329)	(0.0352)	(0.0850)	(0.1574)
Year 2014	0.1569***	0.1974***	0.0978**	0.1862***	0.1212**
	(0.0195)	(0.0262)	(0.0386)	(0.0266)	(0.0476)
N	6386	1763	543	1922	2063
pseudo R^2	0.168	0.180	0.322	0.182	0.153
p	0.0000	0.0000	0.0000	0.0000	0.0000

Source: Authors' Calculations. Note: *** is significant at $p < 0.01$, ** is significant at $p < 0.05$, * is significant at $p < 0.10$. NSCPHGW, NSCPHFT are non-self cluster proportion of households with good water, non-self cluster proportion of households with flush toilet respectively. To account for women without Partners, a category was created for missing husbands under partner's education but coefficient not reported

of health services were significantly positively correlated with 4+ antenatal visits and skilled birth attendants.

As earlier indicated, there are other aspects of the results in Tables 3 and 4 that deserves special mention. For example, the effect of women's secondary and tertiary education on the two RHS is indifferent of the ecological zones. However, returns to primary education is important mostly in the resource poor ecological zones (southern and northern zones). Partners' education follows the same pattern except that returns to partners primary education is significant ($p < 0.05$) only in the northern zone. Additionally, the effect of number of elderly women in a household on use of RHS is also significant mainly in the northern zone. The effect of NSCPHGW (a proxy for access to and availability of health services) is mainly significant in the middle and northern ecological zone for the two RHS. However, the other health service availability and accessibility proxy (NSCPHFT) was significant in the southern and middle zone in the case of 4+ antenatal visits, and the southern zone and Greater Accra in the case of skilled birth

Table 4 Determinants of use of skilled birth attendants in Ghana – marginal effect estimates

Variables	Ecological Zones				
	National	Southern	Gt Accra	Middle	Northern
Woman's_Age	0.0228***	0.0274*	0.0051	0.0293**	0.0002
	(0.0087)	(0.0160)	(0.0103)	(0.0143)	(0.0193)
Woman's age Square	−0.0002*	−0.0003	−0.0000	−0.0003	0.0000
	(0.0001)	(0.0002)	(0.0002)	(0.0002)	(0.0003)
Birth Order: 2nd Birth	−0.1202***	−0.1098**	− 0.0488*	−0.1756***	−0.0899
	(0.0271)	(0.0487)	(0.0292)	(0.0519)	(0.0633)
Birth Order: 3rd Birth	−0.1828***	−0.1603***	−0.1066*	−0.2449***	−0.1285**
	(0.0329)	(0.0594)	(0.0551)	(0.0673)	(0.0573)
Birth Order: 4th Birth	−0.2313***	−0.2586***	−0.0876*	−0.2780***	−0.1579**
	(0.0311)	(0.0600)	(0.0477)	(0.0541)	(0.0704)
Woman's Education: Primary	0.0517***	−0.0141	0.0058	0.0299	0.1649***
	(0.0189)	(0.0378)	(0.0133)	(0.0290)	(0.0458)
Woman's Education: Secondary	0.1460***	0.1208***	0.0939***	0.1124***	0.1383**
	(0.0190)	(0.0334)	(0.0314)	(0.0309)	(0.0564)
Woman's Education: Tetiary	0.2913***		0.0337*		
	(0.0284)		(0.0181)		
Partner Education: Primary	0.0804***	0.0033	−0.1007	0.0512	0.1602***
	(0.0206)	(0.0468)	(0.0847)	(0.0328)	(0.0443)
Partner Education: Secondary	0.0807***	0.0346	−0.0397**	0.0544	0.1464***
	(0.0208)	(0.0396)	(0.0173)	(0.0358)	(0.0399)
Partner Education: Tetiary	0.1617***	0.1422**	−0.0019	0.1432***	0.2039**
	(0.0294)	(0.0595)	(0.0412)	(0.0423)	(0.0895)
Muslim Dummy	−0.0829***	−0.0541	−0.0003	−0.0340	−0.1504***
	(0.0240)	(0.0369)	(0.0167)	(0.0351)	(0.0429)
Ethnicity: Ga/Dangme	−0.0323	0.0317	0.0386***	−0.1217**	
	(0.0449)	(0.0909)	(0.0137)	(0.0556)	
Ethnicity: Ewe and Guan	0.0036	0.0154	0.0136	−0.0619	−0.3282***
	(0.0310)	(0.0405)	(0.0161)	(0.0457)	(0.0540)
Ethnicity: Northern Groups	0.0568*	0.0440	0.0302**	0.0168	−0.4162***
	(0.0330)	(0.0652)	(0.0133)	(0.0351)	(0.0522)
Ethnicity: Others	0.0134	−0.0431	0.0075	0.0203	−0.3974***
	(0.0472)	(0.0854)	(0.0228)	(0.0632)	(0.0330)
Number of Elderly Women in HH	−0.0072	0.0171	0.0023	0.0278	−0.0444*
	(0.0112)	(0.0224)	(0.0041)	(0.0220)	(0.0252)
Wealth Quintile: Poorer	0.0145	0.0568	−0.0676	0.0110	0.0390
	(0.0218)	(0.0409)	(0.0454)	(0.0289)	(0.0508)
Wealth Quintile: Middle	0.0945***	0.1140**	−0.0195	0.1030***	0.2134***
	(0.0232)	(0.0460)	(0.0395)	(0.0308)	(0.0827)
Wealth Quintile: Richer	0.1745***	0.2395***	−0.0129	0.1582***	0.2645***
	(0.0239)	(0.0425)	(0.0329)	(0.0334)	(0.0963)
Wealth Quintile: Richest	0.2197***	0.1724***	0.0311	0.2039***	0.3937***
	(0.0277)	(0.0578)	(0.0390)	(0.0319)	(0.0895)
Eco_Zone: Greater Accra	0.0319				
	(0.0553)				
Eco_Zone: Middle	0.0754***				
	(0.0242)				
Eco_Zone: Northern	0.0019				
	(0.0388)				
Rural Dummy	−0.1455***	−0.1340***	−0.0719	−0.1032***	−0.2030***
	(0.0245)	(0.0386)	(0.0523)	(0.0371)	(0.0717)
NSCPHGW	0.1241***	−0.0679	0.0386	0.0903**	0.3738***
	(0.0355)	(0.0652)	(0.0464)	(0.0426)	(0.0933)
NSCPHFT	0.2588***	0.5073***	0.0633*	0.1851	0.3942
	(0.0891)	(0.1681)	(0.0339)	(0.1270)	(0.3705)
Year 2014	0.2874***	0.2757***	0.0523**	0.2194***	0.4062***
	(0.0242)	(0.0398)	(0.0227)	(0.0366)	(0.0428)
N	6444	1770	547	1944	2045
pseudo R^2	0.284	0.198	0.456	0.232	0.317
p	0.0000	0.0000	0.0000	0.0000	0.0000

Source: Authors' Calculations. Note: *** is significant at p < 0.01, ** is significant at p < 0.05, * is significant at p < 0.10. NSCPHGW, NSCPHFT are non-self cluster proportion of households with good water, non-self cluster proportion of households with flush toilet respectively. To account for women without Partners, a category was created for missing husbands under partner's education but coefficient not reported

attendants. Finally, the results suggest that the probability of using the two reproductive health services increased in 2014 compared to 1998 in all the ecological zones. The northern and southern zones had the highest increase in the probability of using skilled birth attendants and 4+ antenatal visits respectively.

Decomposition results

In this section, we present results of the decomposition as contained in Table 5. The top panel of the table shows the mean probability of use of the relevant reproductive health input for the two periods (Pr_0 = 2014) and (Pr_1 = 1998), the difference between the two probabilities (i.e. labeled "difference") and the proportion of the difference explained by the determinants captured in the regression model (labeled "explained"). From Table 5, the level of increase in the probability of having 4+ antenatal visits between 1998 and 2014 is 0.232 (national), 0.253 (southern zone), 0.159 (Greater Accra), 0.241 (middle zone) and 0.214 (northern zone). The decomposition also

Table 5 A decomposition of changes in 4+ antenatal visits and use of skilled attendants during delivery in Ghana between 1998 and 2014

Determinants	4+ Antenatal Visits					Skilled Delivery Assistance				
	National	Southern	Gt. Accra	Middle	Northern	National	Southern	Gt. Accra	Middle	Northern
Pr_0	0.8771	0.8766	0.9139	0.8976	0.8065	0.7570	0.7352	0.9318	0.8106	0.5355
Pr_1	0.6451	0.6238	0.7544	0.6562	0.5921	0.4565	0.4168	0.7529	0.5350	0.1586
Difference	0.2319	0.2527	0.1596	0.2414	0.2144	0.3006	0.3184	0.1790	0.2756	0.3769
Explained	0.0461	0.0242	0.0224	0.0474	0.0863	0.0991	0.0342	0.1857	0.1243	0.1332
Contributions										
Woman's Age	0.0042	0.0066	0.0118	0.0073	−0.0008	0.0029	0.0054	0.0036	0.0115**	−0.0018
	(0.0030)	(0.0059)	(0.0105)	(0.0057)	(0.0032)	(0.0018)	(0.0043)	(0.0069)	(0.0057)	(0.0019)
%	9.1	27.3	52.7	15.4	−0.9	2.9	15.8	1.9	9.3	−1.4
Birth Order	0.0008	0.0009	0.0205	−0.0009	0.0008	0.0012	0.0027	−0.0033	−0.0044	−0.0004
	(0.0027)	(0.0049)	(0.0130)	(0.0052)	(0.0034)	(0.0020)	(0.0040)	(0.0090)	(0.0055)	(0.0025)
%	1.7	3.7	91.5	−1.9	0.9	1.2	7.9	−1.8	−3.5	−0.3
Woman's Education	0.0062***	0.0078*	−0.0060	0.0024	0.0124***	0.0119***	0.0149***	0.0209	0.0036	0.0153***
	(0.0022)	(0.0043)	(0.0136)	(0.0033)	(0.0043)	(0.0028)	(0.0056)	(0.0138)	(0.0031)	(0.0056)
%	13.4	32.2	−26.8	5.1	14.4	12.0	43.6	11.3	2.9	11.5
Partner's Education	−0.0006	−0.0037	0.0190*	−0.0006	0.0058	0.0030	−0.0030	−0.0022	0.0088**	0.0161***
	(0.0022)	(0.0042)	(0.0104)	(0.0039)	(0.0046)	(0.0025)	(0.0048)	(0.0088)	(0.0044)	(0.0058)
%	−1.3	−15.3	84.8	−1.3	6.7	3.0	−8.8	−1.2	7.1	12.1
Ethnicity	0.0039*	−0.0007	−0.0142	0.0039	0.0005	0.0051***	0.0015	−0.0012	0.0064**	0.0004
	(0.0022)	(0.0023)	(0.0094)	(0.0029)	(0.0025)	(0.0019)	(0.0027)	(0.0110)	(0.0030)	(0.0026)
%	8.5	−2.9	−63.4	8.2	0.6	5.1	4.4	−0.6	5.1	0.3
Muslim Dummy	−0.0002	−0.0029	−0.0034	−0.0015	−0.0036	0.0007	−0.0005	−0.0078	−0.0005	0.0084***
	(0.0006)	(0.0022)	(0.0058)	(0.0016)	(0.0038)	(0.0006)	(0.0032)	(0.0093)	(0.0010)	(0.0032)
%	−0.4	−12.0	−15.2	−3.2	−4.2	0.7	−1.5	−4.2	−0.4	6.3
No. of Elderly Women	0.0000	0.0003	−0.0024	0.0002	−0.0041***	0.0000	−0.0045**	0.0068	−0.0001	−0.0021*
	(0.0003)	(0.0016)	(0.0034)	(0.0011)	(0.0014)	(0.0002)	(0.0022)	(0.0115)	(0.0012)	(0.0011)
%	0	1.2	−10.7	0.4	−4.8	0.0	−13.2	3.7	−0.1	−1.6
Household Wealth	0.0074***	0.0207***	0.0117	0.0049	0.0002	0.0116***	0.0209***	−0.0028	0.0130***	−0.0050
	(0.0025)	(0.0070)	(0.0152)	(0.0030)	(0.0050)	(0.0020)	(0.0073)	(0.0077)	(0.0041)	(0.0044)
%	16.1	85.5	52.2	10.3	0.2	11.7	61.1	−1.5	10.5	−3.8
Eco Zones	−0.0026					−0.0012				
	(0.0027)					(0.0020)				
%	−5.6					−1.2				
Water and Sanitation	0.0298***	0.0037	−0.0110	0.0259**	0.0724***	0.0486***	−0.0114	0.1693***	0.0654***	0.0945***
	(0.0082)	(0.0116)	(0.0398)	(0.0128)	(0.0141)	(0.0088)	(0.0132)	(0.0278)	(0.0162)	(0.0122)
%	64.6	15.3	−49.1	54.6	83.9	49.0	−33.3	91.2	52.6	70.9
Rural Dummy	−0.0028	−0.0086*	−0.0036	0.0058	0.0028	0.0152***	0.0083*	0.0027	0.0208***	0.0081
	(0.0036)	(0.0045)	(0.0076)	(0.0068)	(0.0046)	(0.0038)	(0.0045)	(0.0069)	(0.0073)	(0.0050)
%	−6.1	−35.5	−16.1	12.2	3.2	15.3	24.3	1.5	16.7	6.1
Observations	6386	1809	543	1969	2065	6444	1816	547	1992	2089

Source: Authors' Calculations. Note: *** is significant at p < 0.01, ** is significant at p < 0.05, * is significant at p < 0.10. Contribution estimates are mean values of the decomposition, bootstrapped to 5000 replications. Note that the base group (Pr = 0) is 1998 and the reference group (Pr = 1) is 2014. Note also that the contribution of the error term has been ignored in the current estimates as is common in the literature

suggest that the part of the difference explained by the determinants (i.e. from national to the ecological zones) is between 10% (southern zone) and 40% (northern zone). For delivery assistance, the increase in the average probability of use is 0.301 (national), 0.318 (southern zone), 0.179 (Greater Accra), 0.276 (middle zone) and 0.377 (northern zone).

The second panel of the decomposition results shows individual contributions of the determinants. A positive percentage contribution is indicative that the determinant in question contributed to increasing the probability of use and vice versa for a negative value. The results in Table 5 suggest that the contribution of the woman's age was only significant in the case of skilled delivery for the middle belt. Per the results, women's education constitutes a key variable contributing to the increased probability of using the two RHS. This is because except for Greater Accra and the middle belt, the women's education coefficients are significant across geography and the two RHS. Most importantly, the percentage contribution is highest for both 4+ antenatal visits and skilled attendants at birth in the southern (32.2% and 43.6%) and northern (14.4% and 11.5%) zones respectively.

Additionally, partner's education is significant, contributing about 84.8% to the increased probability of having 4+ antenatal visits in Greater Accra and 7.1% and 12.1% respectively of the increased probability of using skilled birth services in the middle and northern zones. Ethnicity is also significant at the national level and in the middle zone but contributing only a marginal 5.1% in each case to the increased probability of using skilled birth attendants. Being a Muslim is only significant in the northern belt with respect to skilled birth attendants but contributing a marginal 6.3% to the period increase in the probability of using skilled birth attendants. The number of elderly women in a household reduces the usage gap, with the estimates being significant for 4+ antenatal visit in the northern zone (4.8%), skilled birth attendants in the southern (13.2%) and northern zones (1.6%). Household wealth is also important and significant at the national level. However, it most important effect is in the southern zone, where it contributed 86% and 61% respectively to the increased probability of women making 4+ antenatal visits and using skilled birth attendant during childbirth.

The results in Table 5 shows that the contribution of the health facility availability and accessibility proxies to the increased probability (between 1998 and 2014) of a woman having either 4+ antenatal visits or skilled birth attendants is significant at the national level and the middle and southern zones. At the national level, availability and accessibility contributes about 65% and 49% respectively to the increased probability of use of 4+ antenatal visit and skilled birth attendants. At the

ecological zone level, availability and accessibility of health services contributed 54.6% (middle zone) and 85% (northern zone) to the change in 4+ antenatal visits and 91% (Greater Accra), 53% (middle zone) and 71% (northern zone) to the change in the use of skilled birth attendants. As expected, location of residence is a statistically significant contributor to changes in the use of skilled birth attendants between 1998 and 2014. What is however surprising is the fact that living in a rural area significantly contributed positively (i.e. national level: 15%, southern belt: 24% and middle belt: 17%) to the change in the use of skilled birth attendants between 1998 and 2014.

Discussion

Overall the findings of the study suggest that utilization of RHS improved between 1998 and 2014 both at the national and ecological zone levels. From the results, factors such as women's age, being a Muslim, number of elderly women in the household and living in a rural area are all significantly negatively correlated with utlisation of RHS, Also, women and partners education, household wealth and access to and availability of health services are significantly positively correlated utilization of the two RHS. Additionally, women and partners education, household wealth and availability and accessibility to health facilities are key factors influencing changes in utilization of RHS services both at the national and ecological zone levels. Although the northern and southern belts have lower levels of women and partner education and availability and accessibility of health facilities, they nonetheless recorded the greatest improvements both in education and utilization of the two RHS. Thus, the significant contribution of women and partners education and availability and accessibility of health facilities to the increased probability of using the two RHS could be attributed to the marginal efficiency of educational and health infrastructure investments in the two ecological zones. In other words, educational and health infrastructure investments in the northern and southern zones generate higher marginal returns compared to Greater Accra and the middle zone where levels of education and health infrastructure are already high.

The results of the effect of individual, household and community level factors on the use of the two RHS is consistent with the existing literature. For example, women's age has been found to have a quadratic effect on the utilization of reproductive health services [7−10]. Women's education has also been discussed in the RHS literature as a key determinant of use of RHS. It is often argued that the correlation between education and use of health services come from autonomy [27−29] and health production efficiency [30, 31]. Female education in particular is argued to improve women's autonomy through the development of capabilities and confidence that helps women to make decisions about their own health. There is evidence in the bargaining literature that suggests that male education enhances female autonomy and empowerment.

Existing evidence from Ghana [9, 10], Rwanda, Uganda, Turkey, Bangladesh and Thailand [6, 13, 32–34] suggest that household wealth is a key determinant of utilization of RHS. Consistent with the results, prior studies have found a significant positive correlation between household wealth and utilization of RHS. However, given that RHS such as antenatal and delivery care are supposed to be available and free in all public hospitals in Ghana, the relative importance of household wealth may be a confirmation of the argument that the indirect cost of reproductive healthcare (i.e. travel cost and opportunity cost) may be so high in Ghana [10] that free direct prices may not constitute enough incentives for pregnant women to use RHS. The positive correlation between the proxies for accessibility and availability of health services is also consistent with the existing literature. Different measures of health services availability and accessibility such as non-self cluster proportion of health utilisations variables [10, 20], Distance from health facility [7], constraints to seeking care [9] have all been found to be positively correlated with utilization of health services. Consistent with the results, other factors such as ethnicity [35, 36], religion [7–9, 16] and household size [9, 10] have also been argued in the RHS literature as correlates of utilization of RHS.

With respect to the decomposition results, the existing evidence [11–13] suggest that health behavior, education, responsive health systems and availability and accessibility of health services have been key drivers of change in utilization of health services in countries like Ghana, Rwanda and Uganda. The results of the paper emphasizes this fact and more so in the northern zone. The importance of availability and accessibility to health services in the northern zone is due to the fact that it has for some time now been the target of several donors and NGOs for the implementation of several RHS interventions and research. Thus, the progress suggested by the results may well be related to the outcomes of the several studies and RHS interventions on-going in the northern zones. Related to the donor and NGO effect is the fact that the northern zone has benefited immensely from the Ministry of Health's policy to bridge the health outcomes gap between the southern and the northern parts of Ghana. A major intervention in this direction has been the provision of Community Health Planning and Services (CHPS) compounds aimed at improving access to health services especially in the rural and remote parts of the country.[1] For example data from the District Health Information Systems (DHIMS) of the Ghana Health Service (GHS) suggest that about 722 CHPS compounds have been put up in the northern zone.

It is important though to emphasise that the distribution of CHPS facilities in the northern zone is not uniform but skewed (i.e. a higher concentration in Upper East followed by Upper West and the Northern region as shown in Figs. 1 and 2). It is also important to note that other zones such as the middle belt have benefited from the CHPS programme more than the northern and southern zones (see Fig. 1) and yet did not record the kind of improvements in the use of the two RCH as seen in the northern and southern zones. Thus, the recorded improvements in the northern and southern zones may be related to the efficiency of the existing stock of health infrastructure (i.e. marginal efficiency of investments) and not just the numbers.

Policy implications
The results of the study as discussed above, are straightforward and unambiguous. However, there are a couple of issues that needs further emphasis for the purposes of policy development and interventions targeting.

The fact that the resource-poor zones (i.e. southern and northern) recorded the highest levels of improvements in 4+ antenatal visits and skilled birth attendants respectively is instructive. This may be an indication that pro-poor policies implemented by the health sector is yielding results. Thus, there may be the need to scale-up such interventions in order to speed up the rate of progress. Also important is the fact that the two resource-poor zones that seem to have witnessed the greatest improvements in both 4+ antenatal visits and skilled birth attendance also had the greatest improvements in both women and partners education, household wealth and availability and accessibility to health facilities. As it turned out, and also suggested by the decomposition results, these same factors were key in explaining the positive change in the probability of using the two reproductive health services especially in the two resource-poor zones. Even more important is the fact that the marginal efficiency of educational investments was higher in the two resource-poor zones (southern and northern) compared to the others. Given also that primary and secondary education tend to be very important in terms of education's effect on the use of reproductive health services (as per the regression results), policy-makers may have to prioritise and invest more in primary and secondary education, especially in the two resource poor zones. Such investment as the results seem to suggest, may be crucial to further improving reproductive health outcomes in resource-poor regions in Ghana.

Limitations of the study
It is important to emphasise that the study would have benefited from expanding the scope of outcome variables

and countries used. This would have made it possible to generalise the results for RHS in general. Secondly, the cross-sectional nature of the data and the absence of direct measures of health services availability and accessibility could introduce some form of biases in the results. This not withstanding, the data used is nationally representative and the econometric model robust. Above all, the results are consistent with the existing literature.

Conclusion

The results make it clear that resource poor zones in Ghana such as the northern and southern zones lag behind the middle belt and Greater Accra in terms of utilisation of RHS. This not withstanding, improvements in primary and secondary education as well as health related investments have been key to appreciable improvements in the utilisation of RHS from 1998 to 2014. There is therefore the need for policy makers to scale-up investments in existing pro-poor interventions, especially in the area of education (i.e. primary and secondary) and health to improve the levels of utilisation of RHS in general and especially in resource poor zones such as the southern and northern zones in Ghana.

Endnotes

[1]CHPS are lower level health facilities put up and operated by the staff of the Ministry of Health and normally found in the rural areas. The basic idea behind CHPS is enable rural dwellers to have easy access to health facilities and more importantly, reproductive health services for pregnant mothers.

Additional file

Additional file 1: Table S1. Determinants of 4+ Antenatal Visits in Ghana – Log Odds with Confidence Intervals. Contains regression estimates of the determinants of 4+ antenatal visits in Ghana, with the coefficients expressed in log odds and also showing the confidence intervals. **Table S2.** Determinants Use of Skilled Birth Attendants in Ghana – Log Odds with Confidence Intervals. Contains regression estimates of use of skilled birth attendants in Ghana, with the coefficients expressed in log odds and also showing the confidence intervals.

Acknowledgements
The author will like to acknowledge colleague faculty members who read through the manuscript and offered various suggestions to improve the paper. In the same breath, the author will like to acknowledge students and faculty of the School of Public Health in the University of Ghana who offered suggestion to improve the paper when it was presented in one of their seminar series.

Funding
Not Applicable. The paper was self-financed.

Author's contributions
The author solely conceptualised the paper, secured the relevant data, cleaned the data, carried out the empirical estimation and was responsible for writing out all the sections of the paper. The author read and approved the final manuscript.

Competing interests
The author declares that the paper was funded fully from his personal resources and neither are there any political or other interest to declare.

References
1. WHO. Trends in maternal mortality: 1990 to 2013 estimates by WHO, UNICEF, UNFPA, the World Bank and the United Nations population division. Geneva: World Health Organisation. p. 2014.
2. Unicef. Improving child nutrition: the achievable imperative for global progress. New York: UNICEF; 2013.
3. Save the Children. Surviving the first day. In: State of the world's mothers 2013. Westport Connecticut: Save the Children; 2013.
4. Ghana Statistical Service (GSS), Ghana Health Service (GHS), ICF International. The 2014 Ghana demographic and health survey (DHS) key findings. Rockville: GSS, GHS, and ICF International; 2015.
5. Ministry of Health. Independent annual review of the health sector Programme of works for 2007. Accra: Ministry of Health, Ghana; 2008.
6. Celik Y, Hotchkiss DR. The socio-economic determinants of maternal health care utilization in Turkey. Soc Sci Med. 2000;50(12):1797–806.
7. Overbosch GB, Nsowah-Nuamah NNN, van den Boom GJM, Damnyag L. Determinants of antenatal care use in Ghana. J Afr Econ. 2004;13(2):277–301.
8. Abor PA, Abekah-Nkrumah G, Sakyi K, Adjasi CKD, Abor J. The socio-economic determinants of maternal health care utilization in Ghana. Int J Soc Econ. 2011;38(7):628–48.
9. Abekah-Nkrumah G, Guerriero M, Purohit P. ICTs and maternal healthcare utilization. Evidence from Ghana. Int J Soc Econ. 2014;41(7):518–41.
10. Abekah-Nkrumah G, Abor PA. Socioeconomic determinants of use of reproductive health services in Ghana. Heal Econ Rev. 2016;6(1):1.
11. Bosomprah S, Aryeetey GC, Nonvignon J, Adanu RM. A decomposition analysis of change in skilled birth attendants, 2003 to 2008, Ghana demographic and health surveys. BMC Pregnancy Childbirth. 2014;14(1):1.
12. Rutayisire PC, Hooimeijer P, Broekhuis A. Changes in fertility decline in Rwanda: a decomposition analysis. Int J Popul Res. 2014;(2014):10. Article ID 486210. http://dx.doi.org/10.1155/2014/486210.
13. Pariyo GW, Ekirapa-Kiracho E, Okui O, Rahman MH, Peterson S, Bishai DM, Lucas H, Peters DH. Changes in utilization of health services among poor and rural residents in Uganda: are reforms benefitting the poor? Int J Equity Health. 2009;8(1):39.
14. WHO: Antenatal care: report of a technical working group,. In. Geneva, 31 October-4 November: World Health Organization; 1994.
15. WHO. Mother baby-Pakage: implementing safe motherhood in Counries - practical guide. In: Geneva: maternal health and safe motherhood Programme division of family health World health organisation; 1994.
16. Addai I. Determinants of use of maternal and child health Services in Rural Ghana. J Biosoc Sci. 2000;32(01):1–15.
17. Lavy V, Strauss J, Thomas D, de Vreyer P. Quality of health care, survival and health outcomes in Ghana. J Health Econ. 1996;15(3):333–57.
18. Sahn DE. The contribution of income to improved nutrition in cote d'Ivoire. J Afr Econ. 1994;3(1):29–61.
19. Sahn DE, Stifel DC. Parental preferences for nutrition of boys and girls: evidence from Africa. J Dev Stud. 2002;39(1):21–45.
20. Kabubo-Mariara J, Ndenge GK, Mwabu DK. Determinants of Children's nutritional status in Kenya: evidence from demographic and health surveys. J Afr Econ. 2009;18(3):363–87.
21. Christiaensen L, Alderman H. Child malnutrition in Ethiopia: can maternal knowledge augment the role of income? Econ Dev Cult Chang. 2004;52(2):287–312.
22. Blinder AS. Wage discrimination: reduced form and structural estimates. J Hum Resour. 1973;8(4):436–55.
23. Oaxaca R. Male-female wage differentials in urban labor markets. Int Econ Rev. 1973;14(3):693–709.
24. Fairlie RW. The absence of the African-American owned business: an analysis of the dynamics of self-employment. J Labor Econ. 1999;17(1):80–108.

25. Fairlie RW. Race and the digital divide. Contrib Econ Anal Policy. 2004;3(1). ISSN (Online) 1538-0645. https://doi.org/10.2202/1538-0645.1263.

26. Fairlie RW. An extension of the blinder-Oaxaca decomposition technique to logit and probit models. J Econ Soc Meas. 2005;30(4):305–16.

27. Kabeer N. Resources, agency, achievements: reflections on the measurement of Women's empowerment. Dev Chang. 1999;30(3):435–64.

28. Kabeer N. Gender equality and Women's empowerment: a critical analysis of the third millennium development goal. Gend Dev. 2005;13(1):13–24.

29. Gabrysch S, Campbell O. Still too far to walk: literature review of the determinants of delivery service use. BMC Pregnancy Childbirth. 2009;9(1):34.

30. Burgard S. Race and pregnancy-related care in Brazil and South Africa. Soc Sci Med. 2004;59(6):1127–46.

31. Furuta M, Salway S. Women's position within the household as a determinant of maternal health care use in Nepal. Int Fam Plan Perspect. 2006;32(1):17–27.

32. Chakraborty N, Islam MA, Chowdhury RI, Bari W, Akhter HH. Determinants of the use of maternal health services in rural Bangladesh. Health Promot Int. 2003;18(4):327–37.

33. Gebreselassie A. Factors affecting maternal health care seeking behavior in Rwanda. Macro International Inc: Calverton; 2008.

34. Raghupathy S. Education and the use of maternal health care in Thailand. Soc Sci Med. 1996;43(4):459–71.

35. Matsumura M, Gubhaju B. Women's status, household structure and the utilization of maternal health Services in Nepal. Asia-Pac Popul J. 2001;16(1):23-44.

36. Ekman B, Axelson H, Ha DA, Nguyen LT: Use of maternal health care services and ethnicity: a cross-sectional analysis of Vietnam. 2007. *Available at SSRN 993713.*

Waking up every day in a body that is not yours: a qualitative research inquiry into the intersection between eating disorders and pregnancy

Elizabeth A. Claydon[1][*] [iD], Danielle M. Davidov[1], Keith J. Zullig[1], Christa L. Lilly[2], Lesley Cottrell[1,3] and Stephanie C. Zerwas[2,4]

Abstract

Background: Women with eating disorders are more likely to negatively react to finding out they are pregnant, although this difference in attitudes between women with eating disorders and controls disappears at 18-weeks' gestation. Those with anorexia also are twice as likely to have an unplanned pregnancy and those with bulimia have a 30-fold increased chance compared with healthy controls. Therefore, due to these considerations, pregnancy and the transition to motherhood can be an extremely challenging time for these women both psychologically and physically. The purpose of this qualitative descriptive study was to understand the intersection between eating disorders and pregnancy from the lived experience of women who have been pregnant or want to or do not want to become pregnant.

Methods: A total of 15 women with a current or past history of an eating disorder were recruited, including nine women who have had previous pregnancies as well as six nonparous women. Interviews were the primary unit of data collection, in addition to document analysis of diaries or blogs. Data analysis was based on verbatim transcripts from audio recordings. NVIVO 11© was used to manage the data from these interviews and thematic analysis was then conducted for emergence of major and sub themes.

Results: A total of six themes emerged from the iterative process of coding and categorizing. They were: *Control*, *Disclosure to Others*, *Battle between Mothering & Eating Disorder*, *Fear of Intergenerational Transmission*, *Weight and Body Image Concerns*, and *Coping Strategies*. One theme, *Battle between Mothering & Eating Disorder* also had three sub-themes: Decision to Have Child, Emotions Towards Pregnancy, and Focus on Child/Greater Good.

Conclusions: It is hoped that quotes and themes derived from this study will help inform both prenatal and postnatal care and interventions, as well as addressing intergenerational transmission concerns among mothers with eating disorders.

* Correspondence: elizabeth.claydon@hsc.wvu.edu
[1]Department of Social & Behavioral Sciences, West Virginia University School of Public Health, Robert C. Byrd Health Sciences Center, West Virginia University, One Medical Center Drive, P.O. Box 9190, Morgantown, WV 26506-9190, USA

Background

"Waking up every day in a body that is not yours" is a quote that may resonate with many pregnant women, but for a pregnant woman with an eating disorder (ED) or history of an ED, this bodily disconnect is even more pronounced. Although they realize the bodily changes are necessary for the baby to grow, it is harder for women with, or history of, an ED to accept those changes. Instead, the weight and shape changes become constant triggers, making pregnancy a time of particular physical and psychological strain [1].

Women with EDs experience many battles throughout their disease, but considerably more when they face the prospect of pregnancy. Women with EDs are more likely to negatively react to finding out they are pregnant, although this difference in attitudes between women with EDs and controls disappears at 18-weeks' gestation [2]. These negative reactions are thought to be due to several different factors [1]. First, women with anorexia nervosa (AN) are significantly younger at their first pregnancy than comparison groups, making them potentially less emotionally or developmentally prepared for the pregnancy [3, 4]. Another factor is that women with EDs are more likely than women without EDs to experience an unplanned pregnancy. Those with AN, for example, are twice as likely to have an unplanned pregnancy and those with bulimia nervosa (BN) have a 30-fold increased chance compared with healthy controls [5, 6]. It is still not completely clear why there are these considerably elevated rates of unplanned pregnancy among women with eating disorders, however one theory is that it could be due to patients' belief that amenorrhea (cessation of menstruation) or oligomenorrhea (infrequent menstrual periods) are related to fertility and therefore indicate they cannot get pregnant [5]. Due to this mistaken belief of unlikely pregnancy, women with EDs may also be less likely to use adequate contraception. Therefore, with their negative attitudes towards pregnancy and higher risk of unplanned pregnancies, pregnancy and the transition to motherhood can be a traumatic time for these women both psychologically and physically. Understanding that process is critical to helping improve pregnancy outcomes and maternal-fetal bonding among these women, as well as helping improve and tailor prenatal care to their unique needs.

There is limited research on the intersection of EDs and pregnancy [1, 4–7] and very few studies are qualitative in nature [8, 9], which inhibits understanding this connection from a lived experience perspective. Two qualitative studies in particular built upon this gap but have limitations in describing the nature of this experience. For example, Clark et al. [8] described that women found pregnancy experiences (like feeling the baby kick) to be protective against body dissatisfaction during pregnancy, although that body positivity did not extend into postpartum. Tierney et al. [9] identified three types of women in their interviews: women who went into recovery during pregnancy and maintained that ED recovery postpartum, those that temporarily recovered during pregnancy, and those that were unable to give up ED behaviors during pregnancy. Both studies cited a need to be able to provide more information to women with EDs about expected body changes during pregnancy and to provide professional support to overcome issues of control that could inhibit a positive and healthy pregnancy. However, neither of the current qualitative studies compared participants across countries nor included participants from the United States; one was based in the United Kingdom [9] and the other in Australia [8]. Additionally, both studies also specifically included women who were or had been pregnant but did not look at women with EDs who were hoping to become pregnant 1 day, let alone address the concerns such women might have about becoming pregnant.

The purpose of this qualitative study is to describe the experience of pregnancy for women who have a current or past ED. A qualitative study is necessitated for this area of research because the topic is complex and requires participants' perspectives and in-depth insight to truly understand their lived experiences. Only through such rich detail can we hope to understand the intersection between EDs and pregnancy from the experience of women who face those issues.

This study employed Qualitative Description [10]. This design is appropriate for gathering rich information about a topic where relatively little is known and then describing the phenomenon, process, or perspectives from the viewpoint of participants involved in their own language, without a highly theoretical or interpretive rendering of the data [11]. Therefore, interpretation of the data in Qualitative Descriptive research does not move far beyond what is provided to keep the findings closer to the original data [10]. The philosophical underpinning of this study was feminist theory, which addresses the various situations and institutions that women face, shaping their experience of the world [12]. The aim of most feminist theory approaches is to "correct both the invisibility and distortion of female experience in ways relevant to ending women's unequal social position" [13]. A transformative framework also guided our description because it operates under the tenet that knowledge is not neutral but based on a complicated web of power dynamics that reflect social relationships and that therefore, must be used to improve society [14]. This transformative framework is aligned with the purpose of this study – to aid a marginalized population, specifically women with past or present EDs – in order to help people and thus improve society [15].

The specific aims of this study were to: 1) Describe the concerns that women with EDs feel in becoming pregnant, 2) Understand some of the unique barriers in prenatal care that women with EDs face and 3) Learn how women with EDs can be better supported throughout pregnancy to improve both maternal and child health outcomes.

Methods

Personal Lens

Qualitative research requires investigators to provide their own personal lens and background on research in order to check biases and ensure the trustworthiness of the data. This is a topic that the principal investigator (PI), EAC, is very passionate about on a personal level, having struggled with AN for several years. The PI is in recovery now after relapsing twice; however, during her last relapse, she became pregnant, which drastically changed her need and desire to take care of herself for the sake of her child. The PI received extensive support from doctors, psychiatrists, and nutritionists during her pregnancy, had a healthy pregnancy and subsequently, a healthy baby. However, the process of recovering from AN during pregnancy was incredibly challenging on an emotional level and the PI encountered many individuals who did not understand the pregnancy process from the viewpoint of a woman with an ED. Because of this experience, the PI felt it was imperative to understand this experience from women who have been pregnant and also the unique concerns that women have who want to (or do not want to) become pregnant and how their EDs affect these goals. The PI's own experience is the reason for taking a transformative framework approach to this study because she understood the importance of translational research to change practice and prenatal care so that women with EDs are better supported during their pregnancies.

Participants

An exemption was obtained from West Virginia University's Institutional Review Board (IRB), the Office of Research Integrity and Compliance, negating the need for written consent because it was determined that a written consent would be the only documentation connecting them to the study (IRB #: 1602021245). Once that exemption was obtained, participants were recruited via personal referral and Facebook by asking for women (aged 18 and older) who have 1) an eating disorder, or a history of an eating disorder, and 2) have been pregnant or who did or did not want to become pregnant. Inclusion criteria were as follows: current eating disorder or history of an ED, past pregnancy (either planned or unplanned), or desire/lack of desire to have a pregnancy. Individuals who were currently pregnant were excluded due to ethical concerns about enrolling pregnant women with EDs who may be nutritionally deprived. An advertisement was also used in recruitment and all interested participants were provided a cover letter further explaining the study (See Additional file 1 for IRB-approved advertisement and cover letter).

Due to the PI's history of an eating disorder and her transparency on social media about her history, she was well-positioned to have access to individuals who met the inclusionary criteria. Pseudonyms were used to protect the participants' identities and were chosen using a random name generator. A total of 15 participants were interviewed. Eight participants who volunteered to participate were acquaintances or friends of the PI. Another friend acted as a gatekeeper to provide the PI with a total of five women who had been pregnant. Four of the five women were interviewed for this study; the fifth agreed to be in the study and was scheduled, but could not participate due to a family emergency, after which the PI was unable to get back in contact with her. Another co-author (SCZ) suggested two further participants: specifically, mothers who had blogged about their experiences of being pregnant with an ED. Therefore, this was a convenience sample, but purposive since individuals were specifically selected who could help to answer the research questions [16]. Additionally, all participants were made aware that the PI, who conducted all interviews, had a history of an ED and had been pregnant. At the time of the study, the PI had a Master of Public Health and a Master's of Science degree and was completing her doctorate in public health; she also had training and expert guidance from a co-author (DMD) in qualitative research methods.

Ethics and consent to participate

Participants were asked if the sessions could be audio-recorded and were assured that identifying information would be removed and would not be used in any reports or published materials. Any documents (such as diaries or blogs) were also de-identified before quotes were used. This study was filed with West Virginia University's IRB, the Office of Research Integrity and Compliance, and was given an exemption for both interview data and document collection. A copy of the interview protocol including questions and probes can be found in the Additional file 1. A list of resources and referrals for ED treatment and support was created for the purpose of being provided to any women who became distressed during the interviews or who expressed interest in ED resources (see the Additional file 1). None of the participants became distressed, however one expressed a desire for more resources and another mentioned wanting to get treatment at some point; the resource and referral list was sent to both women.

Data collection

Interviews were the primary unit of data collection, which is appropriate given that there was very sensitive and confidential information to be gathered that might not be as readily shared in a group format, such as through focus groups [16]. The PI conducted individual interviews with participants between March and August 2016, each lasting approximately a half-hour. These interviews were conducted by phone or Skype, depending on the participant's convenience and preference. All interviews were conducted from the PI's home, and, to the PI's best knowledge, from the participants' homes. No one else was present with the PI during the interviews, but sometimes a family member or child of an interviewee would be present momentarily on the interviewee's side; the interview was stopped until the other person left. Participants were read a consent script and asked if they consented to participate before interview questions were asked. Participants also completed a one-page demographic form prior to the interview, in order to gather information regarding their age, highest level of education, current weight and height (if women did not feel comfortable providing their weight, they were not required to), number of children and year of first delivery, and current employment (See the Additional file 1). This form was sent out ahead of time to save time during the scheduled interview and to allow for the collection of some sensitive information such as weight that participants might feel more comfortable answering in writing.

Audio recording was conducted using QuickTime Player© for phone interviews and eCamm© for Skype interviews. Field notes were also taken throughout the interview on a printed interview protocol with information written under each pertinent question. Member-checking is a technique commonly used in qualitative research to improve the accuracy, credibility, and internal validity of a study and involves giving the informants the opportunity to check the authenticity of the material that is being collected [16]. In this study, member-checking was conducted by verifying information or repeating statements back to participants during interviews to check the validity of the information being captured. Member-checking was also conducted by circling back through email, or text message if preferred, with participants, post-interview, to clarify any areas that remained unclear.

Women who had been pregnant were asked to share diaries or blogs from the time when they were pregnant to help triangulate their interview data; a total of four participants volunteered to share pertinent diary or blog entries. Therefore, method triangulation was used and quotes from the diaries and blogs were also captured in this study through document analysis (consistent with triangulation recommendations from Creswell [16] to use "multiple and different sources, methods, investigators, and theories to provide corroborating evidence"; p. 251). We also employed source triangulation by drawing perspectives from women who had children as well as nulliparous women.

It is common for the interview protocol to change during qualitative research, which did occur to some extent during the course of this study. During the first two interviews, the topic of intergenerational transmission came up either in relation to the development of the participant's ED or in their fear that their child/future child might have or develop an ED. Therefore, after those first two interviews, we included questions about intergenerational transmission as a probe if not mentioned or as follow up questions if mentioned.

Data analysis

Data analysis was conducted in the form of thematic analysis, which is the act of gleaning major and sub-themes from qualitative data [16]. The analysis was based on 15 verbatim transcripts from audio recordings; transcription of five interviews was conducted by the study's PI using VideoLan's VLC® (Version 2.2.2) multimedia player to slow the audio recordings. The other 10 interviews were transcribed using the transcription service Rev.com. A non-disclosure agreement was put into effect with this service due to the sensitive information within the interviews. All interviews transcribed by Rev.com were then reviewed by the PI while listening to the original audio content.

The coding of the transcripts followed a standard qualitative methodological process starting with an iterative transcript assessment and ending with theme development [16]. For example, each transcript was read post-transcription, and each one was iteratively read once another transcript was complete. In this way, and according to standard practice, transcripts were continually compared and contrasted between each other in order to assist with thematic analysis. Each transcript was also compared to the PI's interview notes. After those initial readings, the PI went through each transcript and inductively assigned codes to sections of text that addressed a similar issue. NVIVO 11© was used facilitate all aspects of data management and coding. Some codes were in vivo using the guiding theories for the study and the rest were based on subjective assessment of the best encompassing descriptor [16]. Once all transcripts were coded, the codes on each transcript were reviewed in light of any new codes that may have emerged. This same process of coding was used after reviewing the transcripts for document analysis for the diaries and blogs.

All codes from the transcripts were tagged and then similar codes were grouped to create categories. Codes and categories that were repeatedly portrayed in transcripts then rose to the level of themes. Codes and categories were reviewed several times by the PI to ensure that codes and categories were collapsed or split as necessary into major themes. During that process – and according to standard qualitative research analysis – a few themes were again collapsed when it appeared that the lines between different themes blended better into one comprehensive theme [17].

A second coder also reviewed a total of four transcripts (26.7% of the sample), after training on the protocol, procedure, and coding system; this proportion of the transcripts is adequate according to Loewen & Plonsky [18] who recommend a second coder to code at least 20% of the sample. This second coder was also trained with two sample interviews prior to coding to ensure inter-rater reliability. Any discrepancies during training were discussed via multiple debriefing sessions and a final coding scheme was developed and agreed upon by both coders. After consensus was reached by both coders on the final coding strategy and structure, each coder used the agreed upon framework to code the remaining transcripts.

Results

Description of participants

Of the 15 participants interviewed, there were nine women with children and six nulliparous women. Participant demographics can be additionally seen in

Tables 1 and 2, but the women will also be briefly described here. Ages listed are ages at time of interview. The nine mothers were named via the random name generator: Amelia, Nancy, Charlotte, Ann, Kathryn, Ruby, Nicole, Rose, and Laura. Amelia, age 27, is a mother of one, the result of an unplanned pregnancy at age 19. She continues to suffer from an Eating Disorder Not Otherwise Specified (EDNOS) – although EDNOS was the self-reported diagnosis, this diagnosis is now classified as 'Other Specified Feeding or Eating Disorder' (OSFED) in Diagnostic and Statistical Manual of Mental Disorders-5th Edition (DSM-5) [19]. Nancy, 38, is a mother of three, with a past history of AN (purging subtype); she was only just in recovery when she became pregnant with her first, at age 28. Charlotte, 30, suffers from BN, which impacted all of her three pregnancies, two of which were unplanned. Ann, age 55, has a history of AN, which influenced both of her pregnancies and continued for several years after her giving birth. Ann's biological mother had AN, but Ann was raised by an adopted family from the age of 18 months. Kathryn, 31, also has a past diagnosis of AN, and had one child after being in recovery for several years. Ruby, also age 31, has a history of BN and had one child while in recovery although experienced some disordered eating symptoms throughout pregnancy. Nicole, 34, has a history of

Table 1 Maternal demographic characteristics

Participant	Amelia	Nancy	Charlotte	Ann	Kathryn	Ruby	Nicole	Rose	Laura
Age	27	38	30	55	31	31	34	32	41
Relationship Status	In a relationship	Married	Married	Married	Married	Married	Married	Married	Divorced
Location	New York, U.S.	Virginia, U.S.	England, UK	California, US	Wisconsin, US	New Jersey, US	Georgia, US	Maryland, US	Massachusetts, US
Race	Slavic/White	Caucasian	White, British	Caucasian	White	White/Caucasian	Caucasian	Caucasian	Caucasian
ED Type	EDNOS[a], current	Past AN (purging type)	Bulimia	Past AN	Past AN	Past BN	Past EDNOS	Past BN	Past AN
ED Active in Pregnancy	No	No	Partially	Yes	No	No	No	No	No
BMI	17.8	26.6	24.2	18.5	21.1	30.7	Height 5'9", weight not provided	21.5	29
Education	High School	College	College	Graduate School	Graduate School	Graduate School	College	Graduate School	Graduate School
No. of Children	1	3	3	2	1	1	2	1	1
Child Sex	F	F, M, M	F, F, F	F, F	F	F	M, F	M	M
1st Child's Birth Year	2009	2006	2005	1986	2014	2015	2012	2016	2013
Current Job	Pharmacy Tech	Digital Marketing Consultant	Not currently employed	Certified Psychotherapist	Research Associate (Postdoc)	Graduate Teaching Assistant	Executive Director	Biologist	Not currently employed

AN anorexia, *BN* bulimia, *BED* binge eating disorder, *EDNOS* eating disorder not otherwise specified

[a]Eating Disorder Not Otherwise Specified, now labeled 'Other Specified Feeding or Eating Disorder' in DSM-5

Table 2 Nulliparous demographic characteristics

Participant	Melissa	Maria	Marilyn	Kimberly	Sarah	Louise
Age	28	29	25	28	25	29
Relationship Status	Living w/partner but ending relationship	In a relationship	Single	Married	Single	Married
Location	Nova Scotia, Canada	San José, Costa Rica	Texas, US	Colorado, US	Delaware, US	TX, US
Race	Caucasian	Hispanic	Caucasian	White	Caucasian/white	Caucasian
ED Type	Bulimia, current	EDNOS, past	Past BED & current BN	Past AN & BN	Bulimia, current	Past AN & BED
BMI	20.8	22.3[a]	27.4	18.8	22.5	22.9
Highest Education	College	Graduate School	College	College	College	Medical School
Current Job	Support worker for individuals w/disabilities	Chief of Staff to Congressman	Paralegal	Romance Writer	Registered nurse	Medical Resident

AN anorexia, *BN* bulimia, *BED* binge eating disorder, *EDNOS* eating disorder not otherwise specified
[a]Since last weighing, but has not varied much

EDNOS, and became pregnant with her first child soon after coming out of inpatient treatment; her pregnancy, although not unplanned, was also not expected to occur so soon after. Rose, 32, had BN when she was much younger and had been in recovery for almost 20 years before having her first child. Laura, 41, also experienced AN when she was younger and had also been in recovery for about 20 years at the time of her pregnancy.

Six participants did not have children and had mixed feelings about future pregnancies due to their EDs; the six are: Melissa, Maria, Marilyn, Kimberly, Sarah, and Louise. Melissa, age 28, had a previous abortion from an unplanned pregnancy in 2014 and continues to suffer from BN. Maria, age 29, with a past history of EDNOS, had recently become engaged and expressed a desire to become pregnant after a few years of marriage. Marilyn, 25, has a history of binge eating disorder (BED) and was currently experiencing BN at the time of this study; due to her ED, she was not actively thinking of becoming pregnant, although theoretically considered surrogacy or adoption. Kimberly, 28, has a history of AN and BN, and does not want to have children, in part because of her ED history. Sarah, 25, has current BN, and is considering potentially adopting a child in the future. Louise, age 29, has a history of AN and BED, and is considering becoming pregnant in the next few years.

Due to the high rates of unplanned pregnancy in the ED population, it is also important to note the prevalence within this group of women. The women reported a total of 17 pregnancies, including two abortions; of those, six were unplanned, including those two abortions, and eleven pregnancies were planned.

Thematic analysis

A total of six themes emerged from the iterative process of coding and categorizing. They were: *Control, Disclosure to Others, Battle Between Mothering & ED, Intergenerational*

Transmission, Weight and Body Image Concerns, and *Coping Strategies*. One theme, *Battle Between Mothering & ED* also had three subthemes. A detailed description of these themes and subthemes can be found in Table 3.

Control

Individuals with EDs often feel that the ED provides them with a sense of control. Typically, when other aspects of their life feel unmanageable, the ED with its behaviors and rules acts as their constant. It is not surprising perhaps, then, that control stood out as a major theme for these women, in terms of how they talked about their eating

Table 3 Themes/Subthemes

Theme/Subtheme	Description
Control	Mentions of control either regarding their eating disorder or pregnancy/future pregnancy
Disclosure to Others	Choice (& decisions in choice) to tell others about their ED, including family/friends or medical professionals
Battle Between Pregnancy & ED	The internal battle expressed between a woman's ED & her mothering instinct
Decision to Have Child	*The factors involved in decided whether to have a future child or keep/abort an unplanned pregnancy*
Emotions Towards Pregnancy	*Emotions towards pregnancy or initial reactions upon becoming pregnant*
Focus on Child/Greater Good	*Focusing on the wellbeing of the child or sacrificing oneself for the 'greater good'*
Intergenerational Transmission	Worry regarding whether their children or future children would also suffer from EDs or body image concerns
Weight & Body Image Concerns	Concerns about body image or weight primarily regarding pregnancy (including pregnancy weight gain & loss, as well as OB weight checks)
Coping Strategies	Ways expressed to cope with the challenges of a past or future pregnancy

disorder and their view on pregnancy and the need to feel an aspect of control going into, or during, pregnancy.

Amelia spoke about the aspects of control that initiated and maintained her eating disorder and how being able to track everything helped her cope with the stress in her life. She also expressed how hard it was to have to give up that level of control because tracking her calories during pregnancy would, in her words, "completely drive me insane":

> That was the hardest for me, because at the end of the day, I didn't have those numbers to look back on. I didn't know how I did that day. I didn't know like any of that so, it was a complete kind of loss of control and having to give that up because otherwise it was going to completely drive me insane. (Amelia, interview data, Spring 2016)

Melissa recounted her dread of not being in control of her body and how her belief that she could control her body by starving it was invalidated when she became pregnant unexpectedly.

> I had that false, grandiose thought that I was in control of my body and I was calling the shots. And I wasn't and it was kind of surprising. It was a humbling experience ... I can't just march ahead and not take any precautions thinking that I can just starve my body into compliance. (Melissa, interview data, 2016)

In contrast, Ann discussed trying to reassert control during her second pregnancy, since she felt she let others dictate what she did during her first pregnancy too much, which limited her ED behaviors and allowed her to gain more weight than she was comfortable with. Ann stated: "I am not doing whatever I did last time. No one's going to tell me how much I can exercise. No one's going to control me. I am never going in that body again."

Disclosure to others

The issue of maintaining secrecy or disclosing information about the disorder relates to the previous theme of control. The women discussed reasons why they kept their disorder secret or when and why they would disclose it to others. Melissa said: "I kind of just latched onto an eating disorder, 'cause [sic] it was my best friend, my little secret, it was just mine." Similarly, Amelia revealed:

> I have never sought treatment and I am incredibly private about it and sort of like my one secret that I've always had and it's sort of one of those things, like they can take everything else away from me, but they can never take this away. (Amelia, interview data, Spring 2016)

Even when women disclosed it to close others, such as their spouses, those partners still were not able to understand the depths of the problem, which still left the women feeling isolated. Ruby shared:

> My husband has no conception of it. He knows a little bit about that I had an eating disorder and that I've yo-yo dieted and things like that, but he really doesn't understand the mental processes that go behind it, and the constantly being, I'm going to say obsessed. (Ruby, interview data, Summer 2016)

This secrecy or disclosure in relation to medical professionals was also pertinent for women who had been pregnant, as well as those who were contemplating a future pregnancy. The decision whether to discuss information about their eating disorder with an obstetrician or midwife was mixed based on their concerns and what they hoped to gain from sharing that information. Some voiced that it was important to be completely open whereas others, like Amelia, expressed: "I wanted no treatment, no therapy, nothing like that. My OBs are physical doctors ... if I could physically take care of it myself, there was no need for me to involve them." Ann also strongly agreed with that sentiment: "My doctor never knew any of this because I kept everything. Everything. No one knew anything. No one in the whole world. Only me."

Meanwhile, Charlotte discussed some of the challenges that were involved in trying to disclose an ED to medical professionals and wanting treatment:

> I certainly felt a lack of ... communication between psychiatric care and maternity care and needing some sort of, it doesn't have to be a specialized midwife but just someone who can cross barriers and help you navigate your way through the pregnancy from both perspectives and not just one or the other. (Charlotte, interview data, Spring 2016)

Battle between pregnancy & ED

One of the most predominant themes for all of the women was the battle between pregnancy and their ED. This battle played out in various different subthemes, including their decision whether to have a child (including whether to keep or abort an unplanned pregnancy), their emotions (both positive and negative) towards pregnancy, and their focus on the child or the greater good of sacrificing themselves or their ED behaviors for a child.

However, the most prevalent theme was the overall internal battle that these women expressed having when trying to balance the demands of pregnancy and mothering with their ED or history of an ED. Many adopted a 'mama bear' standpoint once they became pregnant, which would force them to change their behaviors, but others stated that being pregnant and having an ED or history of an ED could not be mutually exclusive and were bound to interact.

Those who had been pregnant recounted that battle vividly. Amelia stated: "I swear to god, I had like a countdown to when she was born, and I didn't have to eat anymore." And Charlotte expressed frustration because of "the guilt of not being able to get myself together for the sake of the baby."

Ruby also mentioned how it was challenging not to use pregnancy as an excuse to engage in ED behaviors:

It becomes that battle where you're like well, I've got morning sickness. Should I use that as an excuse? I'm not going to say that I didn't do it once or twice, but it was mainly due to the fact that I was already throwing up anyway. (Ruby, interview data, Summer 2016)

Some dealt with this battle by figuratively disconnecting themselves from the pregnancy in order to push away the impact that their actions were having:

Rosie Robot was who carried the babies, but when you think about a robot carrying a baby, they don't have any emotion. There's nothing there. Then there was me who was trying to be me. I tried. I didn't know I was doing this stuff at that time. I had no idea. I never wore any maternity clothes, ever. I wouldn't wear maternity clothes. I hid it. I hid my pregnancy. Our next-door neighbors … didn't know I was pregnant until I was 9 months pregnant. (Ann, interview data, Summer 2016)

Even women who had not been pregnant speculated about their concerns of not being able to win this battle. For example, Kimberly expressed feeling: "so incredibly selfish … I feel like that kind of hidden darkness could be brought out by something like pregnancy, so I don't know how that would work."

Subtheme: Decision whether to have child
Although many women wanted to become pregnant and planned to do so, several women had unplanned pregnancies and ultimately made different decisions about whether to continue with their pregnancies. Marilyn, when asked – like the other nulliparous women about a potential future pregnancy – expressed thinking about adoption or surrogacy because of the effect of pregnancy on the body and her ED.

Melissa recounted her decision to have an abortion:

I just couldn't do 9 months of that. Regardless of the after part, it was the process. So, I scheduled myself for a [dilation and curettage] D&C and had that

procedure done I think the day before Christmas Eve and then went home for Christmas. (Melissa, interview data, Spring 2016)

Ann also had an abortion in college before having two later pregnancies that were planned and carried to term. "I just thought okay, I guess I'm having an abortion. I remember I scheduled my abortion on the day of a final. It was like I had a final at 11:00 and had the abortion at 2:00."

Like Marilyn, Maria had considered surrogacy in the past during her ED, stating that: "I would rather carry my own kids. But at that time, I was … seriously considering it just because I didn't trust myself enough I think to carry them." Sarah agreed, suggesting that she was more in favor of adoption than carrying a child herself.

Kimberly's decision not to have children was partially influenced by her ED history. "By the time I recovered I was well into my twenties and I just was so used to not wanting children that, you know, I didn't start at that point."

Subtheme: Emotions towards pregnancy
Although all women undergo a multitude of both positive and negative emotions towards pregnancies, especially unplanned pregnancies, these emotions can be even more fraught for women with EDs because of the personal struggles they face. The women with unplanned pregnancies described being scared, isolated or having an 'earth-shattering' moment upon finding out they were pregnant, whereas women with planned pregnancies expressed being delighted. Nulliparous women also weighed in on their emotions towards a theoretical future pregnancy.

Amelia, although, faced with an unplanned pregnancy, did recount in her personal diary at 5 months pregnant that she was "Getting kind of obsessed with the idea of being perfect. Perfect lover. Perfect wife. Perfect mother. Perfect anorexic."

Melissa, however, had a different reaction to her unplanned pregnancy:

I'd missed a period, but I didn't really think too much of that because … that was normal for me and so … I took a pregnancy test and it came up positive and it was probably the most earth-shattering moment of my life. (Melissa, interview data, Spring 2016)

Women generally reacted to planned pregnancies with positive attitudes, although some women talked about how their ED affected their responses to pregnancy even during planned pregnancies. For example, during her one planned pregnancy, Charlotte expressed the disconnect between wanting her child and the negative emotions of being unable to change her ED behavior: "She was just very much loved and wanted ... even though I couldn't help but go through the exact same pattern."

Many nulliparous women had concerns about future pregnancies, which Kimberly voiced. "Yeah, I could see ... the whole something being inside your body as a little weird to me. And it kind of gives me that same itchy feeling I would get when I'd like eat food I considered bad."

Subtheme: Focus on child/greater good

Many pregnant women also turn their focus to their baby or make sacrifices for what is seen as the greater good. Even women who did not plan on becoming pregnant described needing to 'bite the bullet' and deal with the challenges for the sake of the baby. This focus on the child or the greater good was what helped or might help them come out of their EDs enough to be able to have healthy pregnancies.

Amelia used her 'mama bear' instinct to force herself to eat or gain weight for the sake of the baby. "You have to keep telling yourself over and over you know ... this isn't about you anymore like it's never going to be about you again; it's about this child."

However, even women who had been in recovery for years had to use their focus on the child to help them through challenges in pregnancy associated with their history of an ED. Kathryn stated: "Eating disorder behaviors really just didn't feel like an option. Kind of like a, 'this isn't about me, this is about someone else.'" Ruby agreed, saying that: "You don't want to not eat because if you don't eat then your baby's not getting nutrition. It's more than just about you at that stage."

Intergenerational transmission

All the women spoke about their concerns revolving around a theme of intergenerational transmission, which is defined here as the transmission of beliefs or norms around dieting, eating, and weight or shape across generations. This theme of intergenerational transmission reflected both the women's recollection of parental comments or actions growing up or their concerns about how their comments or actions could influence their child or a potential child. For example, Amelia described being very careful about trying to create normalcy for her child, to not label foods as good or bad, and to not talk about her body negatively. Still, she was concerned by the body hyper-awareness that her daughter displayed at a young age and was also concerned that she was a hypocrite by promoting advice that she herself did not follow:

I think my hardest thing is I'm a total hypocrite, because I'm telling her you know, well as long as you are healthy, and you drink enough water and you get

enough sleep, and you exercise and everything, you're going to be fine ... while at the same time, I don't do that at all. (Amelia, interview data, Spring 2016)

Melissa expressed her worries about the health ramifications on her child, which influenced her decision to abort her pregnancy. She also felt that it was hard for her to be a support worker for those with disabilities when she had her own struggles:

It's difficult to have an eating disorder and then be in the role that I'm in because I feel you know, it's the imposter syndrome, right like how am I trying to guide these kids into healthy decision making when secretly I'm you know, I'm participating in my own kind of battle? (Melissa, interview data, Spring 2016)

Similarly, Maria divulged concern about having girls in a future pregnancy due to her history of an eating disorder, out of fear that they would be more likely than boys to also develop an eating disorder. "I'm sort of scared of having girls ... I mean like it's a stereotype because guys can also have eating disorders. But like I'm more scared of having girls like, being a mother to girls."

Many women also shared how they felt they had been influenced by their parents' behaviors or weight commentary.

I've done a lot of reading about this, I think part of the reason that I feel like I have a weight problem is because my mother had a weight problem, and I was never really able to accept myself as beautiful. Just from this body image perspective ... I never learned what was healthy. (Ruby, interview data, Summer 2016)

When I started dieting in middle school, she [Louise's mother] actually taught me how to diet. She taught me how to count calories. She taught me how to weigh food, and how to prepare food, and encouraged me in dieting until it became a little more obvious that it was out of hand. I mean obviously, she didn't mean for that to happen. (Louise, interview data, Summer 2016)

Some women also expressed confidence that they would know the warning signs if their child developed an eating disorder and would therefore be able to get them into treatment earlier. Ann discussed a more direct intervention of how her husband stepped in to try to break the cycle for their children:

Fortunately, my husband, when they were in second grade and third grade ... because I was making like bizarre food. He completely took over food. He brought in chips. He normalized food for my girls. I think that probably saved them, considering that my own biological mother had an eating disorder and then I did. (Ann, interview data, Spring 2016)

Weight & body concerns

Weight and body image concerns are central to all eating disorders and so it is understandable that they would feature as a central theme among concerns about pregnancy. A common theme arose that although the women described the weight gain as being for a positive reason, they still could not reconcile it with their fear of weight gain.

A few also mentioned concerns about how to lose the baby weight healthily without triggering their eating disorder again. Maria expressed that, "objectively I know that people gain weight in pregnancy, but I think another fear would be how I would lose it afterward … like how to do it in like the healthiest way possible." Sarah affirmed this fear, stating that "feeling like you have to lose weight is definitely a trigger for an eating disorder."

Weight checks with obstetricians during pregnancy were also an expressed fear, as well as how doctors would deliver information regarding weight gain. Some realized that being weighed at prenatal visits would be very stressful and thought about opting for, or did opt for, blind weighing. Maria thought she would choose that option, because she has chosen not to weigh herself and hoped that "somebody could know and do the checks, but it's information that I'd rather not know." However, the women differed in how they approached that experience. Kathryn was able to frame her weight checks positively, saying that "it didn't feel as revealing the way I think being weighed when not pregnant does … it was kind of a relief … it didn't really mean that I was a big, fat pig."

Many women cited body image concerns as issues that they had or feared they would face during pregnancy. As Amelia's body changed she expressed feeling like she was losing her body or felt trapped in her body. "I feel so fleshy, swollen, flabby, jiggly, sloppy, oily, nasty, just FAT. It's fucking killing me. I miss restricting so badly … this body is like a prison and I want out." ~ Amelia, personal diary, c. 5 months pregnant.

For Louise, projected body image issues included the expectation of the 'ideal' pregnant woman's body and her concern that she would not conform to that ideal.

This is going to sound terrible, but I'm not going to be one of those girls who look pretty when they're pregnant. They've got this nice slender body, and then they just have this little bump … No, mine's going to be one of those like, "Well, I look like a marshmallow," because that's just how my body

carries weight … I know that that's how I'm going to look, and how I'm going to feel, and it scares me. (Louise, interview data, Summer 2016)

Coping strategies

Both Amelia, during her pregnancy, and Maria when thinking about future pregnancy, noted some coping strategies that they did or would employ in order to help them through challenges.

Amelia particularly used distraction as a coping mechanism, as well as reframing the pregnancy as a "temporary medical condition." "I completely threw myself relentlessly into school at that point … because I had to distract myself somehow." She also let go of her accountability with tracking her eating and calorie intake:

I forced myself to not keep track of things anymore … because at the end of day I knew I had to be consuming at least 2300 calories and if I hit that, I'd be upset, but then if I didn't hit that, I'd be upset. So, either way, you're never going to win in that situation … I just had to give up accountability all together and just say fuck it. (Amelia, interview data, Spring 2016)

Maria, however, thought she would rely on professional and social support throughout pregnancy. She believed she would need this help because, she stated: "I don't trust myself to make the best decisions regarding pregnancy. Maybe I would and I'm underestimating myself, but I would rather just have the outside support."

Ruby attempted to avoid engaging in eating disorder behaviors, such as purging, through conscious effort and her knowledge that the behaviors were unhealthy:

I go to the bathroom at the end of the meal and it's like I have to remind myself not to do it. I choose not to because I know it's not healthy, but it's a choice that I make. (Ruby, interview data, Summer 2016)

Discussion

From these conversations with women discussing the intersection between EDs and pregnancy, a total of seven themes rose to the forefront. Some, such as *Weight and Body Image Concerns* and *Control* were expected due to the nature of EDs. However, others like *Intergenerational Transmission* were not. The fact that this theme arose to salience supports the recent research that suggests social or environmental transmission of dieting behavior is something that individuals recall or are concerned about [20]. Additionally, it is critical to note that all these women expressed concerns about intergenerational transmission of their EDs or ED behaviors, even when the prospect of pregnancy was so frightening. For them to all raise this as a concern indicated that despite the *battle between pregnancy and their ED* that had existed or would exist, their focus on the well-being of the child won out.

The women's expressed concern regarding *disclosure* to their doctors indicates an area of potential improvement within prenatal care, but also within the educational systems. Medical professionals could benefit from further training about EDs in order to help provide more sensitive information and care – particularly around weight and weight gain – to women who have or have had an ED. It also would be beneficial to explore these women's *coping strategies* further to help provide psychological or social support on adjusting to pregnancy, especially since many pregnancies in women with EDs are unplanned.

Based on Tierney et al.'s [9] assessment of the three routes women with eating disorders take during and after pregnancy, we also grouped the women who had been pregnant into those categories. Research from large prospective studies shows that remission rates are 78% for purging disorder (PD); 34% for BN for full remission and an additional 29% for BN for partial remission [21]. However, there are no estimates available for AN because there are currently no clear criteria to establish maternal underweight during pregnancy. This study focused on women with a previous pregnancy who had current or past AN, BN, and EDNOS. Kathryn (past AN), Ruby (past BN), Nicole (past EDNOS), Rose (past BN), and Laura (past AN) all went into recovery or were in recovery when they became pregnant and maintained that recovery postpartum. Nancy (with AN purging subtype) and Amelia (with EDNOS) recovered during pregnancy and Amelia went back to ED behaviors immediately postpartum. Nancy was able to maintain her recovery after her first pregnancy and had a minor relapse after her second pregnancy before going back into recovery. Both Charlotte (BN) and Ann (past AN) continued ED behaviors during their pregnancies. Charlotte was able to stop her behaviors when she was 5–6 months pregnant during each of her three pregnancies, but never went into recovery, and went back to behaviors immediately after pregnancy. Ann continued her ED behaviors throughout both her pregnancies and did not go into recovery until years after.

Strengths

The current study overcomes some of the limitations of previous qualitative studies by having a more international perspective, finding common themes across participants from the U.S., the United Kingdom, Canada, and Central America. Additionally, this study captures the experiences of childless women with EDs who did or did not want to become pregnant and how their eating disorder affected that choice. Those women who did

have children also had a mixture of planned and unplanned pregnancies, providing a more nuanced understanding of those experiences.

Given the sensitive nature of these interviews and the personal details that interviewees were asked to share, conducting the interviews over the phone or via audio Skype actually may have facilitated sharing more personal information due to the increased distance between participant and interviewer.

Other strengths of this study were the steps taken to ensure its trustworthiness and internal validity [22]. For example, the method and source triangulation employed ensured credibility and confirmability of findings, as did member-checking to verify that transcripts were accurate and that the themes were representative. We used negative case analysis by including women who had not been pregnant; the fact that they highlighted similar concerns provides additional credibility. We provided a thick description of the methodology employed, allowing for the transferability of these findings. The dependability of the data was enhanced by using a second coder for over 20% of the sample and ensuring training for that coder. Additionally, we reached thematic saturation, reinforcing the internal validity of the selected themes.

Limitations

There are several limitations that need to be acknowledged. First, there is limited method triangulation because only a few (*n* = 4) provided documents for document analysis, so primarily thematic analysis from interviews was used. However, source triangulation was ensured by using both nulliparous women with children, which adds to the trustworthiness of the study and its data. Second, the transferability of the study is limited because the sample is comprised entirely of Caucasians, with only one identifying as Hispanic. Therefore, we cannot know if the results would vary in different racial or ethnic groups. The majority of the women were also highly educated, so again, future studies would need to include different demographic groups to understand the transferability of the results. Finally, we used a qualitative descriptive approach for this study, given the dearth of existing information on the topic and small sample size. A more interpretive and in-depth approach to data analysis, such as Interpretive Description [23], may have allowed us to more fully explore several important themes and sub-themes that emerged in this analysis. For example, issues of "control" clearly emerged in this analysis, and as such we felt it rose to the level of a major theme; however, issues of control underpin EDs in general, and also may cut across or be represented in the other major themes presented here, such as coping strategies. For example, a pregnant woman could be afraid of control being taken away from her during the pregnancy and not disclose her ED to her obstetrician as a form of coping strategy. These preliminary findings lay an important foundation for future interpretive studies to clarify this issue with a larger, theoretically generated samples of women with EDs who have been pregnant, who wish to become pregnant, and those who do not want to become pregnant.

Conclusions

The compelling insights on pregnancy gathered from women who suffer from EDs provide useful areas for future intervention to improve the prenatal, pregnancy, and postpartum period for similar women. Their concerns, challenges, and experiences resonate with each other despite the differences in their situations, lending credence that the themes gathered in this qualitative descriptive study may be generalizable to a larger group of women. Future research will need to explore both racial and cultural differences, as well as differences in socio-economic backgrounds that were not as varied among these 15 women. Additionally, some women mentioned issues such as surrogacy or adoption that stemmed from their ED, which would be valuable to research further. One future area of research would be to more clearly understand what motherhood means to women with EDs or a history of an ED. Amelia discussed her "mama bear" mentality, but more research needs to be done to discern how others conceptualize what being a mother means.

For the PI, from a personal perspective, this research is both critically important, but also emotionally charged. Having experienced a pregnancy while in recovery from an ED, the PI could empathize with these women over their concerns and battles between the strength of their mothering instinct versus the power of their ED. Many of the women interviewed were appreciative of a study on this topic because they felt lost in a society that could not understand the battle that they had undergone or would 1 day face. Maria mentioned her worry that others would think some of her concerns superficial or vain. These are worries that women should not have to have. This research is playing a part in giving a voice to this population's concerns in order to help them through such an emotionally and physically challenging process.

Abbreviations

AN: Anorexia nervosa; BED: Binge eating disorder; BN: Bulimia nervosa; D&C: Dilation and curettage; DSM-5: Diagnostic and Statistical Manual of Mental Disorders-5th Edition; ED: Eating disorder; EDNOS: Eating disorder not otherwise specified; EDs: Eating disorders; IRB: Institutional review board; OSFED: Other specified feeding & eating disorder

Acknowledgements

First and foremost, we want to offer heartfelt gratitude to the women who bravely shared their personal stories and struggles in an effort to help others facing similar circumstances. We would also like to express our extensive gratitude to Mary Quattlebaum of University of North Carolina Chapel Hill for her excellent assistance as second coder for the qualitative data.

Funding

This research was supported, in part, by grant #5R49CE002109 from the National Center for Injury Prevention and Control, CDC, to the West Virginia University Injury Control Research Center. Contents are solely the responsibility of the authors and do not represent official views of the CDC. This funding provided stipend support to the primary author, EAC, while completing this research as part of her dissertation.

Authors' contributions

All authors included contributed significantly to the writing and editing of this manuscript and have approved the final version. Additionally, this research was part of a dissertation and all co-authors were part of the dissertation committee for EAC; therefore, they were integrally involved at each step of the process. EAC planned and developed the research study, prepared and submitted the IRB protocol, recruited participants, interviewed all participants, transcribed five interviews (and coordinated the transcription of the rest), coded transcripts, conducted the thematic analysis, selected representative quotes for inclusion in the manuscript, and was the lead writer for the manuscript. DMD was the qualitative expert for consultation and helped with the planning and development of the study as well as helping to prepare and submit the IRB protocol and the interview protocol; she also helped EAC select representative quotes for inclusion in the manuscript and helped revise the manuscript in many stages of its development. KJZ assisted with the planning and development of the study and took accountability for the integrity and accuracy of the data; he also played a significant role in revising the manuscript in many iterations. CLL assisted with planning and developing the research study and came from a quantitative perspective, which encouraged further explanation of qualitative processes within the manuscript; she also revised the manuscript throughout the process. LC provided an obesity prevention and childhood psychology lens to the study, helped plan and develop the study, and significantly revised the manuscript. SCZ provided the necessary additional eating disorder expertise for this research, assisted with planning and developing the study, connected the PI with a second-coder to ensure the reliability of coding, and significantly revised the manuscript.

Competing interests

The authors declare that they have no competing interests.

Author details

[1]Department of Social & Behavioral Sciences, West Virginia University School of Public Health, Robert C. Byrd Health Sciences Center, West Virginia University, One Medical Center Drive, P.O. Box 9190, Morgantown, WV 26506-9190, USA. [2]Department of Biostatistics, West Virginia University School of Public Health, Morgantown, WV, USA. [3]Department of Pediatrics, West Virginia University School of Medicine, Morgantown, WV, USA. [4]Department of Psychiatry, UNC School of Medicine, Chapel Hill, NC, USA.

References

1. Zerwas S, Claydon E. Eating disorders across the lifespan: from menstruation to menopause. In: Barnes DL, editor. Women's reproductive mental health across the lifespan. New York: Springer Publishing; 2014. p. 237–61.
2. Easter A, Treasure J, Micali N. Fertility and prenatal attitudes towards pregnancy in women with eating disorders: results from the Avon longitudinal study of parents and children. BJOG. 2011;118(12):149–8. https://doi.org/10.1111/j.1471-0528.2011.03077.x
3. Bulik CM, Von Holle A, Siega-Riz AM, Torgersen L, Lie KK, Hamer RM, et al. Birth outcomes in women with eating disorders in the Norwegian mother

and child cohort study (MoBa). Int J Eat Disord. 2009;42(1):9–18. https://doi.org/10.1002/eat.20578.

4. Micali N, Treasure J, Simonoff E. Eating disorders symptoms in pregnancy: a longitudinal study of women with recent and past eating disorders and obesity. J Psychosom Res. 2007;63(3):297–303. https://doi.org/10.1016/j.jpsychores.2007.05.003.

5. Bulik CM, Hoffman ER, Von Holle A, Torgersen L, Stoltenberg C, Reichborn-Kjennerud T. Unplanned pregnancy in women with anorexia nervosa. Obstet Gynecol. 2010;116(5):1136–40. https://doi.org/10.1097/AOG.0b013e3181f7efdc.

6. Morgan JF, Lacey JH, Chung E. Risk of postnatal depression, miscarriage, and preterm birth in bulimia nervosa: retrospective controlled study. Psychosom Med. 2006;68(3):487–92. https://doi.org/10.1097/01.psy.0000221265.43407.89.

7. Abraham SF, Pettigrew B, Boyd C, Russell J, Taylor A. Usefulness of amenorrhoea in the diagnoses of eating disorder patients. J Psychosom Obstet Gynaecol. 2005;26(3):211–5. https://doi.org/10.1080/01674820500064997.

8. Clark A, Skouteris H, Wertheim EH, Paxton SJ, Milgrom J. My baby body: a qualitative insight into women's body-related experiences and mood during pregnancy and the postpartum. J Reprod Infant Psychol. 2009;27(4):330–45. https://doi.org/10.1080/02646830903190904.

9. Tierney S, Fox JRE, Butterfield C, Stringer E, Furber C. Treading the tightrope between motherhood and an eating disorder. Int J Nurs Stud. 2011;48:1223–33.

10. Sandelowski M. What's in a name? Qualitative description revisited. Res Nurs Health. 2009;33:77–84.

11. Bradshaw C, Atkinson S, Doody O. Employing a qualitative description approach in health care research. Glob Qual Nurs Res. 2017;4:2333393617742282.

12. Olsen V. Feminist qualitative research in the Millenium's first decade: developments, challenges, prospects. In: Denzin NK, Lincoln YS, editors. The SAGE handbook of qualitative research. 4th ed. Thousand Oaks: Sage Publications; 2011. p. 129–46.

13. Lather P. Getting smart: feminist research and pedagogy with/in the postmodern. New York: Routledge; 1991.

14. Mertens DM. Mixed methods and the politics of human research: the transformative-emancipatory perspective. In: Tashakkori A, Teddlie C, editors. Handbook of mixed methods in social and behavioral research. Thousand Oaks: Sage Publications; 2003. p. 135–64.

15. Mertens DM. Transformative research and evaluation. New York: Guilford Press; 2009.

16. Creswell JW. Qualitative inquiry and research design: choosing among five approaches. 3rd ed. Thousand Oaks: Sage Publications; 2013.

17. Saldāna J. The coding manual for qualitative researchers. London: Sage Publications; 2009.

18. Loewen S, Plonsky L. An A-Z of applied linguistics research methods. 1st ed. Basingstoke: Palgrave Macmillan; 2015.

19. American Psychiatric Association. Diagnostic and statistical manual of mental disorders. 5th ed. Arlington: American Psychiatric Publishing; 2013.

20. Claydon EA, Zullig KJ, Lilly CL, Zerwas SC, Davidov DM, Cottrell L, White MA. An exploratory study on the intergenerational transmission of obesity & dieting proneness. Eat Weight Disord. 2018:1–9. https://doi.org/10.1007/s40519-018-0478-1.

21. Bulik CM, Von Holle A, Hamer R, Knoph Berg C, Torgersen L, Magnus P, et al. Patterns of remission, continuation and incidence of broadly defined eating disorders during early pregnancy in the Norwegian mother and child cohort study (MoBa). Psychol Med. 2007;37(8):1109–18. https://doi.org/10.1017/S0033291707000724.

22. Lincoln YS, Guba EG. Naturalistic inquiry. Newbury Park: Sage Publications; 1985.

23. Thorne S, Kirkham SR, MacDonald-Emes J. Interpretive description: a noncategorical qualitative alternative for developing nursing knowledge. Res Nurs Health. 1997;20(2):169–77.

Examining trends in inequality in the use of reproductive health care services in Ghana and Nigeria

Oluwasegun Jko Ogundele[1][*] [iD], Milena Pavlova[1] and Wim Groot[1,2]

Abstract

Background: Equitable use of reproductive health care services is of critical importance since it may affect women's and children's health. Policies to reduce inequality in access to reproductive health care services are often general and frequently benefit the richer population. This is known as the inverse equity situation. We analyzed the magnitude and trends in wealth-related inequalities in the use of family planning, antenatal and delivery care services in Ghana and Nigeria. We also investigate horizontal inequalities in the determinants of reproductive health care service use over the years.

Methods: We use data from Ghana's (2003, 2008 and 2014) and Nigeria's (2003, 2008 and 2013) Demographic and Health Surveys. We use concentration curves and concentration indices to measure the magnitude of socioeconomic-related inequalities and horizontal inequality in the use of reproductive health care services.

Results: Exposure to family planning information via mass media, antenatal care at private facilities are more often used by women in wealthier households. Health worker's assistance during pregnancy outside a facility, antenatal care at government facilities, childbirth at home are more prevalent among women in poor households in both Ghana and Nigeria. Caesarean section is unequally spread to the disadvantage of women in poorer households in Ghana and Nigeria. In Nigeria, women in wealthier households have considerably more unmet needs for family planning than in Ghana. Country inequality was persistent over time and women in poorer households in Nigeria experienced changes that are more inequitable over the years.

Conclusion: We observe horizontal inequalities among women who use reproductive health care. These inequalities did not reduce substantially over the years. The gains made in reducing inequality in use of reproductive health care services are short-lived and erode over time, usually before the poorest population group can benefit. To reduce inequality in reproductive health care use, interventions should not only be pro-poor oriented, but they should also be sustainable and user-centered.

Keywords: Concentration index, Inequality, Inequity, Reproductive services, Ghana, Nigeria

Background

Equitable provision of reproductive health care services is of critical importance since it affects, among others, individual and economic development and bears on universally recognized human rights. The loss of healthy life years due to morbidity or mortality resulting from reproductive ill-health among pregnant women is highest in Sub-Saharan Africa [1]. This increases poverty and impedes the economic growth of nations since it impacts on child development and women's labor force participation [2–4]. In Sub-Saharan Africa countries, reproductive health care services are not affordable to everyone in need, leading to unequal access to care [5–7].

Policies to reduce inequality in access to reproductive health care services, particularly in Sub-Saharan African countries, often have unintended and unwanted consequences. Such as health providers preference for urban

* Correspondence: j.ogundele@maastrichtuniversity.nl
[1]Department of Health Services Research, CAPHRI, Maastricht University Medical Center, Faculty of Health, Medicine and Life Sciences, Maastricht University, PO Box 616, 6200MD Maastricht, The Netherlands

and educated clients and the language barrier between provider and client [8]. Likewise, due to the inefficient distribution of health resources, policies often fail the poorest population, inadvertently widening the poor-rich gap [9]. This is often referred to as the inverse equity hypothesis [10]. Evidence on the relationship between government policies and access to services suggests that service delivery usually undermine benefits to the poor. For example, public health spending even though adequate can be allocated inefficiently and further precipitate between-group inequalities [11, 12]. Other studies have confirmed that access to healthcare innovations can be unequally distributed and to the advantage of richer households creating stratification in favor of the higher socioeconomic groups [13–19]. Pre-sustainable development goals era, research showed that interventions that address family planning, as well as maternal health care, are inequitable [20].

In light of this, low- and middle-income countries have implemented pro-poor initiatives with the goal to advance equitable access to quality reproductive health-care services. One example is the reproductive care services information channels in Nigeria [21]. Another is the provision of insurance schemes and community-based health programs in Ghana [22, 23]. Some of such successful interventions have been scaled-up, however with non-replicable successes [24, 25]. Both countries have put in place different health promotion schemes to attain a common goal of reducing inequities associated with the delivery of reproductive health care service such as the fee exemption for maternity care in Ghana [26, 27] and the national health insurance scheme in Nigeria [28]. This study contributes to the literature by investigating the underlying mechanisms of inverse equity for subsequent initiatives for underserved populations [10]. Ghana and Nigeria, through the sustainable development agenda, have agreed to foster equitable access to reproductive health care services [29].

The study analyzes the magnitude and trends in wealth-related inequality in the use of reproductive health care services (family planning and maternal care) in Ghana and Nigeria and provides insight into horizontal inequalities by describing the changes in the determinants of inequalities in the access to reproductive health care services over the years. An assessment of equity changes is essential to establish if policies addressing socioeconomic inequality improve the use of care.

In 2003, the fee exemption for maternity care commenced in four regions of Ghana (The Central, Northern, Upper West, and Upper East Regions), chosen due to the high poverty and maternal mortality levels and the low levels of supervised deliveries [26]. This policy was expanded in 2005 to cover the other six regions of Ghana. Thus all pregnant women in Ghana

are exempted from payments for maternity care services such as prenatal visits, childbirth care (physiological childbirth and childbirth with medical assistance), caesarian section, and postnatal visit in all facilities [27]. Health insurance is compulsory for formal sector workers and voluntary for informal-sector workers and is reported to cover 65% of the population [30, 31]. The insurance premiums vary geographically and are ambiguously based on ability to pay with no clear guideline to determine premium levels [32]. However, significant differences in the use of maternity care persist [32–36]. In a concurrent effort to promote access to health care, reproductive care services included, the community-based health planning services in Ghana provide community-level services targeted at poor mothers and provide services including family planning, supervising delivery and maternity care [25]. The community-based health planning services have been introduced to all districts/regions to facilitate access, especially for the population living further away from health care services.

Nigeria's national health insurance scheme, initiated in 1999 and kicked off in 2005, is a social health insurance scheme aimed at improving access to health care and reducing associated cost. It was piloted in six regions among civil servants and formal sector employees, targeting 5 percent of the population [28]. Coverage through the NHIS remains less than 5% of the Nigerian population (NHIS, 2011). To broaden coverage, the community-based health insurance scheme, flagged off in 2008, was made available to the general population and subsidized for households, particularly in rural communities. The scheme is organized by community members and covers family planning services, antenatal care, as well as vaginal childbirth [37]. The community-based health insurance scheme allows for differences in premium rates, enrolment, and uptake of varied sexual and reproductive health care services across the country [37, 38]. Access to reproductive health care services in Nigeria remains underdeveloped and a large proportion of the population has no health coverage living most of the health expenditure to be borne by households.

The midwives service scheme was implemented in 2009 throughout the country as part of efforts to reach the rural communities and facilitate the adoption of skilled care among the populations by improving the capacity of public primary health facilities [38]. Allocation of midwives service scheme facilities is determined using geographic location as the factor with northeast and northwest regions emerging as a top priority, in part due to high maternal mortality rate and low access to services [24]. Though deemed to be making developments in implementation, highlighted setbacks include the non-availability of qualified midwives and retention of midwives [39]. Reports of horizontal variation in the use of reproductive health in the achievements of the midwives service scheme were reported [24].

Nigeria and Ghana were selected based on their governments having introduced a national health insurance program and other health promotion programs to address the inaccessibility of reproductive health care services [21, 25]. The introductions of these programs have met with different success and have contributed to differences in access and use of reproductive health care services between the two countries. The differences and similarities in the progress towards equality will provide information on constraints to access to services among the poor and improve policies that address these. Research on the equity effect of reproductive health care policies is limited.

Methods

Data

We used secondary data from the Demographic and Health Surveys (DHS). The surveys are conducted under an international program implemented by ICF International and funded by the USAID with contributions from UNICEF, UNFPA, WHO, and UNAIDS [40]. The DHS are cross-sectional and nationally representative surveys in low- and middle-income countries. The DHS adopt a multi-stage cluster design and samples selected for enumeration are ensured to be representative and comparative across countries. The DHS involves a two-stage cluster and systematic sampling design with households selected at random. In both countries, the sampling accounted for differences in population distribution regionally as well as for the urban-rural spread. Designated households were enumerated without allowance for a change or replacement to prevent bias. Respondents were selected on the basis of being female (for the female survey) or male (for the male survey), aged 15-49 and whether the respondent was a usual member of the household or having spent the night prior the survey in the household. These surveys employed standard Demographic Health Surveys (DHS) questionnaires and techniques for data collection [40]. All eligible women aged 15–49 were interviewed with the Women's Questionnaire. Eligible women are all women aged 15–49 who stayed in a selected household the night before the interview, irrespective of whether they were usual residents in the household or not. The Women's Questionnaire was used to collect respondent's individual characteristics including age, marital status, occupation, residence as well as other information on topics including; reproductive history; contraceptive knowledge and use; antenatal, delivery and postnatal care; marriage; attitudes about family planning.

Analyses were performed using data from the women's response file, from the full DHS dataset of Ghana (2003,

2008, and 2014) and Nigeria (2003, 2008, and 2013). We use data from women who have had at least one birth in the 5 years prior to the survey. A summary of indicators used and information on missing data is available in Additional file 1.

Measurement

We consider family planning, antenatal care, and delivery care services as essential aspects of reproductive healthcare. The dependent variables to indicate exposure to or use of family planning, antenatal care, and delivery care services were grouped in similar themes based on the WHO recommendations [41]. Table 1 shows the definition of the indicators used in the intervention areas examined. Responses to questions on the use of similar reproductive health care services were aggregated to produce one outcome variable (see Additional file 1 for grouping description). This was done to capture the different types of health care used during pregnancy. All dependent variables are dichotomized, taking the value 1 when a woman answered "Yes" to the questions and "0" if otherwise. The dependent variable indicating a woman's unmet need for family planning is coded as 1 when a woman answered "No" to the question if she wanted last birth and "0" if she answered "Yes". Control variables include a woman's age, marital status, occupation, location, and region of residence. Coding of the dependent and control variables used are indicated in Additional file 1.

Household Wealth

To measure household wealth, asset ownership and living conditions available in each DHS dataset were used. Wealth was measured by ownership of some or all consumer items and residence characteristics including electricity, radio, television, refrigerator, bicycle, motorcycle, car or truck, non-mobile phone, water source, type of toilet facility, flooring, wall, and roofing materials. These were used to create a wealth index score by adopting D Filmer and LH Pritchett [42] principal component analysis approach to generate the indicator weights for the household assets and subsequently weighted scores for all assets that were summed to create a household wealth index. The types of assets owned were similar between Ghana and Nigeria, though local context implied differences in the consumer items and residence characteristics used in the index. The asset includes weights that varied between countries. This has been described as the local perception of wealth approach.

Equity analysis

To measure household wealth inequality in access to family planning, antenatal care, and delivery care services in Ghana and Nigeria over time, we use the concentration

Table 1 Definition of indicators by intervention area used for the equity analysis

Indicators for family planning	
Family planning info: Health facility	Percentage of women told of family planning at a health facility
Family planning worker visit	Percentage of women who were visited by FP worker last 12 months
Family planning: TV	Percentage of women who heard family planning information on TV last months
Family planning: Print	Percentage of women who got family planning information on a newspaper last months
Modern contraceptive	Percentage of women who currently use by a modern method of contraceptive
Information on pregnancy complication	Percentage of women who were told about pregnancy complications
Family planning: unmet need	Percentage of women who wanted the last child later / wanted no more
Indicators for antenatal care	
Health worker's (HW) assistance during pregnancy outside a facility	Percentage of pregnant women who had care at an informal setting
ANC: nurse assisted	Percentage of pregnant women who got assistance from a nurse/ midwife during pregnancy
ANC: government health facility	Percentage of pregnant women who received antenatal care at a form of government/public health care center
ANC: Private health facility	Percentage of pregnant women who received antenatal care at a form the private healthcare center
ANC: 1st trimester	Percentage of pregnant women who received antenatal care in the first 12 weeks of pregnancy
ANC: 4+ tetanus injection	Percentage of pregnant women who received tetanus injections before birth
ANC: Home	Percentage of pregnant women who had antenatal care at a home
Indicators for delivery care	
Delivery: home	Percentage of pregnant women who had childbirth at a home
Delivery: government health facility	Percentage of pregnant women who had childbirth at a form of government/public health care center
Delivery: private health facility	Percentage of pregnant women who had childbirth at a form of a private health care center
Birth assistance: Doctor	Percentage of pregnant women who had childbirth assisted by a Doctor
Caesarean section	Percentage of pregnant women who had Caesarean section childbirth

curve and associated index. The concentration curve plots the cumulative percentage of use of various health care services on the vertical axis (y-axis) against the cumulative percentage of women ranked by their household wealth on the horizontal axis (x-axis), beginning with the poorest and ending with the richest households. The equality line runs diagonally across the figure when women, irrespective of economic status have the same access to health care service, that is, all values on the x-axis equals all values on the y-axis [43]. A curve that lies below the equality line indicates that access to the health care service is concentrated among wealthier households. If the curve lies above the line of equality it implies the presence of inequity, that is, use of the health care service is concentrated among poorer households.

Concentration indices were used to assess the magnitudes and trend of horizontal inequity. Analyses were performed to measure absolute inequality in reproductive healthcare use. Concentration index (CI) range from -1.0 to +1.0; negative values of the CI indicate that the use of reproductive health care services is concentrated in poor households, positive values indicate among wealthy households, and 0 indicates the absence of household-wealth related inequality [43, 44]. For computation, a more convenient formula for the concentration index defines it in terms of the covariance between the healthcare outcome and the fractional rank in the household wealth distribution.

$$\text{CI} = \frac{2}{\mu} \; cov\,(h,r) \qquad (1)$$

where h is the healthcare outcome of interest, μ is the mean of h and r is the fractional rank of an individual in the household wealth distribution. Additional analyses performed test the null hypothesis of equality across groups to measure horizontal inequality, which is the hypothesis that the index is the same within a group. Comparison of the concentration indices within socioeconomic groups, including age, marital status, maternal occupation, location (rural or urban), and region of residence, was done using the homogeneity test as provided by O O'Donnell, S O'Neill, T Van Ourti and B Walsh [45].

We used sampling weights for all statistical analysis. Data analyses were performed using STATA version 15.1.

Results

Figures 1, 2 and 3 show the concentration curves of reproductive health care service use. At the end of the observed years, it appears that reproductive health care services are being used less by women in Nigeria compared with Ghana. The distribution of the outcome variables in the poorest 20 percent, richest 20 percent and

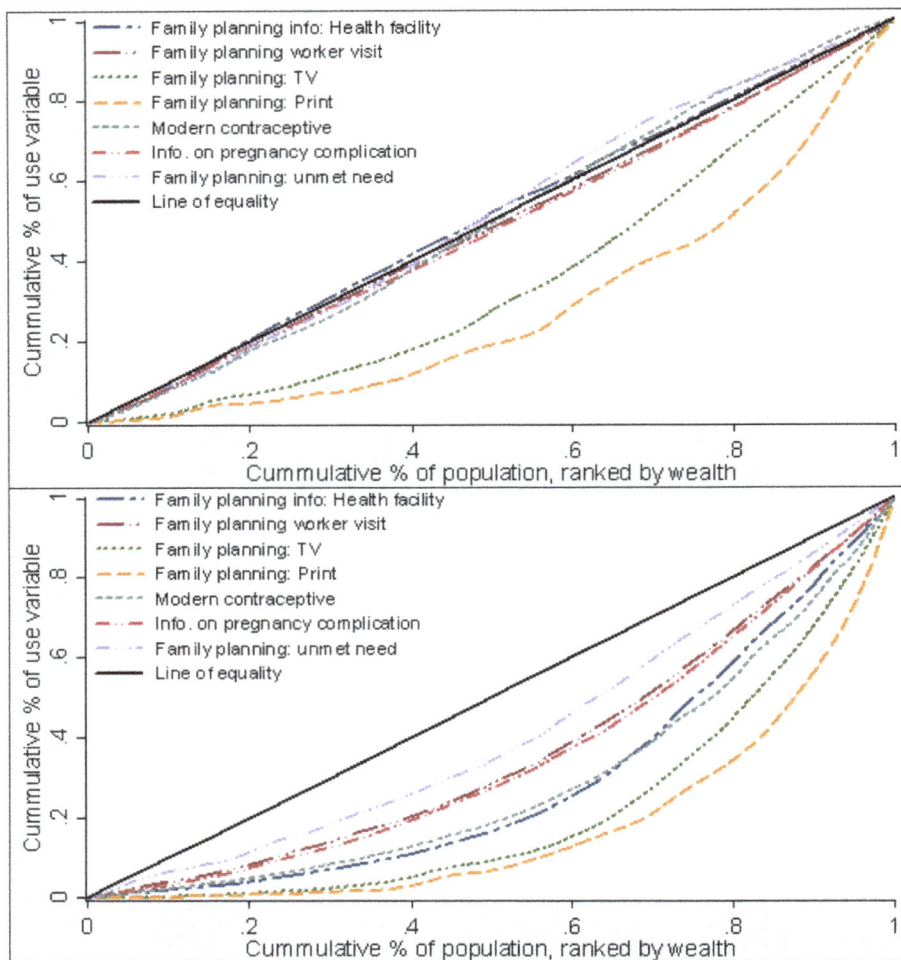

Fig. 1: Concentration curves of use of family planning Ghana (2014) above and Nigeria (2013) below

all women included in the analysis in Ghana and Nigeria (in Additional file 1) suggests changes in the proportion of women using reproductive services in both countries is irregular through the years. Additionally, the data suggest that the use of reproductive health services did not increase substantially among women in the poorest households.

Concentration curve of household wealth-related inequality in use of reproductive health care services

In Figure 1, the top image indicates that the curves of family planning information via print and TV lie distinctively furthest away from the line of equality over the observed years in Ghana, suggesting that these services are to the disadvantage of women in poor households. The bottom image of Fig. 1 shows that all the curves describing the use of family planning services including the use of modern contraceptive lie below the line of equality observed in Nigeria. Lastly, the curve of unmet needs for family planning lies below the equality line and increased

over the periods observed in Nigeria unlike in Ghana where the curve lies closely to the equality line all through (Additional files 2 and 3: Figures S1 and S2).

Figure 2 shows that in Ghana (top image), the concentration curve of antenatal care at private hospitals is below and furthest away from the equality line. Figure 2 (bottom image) suggests that all the examined antenatal care services are distributed to the disadvantage of women in poor households in Nigeria since the curve lies below the equity line. Other concentration curves depicting a woman's use of antenatal care lie close to the equality line (Additional files 4 and 5: Figures S3 and S4).

Figures 3 (top and bottom images) show a clear picture of the curves for indicators associated with delivery care across the years in Ghana and Nigeria respectively. The curve of home births lies above the line of equality in both countries throughout the periods observed, indicating predominance among poor households (Additional files 6 and 7: Figures S5 and S6). Also, the curves depicting the use of private facility, Caesarean section, and assistance by

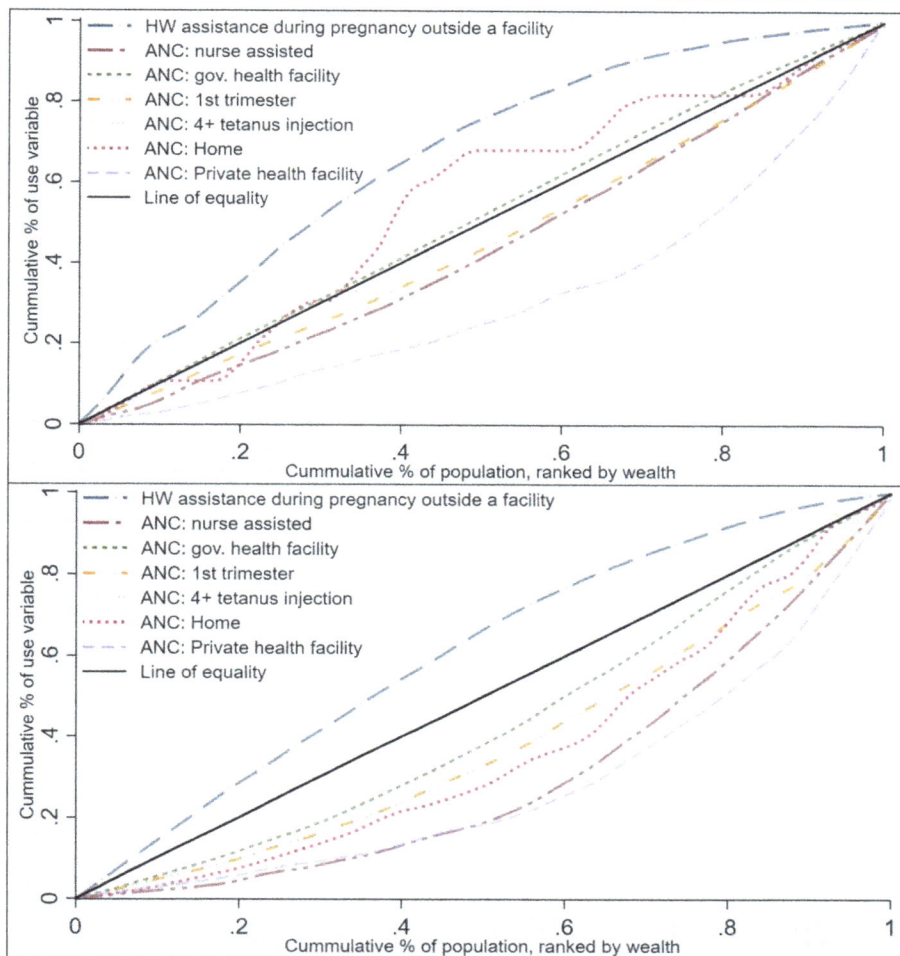

Fig. 2: Concentration curves of use of antenatal care Ghana (2014) above and Nigeria (2013) below

a doctor during child delivery appears to follow a similar pattern and lie furthest away below the equity line throughout the years observed (Additional files 6 and 7: Figures S5 and S6).

Concentration indices of household wealth-related inequality in the use of reproductive health care services

Table 2 shows that the value of the CI declined and remained positive for indicators of family planning information via TV (+0.37 to +0.28), and print (+0.54 to +0.42) from 2003 to 2014 in Ghana. Examination of these indicators by maternal individual characteristics shows that CI values are positive and largest among women who are currently or previously married, agrarians, or live in the Upper East region of Ghana. Concentration indices for indicators of use of family planning information via TV or print medium are positive and high, above +0.43, throughout the years observed in Nigeria, indicating concentration among wealthier households. CI values for visits to health facilities or visits by family planning workers are negative between

2003 and 2014 in Ghana. Women who wanted to give birth no more or later indicated as unmet needs for family planning were insignificant across the years in Ghana. In Nigeria, CI values of unmet needs for family planning were positive and significant over the years. Individual estimates suggest that the degree of inequality associated with unmet needs for family planning is greatest among women in more wealthy households who are not working or in rural residence in Nigeria. Additional test results for group differences indicate that the magnitude of inequality of unmet needs for family planning is significantly different across occupation or residence types in the observed years.

Table 3 presents the values of the concentration indices of indicators of antenatal care services. Values show that the CI of health worker's assistance during pregnancy outside a facility declined slightly from -0.25 in 2003, to -0.21 in 2008 and peaked at -0.27 in 2014 in Ghana. Comparison across groups show that the use of health worker's assistance during pregnancy outside a facility was significantly different between occupation,

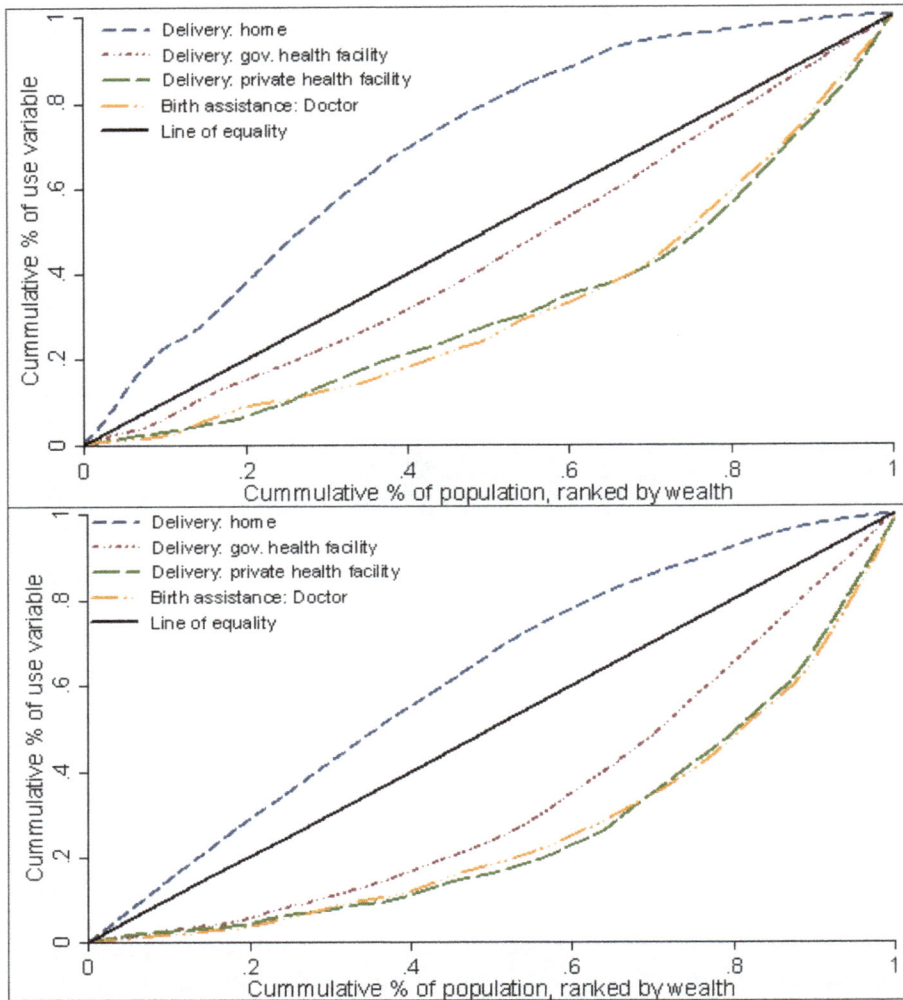

Fig. 3: Concentration curves of use of delivery care Ghana (2014) above and Nigeria (2013) below

residence, and region in Ghana for years 2003 and 2014; women in poor households in the professional / sales occupational category, urban residence, or live in Greater Accra had the greatest negative CI values. In Nigeria, for health worker's assistance during pregnancy outside a facility, the values of CI indicate an increase from -0.17 in 2003 to -0.21 in 2008 and 2013. Test results show significant differences between age and occupational groups, residence type as well as the region of residence; women who are 25-49 years, professional / sales occupation, in urban residences, or live in the South East region of Nigeria consistently have the greatest negative CI values. For the observed years, CI values of antenatal care in government hospitals increased from -0.02 to -0.04 in Ghana, from -0.04 to -0.07 in Nigeria. Urban-rural differences among women became insignificant after 2003 in Ghana and significant from 2008 in Nigeria. A similar increase in CI values is observed for antenatal

care at private hospitals from +0.24 to +0.36 in Ghana and +0.20 to +0.27 in Nigeria. Over the observed years, the CI magnitude of home antenatal care indicator declined and remained negative in Ghana. However, a change in Nigeria from negative to positive was noted, -0.23, -0.15 and +0.05. Results show that in the observed years, CI values increased for nurse assisted antenatal care in Nigeria, +0.33 to +0.39, while it reduced in Ghana, +0.29 to +0.11.

Table 4 quantifies the degree of household wealth-related inequality in the use of delivery care services. Values of the concentration indices of home delivery declined in Ghana, increased in Nigeria, but remained negative in both countries. Closer observation reveals that the magnitude of inequality associated with the use of home delivery in Ghana was significant between regions in years 2003 and 2014. Significant differences in the six regions of Nigeria were also observed, and point estimates show that that the magnitude of inequality is

Table 2: Concentration Indices with Covariates: Ghana (years 2003, 2008 & 2014) and Nigeria (years 2003, 2008 & 2013)

Service type / covariate	Ghana			Nigeria		
	2003	2008	2014	2003	2008	2013
Family planning info: health facility	-0.01	-0.04	-0.04*	0.14*	0.14*	0.15*
Age group						
15-24	0*	0.05	-0.02	0.14	0.18*	0.18*
25-49	-0.01	-0.06	-0.05*	0.13*	0.12*	0.14*
Marital status						
Never	-0.02	-0.06	-0.01	0.04	0.06	0.03
Currently / previously	-0.01	-0.04	-0.04*	0.14*	0.14*	0.16*
Maternal occupation						
Not working	0.05	0	0	0.2	0.18*	0.21*
Professional / sales	0	-0.04	-0.07*	0.14*	0.09*	0.12*
Agriculture	-0.01	-0.05	0	0.06	0.11*	0.08
Others	-0.02	0.02	-0.01	0.13	0.16*	0.14*
Location						
Urban	-0.02	-0.01	-0.02	0.02	0.08*	0.05*
Rural	-0.02	-0.01	-0.01	0.15	0.16*	0.19*
Family planning worker visit	-0.09*	-0.02	-0.05	0.25*	0.39*	0.4*
Age group						
15-24	0.01	0.05	0.01	0.22	0.49*	0.43*
25-49	-0.11*	-0.04	-0.06	0.25*	0.35*	0.38*
Marital status						
Never	-0.1	0.09	0.03	-0.03	-0.04	0.01
Currently / previously	-0.09*	-0.02	-0.06	0.26*	0.4*	0.41*
Maternal occupation						
Not working	0.07	0.15	-0.03	0.43*	0.51*	0.44*
Professional / sales	-0.18*	-0.08	0.02	0.27*	0.32*	0.37*
Agriculture	-0.06	-0.14*	0.02	0.07	0.25*	0.2*
Others	-0.15	0.06	-0.13	0.31	0.4*	0.36*
Location						
Urban	-0.15*	-0.01	0	0.18*	0.2*	0.14*
Rural	-0.04	-0.02	0	0.22	0.39*	0.42*
Family planning: TV	0.37*	0.4*	0.28*	0.5*	0.58*	0.56*
Age group						
15-24	0.3*	0.37*	0.26*	0.44*	0.6*	0.61*
25-49	0.39*	0.41*	0.29*	0.51*	0.56*	0.53*
Marital status						
Never	0.2*	0.22*	0.2*	0.12	0.29*	0.31*
Currently / previously	0.37*	0.42*	0.29*	0.51*	0.59*	0.57*
Maternal occupation						
Not working	0.33*	0.4*	0.24*	0.52*	0.64*	0.65*
Professional / sales	0.23*	0.27*	0.15*	0.45*	0.48*	0.5*
Agriculture	0.32*	0.46*	0.32*	0.51*	0.41*	0.32*
Others	0.27*	0.26*	0.21*	0.42*	0.51*	0.49*
Location						

Table 2: Concentration Indices with Covariates: Ghana (years 2003, 2008 & 2014) and Nigeria (years 2003, 2008 & 2013) *(Continued)*

Service type / covariate	Ghana			Nigeria		
	2003	2008	2014	2003	2008	2013
Urban	0.17*	0.19*	0.13*	0.29*	0.28*	0.25*
Rural	0.32*	0.44*	0.35*	0.39*	0.63*	0.63*
Family planning: print	0.54*	0.52*	0.42*	0.43*	0.65*	0.64*
Age group						
15-24	0.5*	0.56*	0.25	0.4*	0.63*	0.62*
25-49	0.55*	0.51*	0.44*	0.44*	0.64*	0.62*
Marital status						
Never	0.28	0.5	0.36	0.22	0.36*	0.26
Currently / previously	0.55*	0.52*	0.43*	0.45*	0.66*	0.65*
Maternal occupation						
Not working	0.45*	0.46*	0.14	0.42*	0.7*	0.73*
Professional / sales	0.4*	0.43*	0.31*	0.4*	0.57*	0.56*
Agriculture	0.43*	0.55*	0.32	0.47	0.42*	0.5*
Others	0.43*	0.37*	0.19	0.38*	0.57*	0.59*
Location						
Urban	0.31*	0.36*	0.26*	0.34*	0.39*	0.36*
Rural	0.45*	0.54*	0.45*	0.3*	0.67*	0.67*
Modern contraceptive	0.01	-0.05	-0.06*	0.03	-0.04*	-0.02
Age group						
15-24	0.01	-0.05	-0.08*	0.06	0.02	0.02
25-49	0.01	-0.04	-0.05*	0.03	-0.05*	-0.02
Marital status						
Never	0.04	-0.17	-0.06	0.07	0.05	0.07*
Currently / previously	0.01	-0.04	-0.06*	0.03	-0.04*	-0.02
Maternal occupation						
Not working	-0.01	-0.08	-0.05	0.05	-0.05	-0.03
Professional / sales	0.02	-0.04	-0.08*	0.02	-0.03	-0.01
Agriculture	0.01	-0.07*	0	0.04	-0.09*	-0.03
Others	-0.02	-0.01	-0.07*	-0.02	0	-0.05
Location						
Urban	-0.02	-0.06	-0.07*	0.02	-0.02	0
Rural	0.02	-0.05	-0.02	0.03	-0.04*	-0.03
Information on pregnancy complication	0.08*	0.07*	0.02*	0.13*	0.12*	0.1*
Age group						
15-24	0.06*	0.06*	0	0.16*	0.12*	0.1*
25-49	0.09*	0.07*	0.02*	0.11*	0.11*	0.09*
Marital status						
Never	0.15*	0.1	0	0.1	0.1	0.08*
Currently / previously	0.08*	0.07*	0.02*	0.13*	0.12*	0.1*
Maternal occupation						
Not working	0.15*	0	0	0.17*	0.15*	0.1*
Professional / sales	0.06*	0.04*	0	0.11*	0.09*	0.09*
Agriculture	0.1	0.06*	0	0.1	0	0.07*

Table 2: Concentration Indices with Covariates: Ghana (years 2003, 2008 & 2014) and Nigeria (years 2003, 2008 & 2013) *(Continued)*

Service type / covariate	Ghana			Nigeria		
	2003	2008	2014	2003	2008	2013
Others	0.1	0	0.03*	0.11*	0.11*	0.08*
Location						
Urban	0	0	0.02*	0.08*	0.07*	0.05*
Rural	0.07*	0.07*	0	0.09*	0.1*	0.08*
Family planning: unmet need	0.01	0.01	-0.02	0.05	0.18*	0.18*
Age group						
15-24	0.08*	0.06	0.05	0.11	0.25*	0.22*
25-49	-0.02	-0.01	-0.03	0.03	0.17*	0.17*
Marital status						
Never	-0.03	0.09*	-0.03	0.03	0.04	0
Currently / previously	0.01	-0.01	-0.02	0.05	0.19*	0.19*
Maternal occupation						
Not working	0.06	0.03	-0.04	0.08	0.21*	0.29*
Professional / sales	-0.04	-0.09*	-0.11*	0.07	0.16*	0.21*
Agriculture	0.07*	0.09*	0.08	0.06	0.12*	0.01
Others	-0.02	-0.06	-0.07	0.11	0.3*	0.19*
Location						
Urban	-0.02	-0.08	-0.11*	0.07	0.04	0.02
Rural	0.07*	0.07*	0.06	0.03	0.22*	0.21*

Note: Magnitudes of regional variation is available in Additional file 1

$*p \leq 0.01$

not the same across geographical regions. In addition, results from Ghana data show the concentration of home delivery among poor households in rural and urban residences over the years. After 2008, there was no significant urban-rural differential in the magnitude of inequality in Ghana. However, in Nigeria, urban-rural inequality persisted. Though of equivalent magnitude, -0.09, the tests of the null hypothesis of equality indicate a significant difference in between women in rural and urban areas of Nigeria through the years. In 2008, the CI magnitude in Caesarean section increased in Nigeria from +0.49 to +0.58 but a decline in the CI magnitude was noted in Ghana from +0.45 to +0.30 for the same period. Significant differences between age groups were noted in Ghana and Nigeria after 2008; women who are 25-49 years consistently have greater CI magnitude in Caesarean section.

Discussion

The concentration curve and associated indices estimated in this study permit the investigation of the progress made in reducing inequalities in access to reproductive health care services among women in Ghana and Nigeria. These indicators of use of family planning services, antenatal and delivery care services show that the use of some services is inequitably distributed and

that there are differences in the size of inequality within socioeconomic groups of women. Specifically, the use of antenatal care at government facilities, health worker's assistance during pregnancy outside a facility, childbirth at home is distributed unequally and advantaging women in poor households, while the use of family planning information via TV or print media, antenatal care at private facilities are advantaging women in wealthier households in both Ghana and Nigeria. In Nigeria alone, women in richer households have considerably more unmet needs for family planning.

The variation in the magnitudes of inequality across socioeconomic groups within and between the countries (measured by the concentration indices), is also necessary to understand how the determinants of inequalities differ. We find that nearly all indicators of use of reproductive health care services in Ghana indicated a shift towards the equity line, indicating a decline in inequality. However, equity improvement was not observed in doctor-assisted births, antenatal care provided at non-facility formations, government and private facilities. In Nigeria, indicators examined showed mixed shifts, with mostly non-pro-poor changes over the years observed. This was specifically the case for antenatal care at private facilities, antenatal care in government facilities, non-facility formations for antenatal

Table 3: Concentration Indices with Covariates: Ghana (years 2003, 2008 & 2014) and Nigeria (years 2003, 2008 & 2013)

Service type / covariate	Ghana			Nigeria		
	2003	2008	2014	2003	2008	2013
Health worker's assistance during pregnancy outside a facility	-0.25*	-0.21*	-0.27*	-0.17*	-0.21*	-0.21*
Age group						
15-24	-0.23*	-0.06	-0.19*	-0.13*	-0.14*	-0.15*
25-49	-0.26*	-0.25*	-0.29*	-0.19*	-0.23*	-0.23*
Marital status						
Never	-0.21*	-0.2	-0.2	-0.23	-0.15*	-0.17*
Currently / previously	-0.25*	-0.21*	-0.28*	-0.17*	-0.21*	-0.21*
Maternal occupation						
Not working	-0.29*	-0.32*	-0.2*	-0.16*	-0.17*	-0.17*
Professional / sales	-0.35*	-0.2*	-0.29*	-0.19*	-0.28*	-0.26*
Agriculture	-0.07*	-0.03	-0.08	-0.14*	-0.09*	-0.1*
Others	-0.29*	-0.24*	-0.23*	-0.18*	-0.23*	-0.23*
Location						
Urban	-0.3*	-0.18*	-0.19*	-0.22*	-0.27*	-0.24*
Rural	-0.09*	-0.07*	-0.17*	-0.1*	-0.13*	-0.11*
ANC: nurse assisted	0.29*	0.24*	0.11*	0.33*	0.4*	0.39*
Age group						
15-24	0.26*	0.19*	0.11*	0.32*	0.4*	0.39*
25-49	0.3*	0.25*	0.11*	0.33*	0.39*	0.39*
Marital status						
Never	0.1	0.11*	0.09*	0.15	0.23*	0.16*
Currently / previously	0.29*	0.24*	0.11*	0.34*	0.4*	0.4*
Maternal occupation						
Not working	0.26*	0.2*	0.08*	0.46*	0.49*	0.47*
Professional / sales	0.16*	0.14*	0.04*	0.3*	0.35*	0.38*
Agriculture	0.21*	0.26*	0.12*	0.28*	0.26*	0.2*
Others	0.21*	0.14*	0.08*	0.29*	0.4*	0.38*
Location						
Urban	0.06*	0.06*	0.02	0.16*	0.17*	0.12*
Rural	0.24*	0.24*	0.12*	0.31*	0.41*	0.43*
ANC: government health facility	-0.02*	-0.03*	-0.04*	-0.04	-0.07*	-0.07*
Age group						
15-24	-0.01	-0.01	-0.02	-0.04	-0.05*	-0.06*
25-49	-0.02*	-0.04*	-0.05*	-0.04	-0.07*	-0.07*
Marital status						
Never	-0.08*	0.02	0	-0.15	-0.03	-0.05
Currently / previously	-0.02*	-0.03*	-0.04*	-0.04	-0.07*	-0.07*
Maternal occupation						
Not working	-0.01	-0.04*	-0.03*	-0.02	-0.08*	-0.08*
Professional / sales	-0.02	-0.02	-0.05*	-0.05*	-0.08*	-0.08*
Agriculture	0	-0.01	0	-0.06	0	-0.01
Others	-0.03	-0.05*	-0.02	-0.07	-0.1*	-0.09*
Location						

Table 3: Concentration Indices with Covariates: Ghana (years 2003, 2008 & 2014) and Nigeria (years 2003, 2008 & 2013) *(Continued)*

Service type / covariate	Ghana			Nigeria		
	2003	2008	2014	2003	2008	2013
Urban	-0.03*	-0.01	-0.04*	-0.03	-0.1*	-0.07*
Rural	0	-0.02*	-0.02*	-0.03	-0.03*	-0.03*
ANC: private health facility	0.24*	0.3*	0.36*	0.2*	0.23*	0.27*
Age group						
15-24	0.15	0.05	0.21	0.23*	0.21*	0.27*
25-49	0.27*	0.34*	0.38*	0.19*	0.23*	0.25*
Marital status						
Never	0.44*	-0.1	0.26	0.37*	0.17	0.17*
Currently / previously	0.23*	0.33*	0.36*	0.19*	0.23*	0.27*
Maternal occupation						
Not working	0.12	0.42*	0.27*	0.24*	0.35*	0.37*
Professional / sales	0.17*	0.16	0.32*	0.18*	0.23*	0.27*
Agriculture	0.15	0.12	-0.08	0.2	0.01	0.01
Others	0.19*	0.32*	0.27*	0.24*	0.26*	0.33*
Location						
Urban	0.17*	0.11	0.26*	0.14*	0.21*	0.17*
Rural	0.09	0.32*	0.26*	0.18	0.15*	0.21*
ANC: 1st trimester	0.09*	0.09*	0.07*	-0.01	0.03	0.04
Age group						
15-24	0.08*	0.08	0.05	0.05	-0.03	0.01
25-49	0.09*	0.09*	0.07*	-0.03	0.04*	0.04
Marital status						
Never	0.03	0.01	0.08*	0.24	-0.06	0.02
Currently / previously	0.09*	0.1*	0.07*	-0.02	0.03	0.04
Maternal occupation						
Not working	0.13*	0.1*	0.08*	0.07	0.02	0.06
Professional / sales	0.07*	0.07*	0.05*	-0.05	0.06*	0.04
Agriculture	0.06*	0.06	0.02	0	0.01	-0.06
Others	0.04	0.04	0.05*	-0.03	0.1*	0.11*
Location						
Urban	0.06*	0.08*	0.07*	0.07	0.1*	0.09*
Rural	0.06*	0.08*	0.07*	-0.06	0.01	0.04*
ANC: +4 tetanus injection	0.05*	0.03*	0.02*	0.23*	0.27*	0.22*
Age group						
15-24	0.05*	0.04*	0.02*	0.24*	0.28*	0.22*
25-49	0.05*	0.03*	0.02*	0.23*	0.25*	0.22*
Marital status						
Never	0.01	0.07*	0.02	0.08	0.1*	0.07*
Currently / previously	0.05*	0.03*	0.02*	0.24*	0.27*	0.23*
Maternal occupation						
Not working	0.04	0.06*	0.01	0.33*	0.35*	0.29*
Professional / sales	0.02*	0.02*	0.01	0.24*	0.23*	0.21*
Agriculture	0.05*	0.02	0.01	0.14*	0.18*	0.1*

Table 3: Concentration Indices with Covariates: Ghana (years 2003, 2008 & 2014) and Nigeria (years 2003, 2008 & 2013) *(Continued)*

Service type / covariate	Ghana			Nigeria		
	2003	2008	2014	2003	2008	2013
Others	0.03*	0.03*	0.01	0.21*	0.27*	0.19*
Location						
Urban	0.01	0.02*	0.01	0.11*	0.09*	0.06*
Rural	0.03*	0.03*	0.02*	0.2*	0.28*	0.23*
ANC: home	-0.26*	-0.25*	-0.1	-0.23*	-0.15*	0.05
Age group						
15-24	-0.07	-0.23	0.15	-0.23	-0.08	0.21*
25-49	-0.3*	-0.26	-0.19	-0.24*	-0.17*	0.01
Marital status+						
Never	0.08	-	-0.34	-0.31	-0.08	-0.02
Currently / previously	-0.27*	-	-0.07	-0.22*	-0.16*	0.06
Maternal occupation+						
Not working	-0.22	-	0.21	-0.33	-0.22*	0.05
Professional / sales	-0.27	-	-0.13	-0.22	-0.14*	0.09
Agriculture	-0.24	-	-0.06	0.05	0.01	0.11
Others	-0.43	-	-0.53	-0.24	-0.07	0.13
Location+						
Urban	-0.41	-	-0.18	-0.29*	-0.13	-0.02
Rural	-0.1	-	0.03	-0.12	-0.09*	0.11

Note: Magnitudes of regional variation is available in Additional file 1.
*$p \leq 0.01$
+In 2008 the mean value of outcome is undefined.

care, family planning information via TV or print media, unmet needs for family planning, and childbirth at home. The most substantial change in the magnitude of inequality, a decrease, was noted for the use of modern contraceptives during years 2003 – 2008 in both Ghana and Nigeria. The most substantial change in antenatal care was observed in 2003 – 2008 for the indicators antenatal care at government health facilities in Ghana and antenatal care in the 1st trimester in Nigeria. Among indicators of delivery care, the most substantial change in the magnitude of inequality in home delivery in Ghana occurred among women in poor households in the period 2008 – 2014. In Nigeria, a change in the magnitude of inequality was most evident in delivery at a government health facility and private health facility during the period 2003-2008.

Family planning services
We find that use of family planning information via TV or print media is unequally distributed in favor of women in wealthy households of Ghana, specifically, those with agricultural livelihood and women who live in Upper East region. This is unsurprising since wealth is correlated with education which facilitates access and assimilation of information [46]. This finding supports

previous research that showed that higher socioeconomic status improves the use of family planning media messages [47]. Although studies show that few people get family planning information via media messages [48]. Another study found that access to family planning information via television or print medium is in disfavor of women in lower socioeconomic strata [49]. However, access to family planning information via media messages about reproductive health care services has mixed results in promoting access in Africa [23, 49, 50]. We also find that unwanted births, indicated by unmet needs for family planning, are concentrated in wealthy households of Nigeria and occur most among women who are not working or living in rural residences. This finding suggests that there is a high need for contraception among women in rural economically advantaged households. Studies show that wage-earning or economically self-sufficient women are more likely to seek contraception, though modern means of preventing unwanted births could be inaccessible in cultural and religious societies [48, 51]. Finally, regarding access to family planning services, while economic status does preclude women from making sole reproductive decisions it could, however, initiate a demand for contraception [52–54].

Table 4: Concentration Indices with Covariates: Ghana (years 2003, 2008 & 2014) and Nigeria (years 2003, 2008 & 2013)

Service type / covariate	Ghana			Nigeria		
	2003	2008	2014	2003	2008	2013
Delivery: home	-0.14*	-0.13*	-0.1*	-0.12*	-0.15*	-0.14*
Age group						
15-24	-0.13*	-0.09*	-0.07*	-0.09*	-0.12*	-0.11*
25-49	-0.15*	-0.14*	-0.1*	-0.12*	-0.16*	-0.15*
Marital status						
Never	-0.1*	-0.1*	-0.07*	-0.09*	-0.09*	-0.09*
Currently / previously	-0.14*	-0.13*	-0.1*	-0.11*	-0.15*	-0.14*
Maternal occupation						
Not working	-0.14*	-0.11*	-0.07*	-0.11*	-0.14*	-0.13*
Professional / sales	-0.12*	-0.09*	-0.06*	-0.13*	-0.17*	-0.16*
Agriculture	-0.06*	-0.09*	-0.06*	-0.08*	-0.08*	-0.06*
Others	-0.13*	-0.1*	-0.08*	-0.11*	-0.17*	-0.15*
Location						
Urban	-0.07*	-0.05*	-0.04*	-0.09*	-0.12*	-0.09*
Rural	-0.07*	-0.1*	-0.07*	-0.08*	-0.11*	-0.09*
Delivery: government health facility	0.10*	0.10*	0.06*	0.05*	0.07*	0.08*
Age group						
15-24	0.08*	0.07*	0.06*	0.04*	0.06*	0.07*
25-49	0.11*	0.11*	0.07*	0.06*	0.08*	0.08*
Marital status						
Never	0.04	0.1*	0.06*	0.01	0.03	0.03
Currently / previously	0.11*	0.1*	0.07*	0.05*	0.07*	0.08*
Maternal occupation						
Not working	0.08*	0.06*	0.04*	0.06*	0.07*	0.08*
Professional / sales	0.09*	0.07*	0.03*	0.05*	0.08*	0.08*
Agriculture	0.04*	0.07*	0.06*	0.03	0.05*	0.04*
Others	0.11*	0.07*	0.06*	0.05*	0.07*	0.07*
Location						
Urban	0.04*	0.03*	0.01	0.03	0.03*	0.03*
Rural	0.05*	0.08*	0.06*	0.03*	0.06*	0.06*
Delivery: private health facility	0.04*	0.03*	0.03*	0.06*	0.08*	0.07*
Age group						
15-24	0.04*	0.02	0.01	0.05*	0.05*	0.05*
25-49	0.04*	0.03*	0.03*	0.07*	0.09*	0.07*
Marital status						
Never	0.06	0	0.01	0.09*	0.06*	0.05*
Currently / previously	0.04*	0.03*	0.03*	0.06*	0.08*	0.07*
Maternal occupation						
Not working	0.06*	0.06*	0.03	0.06*	0.06*	0.05*
Professional / sales	0.03*	0.02	0.04*	0.07*	0.09*	0.08*
Agriculture	0.01*	0.02*	0	0.06*	0.03*	0.01
Others	0.02*	0.02	0.02	0.06*	0.09*	0.07*
Location						

Table 4: Concentration Indices with Covariates: Ghana (years 2003, 2008 & 2014) and Nigeria (years 2003, 2008 & 2013) *(Continued)*

Service type / covariate	Ghana			Nigeria		
	2003	2008	2014	2003	2008	2013
Urban	0.03	0.01	0.03*	0.06*	0.09*	0.06*
Rural	0.01*	0.02*	0.01	0.04*	0.04*	0.03*
Birth assistance: doctor	0.03*	0.04*	0.05*	0.04*	0.06*	0.05*
Age group						
15-24	0.03*	0.01	0.02	0.03*	0.03*	0.03*
25-49	0.04*	0.05*	0.06*	0.04*	0.06*	0.06*
Marital status						
Never	0.06	0.03	0.04*	0.11*	0.03*	0.03*
Currently / previously	0.03*	0.04*	0.05*	0.03*	0.06*	0.05*
Maternal occupation						
Not working	0.05*	0.06*	0.03*	0.03*	0.05*	0.04*
Professional / sales	0.04*	0.04*	0.06*	0.05*	0.07*	0.06*
Agriculture	0.01*	0.01	0.01	0.04	0.01*	0.02*
Others	0.04*	0.04*	0.06*	0.03*	0.06*	0.05*
Location						
Urban	0.04*	0.04*	0.05*	0.05*	0.08*	0.07*
Rural	0.01	0.02*	0.03*	0.01*	0.02*	0.02*
C Section	0.45*	0.30*	0.31*	0.49*	0.58*	0.49*
Age group						
15-24	0.37	0.05	0.07	0.22	0.46*	0.33*
25-49	0.47*	0.34*	0.32*	0.54*	0.59*	0.52*
Marital status						
Never	0.38	0.26	0.2	0.53	0.57*	0.27
Currently / previously	0.45*	0.31*	0.32*	0.48*	0.58*	0.5*
Maternal occupation						
Not working	0.36	0.26	0.15	0.5*	0.6*	0.59*
Professional / sales	0.45*	0.19*	0.28*	0.44*	0.55*	0.49*
Agriculture	0.14	0.28	0.11	0.61	0.19	0.28
Others	0.43	0.25	0.27*	0.45	0.46*	0.43*
Location						
Urban	0.36*	0.11	0.19*	0.36*	0.41*	0.36*
Rural	0.14	0.38*	0.3*	0.29	0.52*	0.37*

Note: Magnitudes of regional variation is available in Additional file 1.
*$p \leq 0.01$

Antenatal care services

We find that, in both Ghana and Nigeria, women in poor households have increasingly become disadvantaged as inequality in use of antenatal care at private facilities increased in favor of their counterparts in wealthy households. A study carried out in Ghana using DHS data from years 1988 – 2008 found a similar increase. However, this study did not disaggregate antenatal care by type of provider [36]. It is reported that wealthier women are better able to overcome barriers of informal payments of cash or kind and are less likely to

encounter negative health workers attitudes often seen in private health care facilities [55, 56]. Other studies have shown that wealth-related inequalities in the use of antenatal care have increased in the past years [36, 57]. Results from our study further suggest that the use of health worker's assistance during pregnancy outside a facility in both countries became less equitable; women in poor households in urban areas or with professional/ sales occupation use such assistance more frequently. Professional occupation and urban area residents are generally thought to have better access to good quality reproductive health care services, given their knowledge and the service availability accessible to these women to draw from [58–61]. Our finding deviates from other studies which suggest that women in these groups access better antenatal care services. To explain the variation in the use of health worker's assistance during pregnancy outside a facility, studies have also shown that transport and health facilities waiting time may facilitate the use of such assistance or deter the use of modern antenatal care services among women in these categories [60, 62–65]. Specifically, the observed change in home antenatal care from prominence among poor to richer households in Nigeria is unexpected. AF Fagbamigbe and ES Idemudia [66] also noted non-use of antenatal care among the wealthier women during pregnancy and suggest that not only poverty but also other factors like personality and view on the quality of services are relevant. It is also plausible that these are a response to increased pressure on resources in government or other maternal care formations [64]. Unfortunately, there is no information on the quality of care in the DHS data.

The finding that antenatal care in government facilities in both countries is pro-poor and consistently changing to the advantage of women in poor households was observed in different years. No effect was observed among women in the agrarian sector, however. One study report that the use of antenatal care improved among women in Ghana, and, though economic challenges are being surmounted, it may be delayed among women in agricultural occupations [36]. Other studies report pro-wealthy inequality changes in antenatal care use among women in Ghana and Nigeria between 2003 and 2008 [19, 57]. In addition, urban-rural inequality in the use of antenatal care at government facilities was observed in the later years in Nigeria but diminished in Ghana. In Nigeria, we find no evidence that rural women in poor households seek antenatal health care services at government facilities. Other studies found unequal use of antenatal care services to the detriment of women in rural households [62, 66]. A study of Nigeria's midwives service scheme found insignificant success in rural areas attributable to pro-wealthy resource distribution [24]. Nonetheless, the observed diminished urban-rural differential to benefit women in poor households in Ghana has been partially credited to improvements in infrastructure and maternal health care services [36].

Delivery care services

Our study finds that childbirth at home persists among women in poor households although overall inequality magnitude appears to have declined in Ghana while it has increased in Nigeria, there are substantial geographical variations. It appears that by 2014 inequality became notable among women in all seven regions of Ghana. In

a 2005 research on the free delivery care policy in Central and Volta regions of Ghana, an increase in facility delivery and a decline in home delivery was reported [26]. Another study found that coverage of the doorstep community-based health planning and services program in Ghana was substantial in mainly the Upper East region [23]. A separate study carried out among Nigerian women in 2004 did not find a substantial increase in institutional delivery facilities in Nigeria despite the midwives service scheme [24]. Evidence of substantial pro-rich inequality between the Northern and Southern regions was observed in Nigeria, while delivery at government health facilities favored women in the Northern regions. Delivery at a private health facility is more inequitable among the richer households in the Southern regions. We find persisting rural-urban disparities associated with childbirth at a government health facility in Nigeria, but not in the later years in Ghana, that is 2008 and 2014. Other research did not find evidence of rural-urban differences in the shift from home to health facilities in Ghana and Nigeria [67]. The observed inequalities among women who have childbirth at home suggest that implemented health policies such as the community-based health planning and services initiative in Ghana, a free delivery scheme in Ghana, the midwives service scheme in Nigeria and insurance schemes in both counties have not substantially reduced inequality in home birth among women. This is also confirmed in other studies [16, 36, 57].

The finding that Caesarean section in both Ghana and Nigeria is pro-wealthy is not surprising. Our findings are in line with the findings of previous studies that Caesarean section remains under-provided for women in poor households in both countries [16]. The trend suggests that coverage gap in both countries remains relatively high. In addition, the equity trend observed in Nigeria suggests top inequity, indicating that the increase in the CI magnitude related to Caesarean section is extremely high.

Study limitation

The cross-sectional design of the study implies that we can show associations without concluding about causal relationships. Other methodological limitations of the study include recall bias since the survey collects events over a five-year period. A limitation regarding the country comparisons concerns the fact that inequalities were investigated based on the position of women in the distribution of household wealth in their own country. We recognize that a woman who is poor by Ghana standards may be better off in Nigeria. Also, we recognize that measures of coverage gap [68], which we have not analyzed, are as equally important as the equity gap evidenced in this paper. Coverage gap refers to the difference between the targeted and actual use of essential health care services by the population, while equity gap indicates the distribution of the services use across the wealth-based population groups [68]. Thus, the underutilization of reproductive care is not directly addressed in our equity study. However, the study has some strengths as well. In particular, the merging of important indicators of maternal care improved the ability to capture the different categories of reproductive care. In addition, we use a generalized concentration index as a measure of inequality, which is not sensitive to outcome measures because it quantifies the absolute differences in health between income groups. Finally, the measurement of the magnitudes of inequalities over different years gives indications about the changing horizontal inequalities which are country and time specific.

Conclusion

Inequality in the use of family planning, antenatal and delivery care services among women of reproductive health care services in both Ghana and Nigeria have persisted over the years despite efforts and have provided little improvement for women in poor households. The results show that inequality increased in case of antenatal care at private facilities, health worker's assistance during pregnancy outside a facility, antenatal care in government facilities, home births, aspects of reproductive health care services in both Ghana and Nigeria, and unmet need for family planning in Nigeria. Changes in inequality were mostly to the disadvantage of women in poorer households in Nigeria but less in Ghana. The changes in inequality had little effect on improving the use of quality reproductive health care services among women particularly those in poor households. Furthermore, the disambiguation of indicators of the use of reproductive health services shows the extent of the progress made in eliminating unequal access among sociodemographic groups. Also, disaggregation of determinants of access indicated notable horizontal inequalities among women of different socioeconomic groups in Ghana and Nigeria.

The gains made in reducing inequality access to reproductive health care services have eroded over time. This implies that the sustainability of health initiatives to reduce inequalities needs to be addressed. Ghana's health initiatives need to take a pro-poor concept and Nigeria's an accelerated implementation across the population to bring about the decline in inequality in access.

Additional files

Additional file 1: Examining the trend of inequality. A1 - Definition of indicators used in the analysis, Ghana. Grouping description of outcome variable. A2 - Definition of indicators used in the analysis, Nigeria.

Grouping description of outcome variable. A3 - Definition of independent variables used in the analysis. Coding of the dependent and control variables. A4 - Socio-demographic characteristics: Ghana (years 2003, 2008 & 2014) and Nigeria (years 2003, 2008 & 2013). Distribution of the independent variables. B - Supplementary data: Distribution of outcome variables (poorest 20%, richest 20% and total number of women). Distribution of the control variables. C - Concentration Indices with Covariates: Ghana (years 2003, 2008 & 2014) and Nigeria (years 2003, 2008 & 2013). Concentration Indices with Covariates and F-test result. D – Concentration Indices with Covariates: Ghana (years 2003, 2008 & 2014) and Nigeria (years 2003, 2008 & 2013). Concentration Indices with Covariates and F-test result. E – Concentration Indices with Covariates: Ghana (years 2003, 2008 & 2014) and Nigeria (years 2003, 2008 & 2013). Concentration Indices with Covariates and F-test result.

Additional file 2: Figure S1. Concentration curves of use of family planning Ghana (Years 2003, 2008, 2014).

Additional file 3: Figure S2. Concentration curves of use of family planning Nigeria (Years 2003, 2008, 2013).

Additional file 4: Figure S3. Concentration curves of use of Antenatal care, Ghana (Years 2003, 2008, 2013).

Additional file 5: Figure S4. Concentration curves of use of Antenatal care, Nigeria (Years 2003, 2008, 2014).

Additional file 6: Figure S5. Concentration curves of use of Delivery care, Ghana (Years 2003, 2008, 2014).

Additional file 7: Figure S6. Concentration curves of use of delivery care, Nigeria (Years 2003, 2008, 2013).

Acknowledgements
Not applicable

Funding
Not applicable.

Authors' contributions
JO and MP designed the study. JO analyzed the data and drafted the manuscript. JO, MP and WG subsequently revised the manuscript and approved the final draft for submission.

Competing interests
The authors declare that they have no competing interests.

Author details
[1]Department of Health Services Research, CAPHRI, Maastricht University Medical Center, Faculty of Health, Medicine and Life Sciences, Maastricht University, PO Box 616, 6200MD Maastricht, The Netherlands. [2]Top Institute Evidence-Based Education Research (TIER), Maastricht University, Maastricht, The Netherlands.

References
1. Alkema L, Chou D, Hogan D, Zhang SQ, Moller AB, Gemmill A, Fat DM, Boerma T, Temmerman M, Mathers C, et al. Global, regional, and national levels and trends in maternal mortality between 1990 and 2015, with scenario-based projections to 2030: a systematic analysis by the UN Maternal Mortality Estimation Inter-Agency Group. Lancet. 2016;387(10017):462–74.
2. AbouZahr C, Vaughan JP. Assessing the burden of sexual and reproductive ill-health: questions regarding the use of disability-adjusted life years. Bulletin of the World Health Organization. 2000;78(5):655–66.
3. Kabeer N. Women's economic empowerment and inclusive growth: labour markets and enterprise development. International Development Research Centre. 2012;44(10):1–70.

4. Canning D, Schultz TP. The economic consequences of reproductive health and family planning. Lancet. 2012;380(9837):165–71.

5. Borghi J, Hanson K, Acquah CA, Ekanmian G, Filippi V, Ronsmans C, Brugha R, Browne E, Alihonou E. Costs of near-miss obstetric complications for women and their families in Benin and Ghana. Health Policy and Planning. 2003;18(4):383–90.

6. Honda A, Randaoharison PG, Matsui M. Affordability of emergency obstetric and neonatal care at public hospitals in Madagascar. Reprod Health Matters. 2011;19(37):10–20.

7. Arsenault C, Fournier P, Philibert A, Sissoko K, Coulibaly A, Tourigny C, Traore M, Dumont A. Emergency obstetric care in Mali: catastrophic spending and its impoverishing effects on households. Bull World Health Organ. 2013;91(3):207–16.

8. Mayhew SH. Integration of STI services into FP/MCH services: health service and social contexts in rural Ghana. Reprod Health Matters. 2000;8(16):112–24.

9. Gilson L, Kalyalya D, Kuchler F, Lake S, Oranga H, Ouendo M. Strategies for promoting equity: experience with community financing in three African countries. Health Policy. 2001;58(1):37–67.

10. Victora CG, Vaughan JP, Barros FC, Silva AC, Tomasi E. Explaining trends in inequities: evidence from Brazilian child health studies. Lancet. 2000; 356(9235):1093–8.

11. Mills A, Ataguba JE, Akazili J, Borghi J, Garshong B, Makawia S, Mtei G, Harris B, Macha J, Meheus F, et al. Equity in financing and use of health care in Ghana, South Africa, and Tanzania: implications for paths to universal coverage. Lancet. 2012;380(9837):126–33.

12. Demery L. Benefits incidence: a practitioner's guide. In: Poverty and Social Development Group, Africa Region. Washington: World Bank; 2000.

13. Castro-Leal F, Dayton J, Demery L, Mehra K. Public Social Spending in Africa: Do the Poor Benefit? The World Bank Research Observer. 1999;14(1):49–72.

14. Mutangadura G, Gauci A, Armah B, Woldemariam E, Ayalew D, Egu B. Health inequities in selected African countries: Review of evidence and policy implications. Economic Commission for Africa 2007. 2009;14(51):29.

15. Makinen M, Waters H, Rauch M, Almagambetova N, Bitran R, Gilson L, McIntyre D, Pannarunothai S, Prieto AL, Ubilla G, et al. Inequalities in health care use and expenditures: empirical data from eight developing countries and countries in transition. Bulletin of the World Health Organization. 2000;78(1):55–65.

16. Zere E, Kirigia JM, Duale S, Akazili J. Inequities in maternal and child health outcomes and interventions in Ghana. BMC Public Health. 2012;12:252.

17. Zere E, Moeti M, Kirigia J, Mwase T, Kataika E. Equity in health and healthcare in Malawi: analysis of trends. BMC Public Health. 2007;7(1):78.

18. Okpani AI, Abimbola S. The midwives service scheme: a qualitative comparison of contextual determinants of the performance of two states in central Nigeria. Glob Health Res Policy. 2016;1(1):16.

19. Johnson FA, Frempong-Ainguah F, Padmadas SS. Two decades of maternity care fee exemption policies in Ghana: have they benefited the poor? Health Policy Plan. 2016;31(1):46–55.

20. Barros AJ, Ronsmans C, Axelson H, Loaiza E, Bertoldi AD, Franca GV, Bryce J, Boerma JT, Victora CG. Equity in maternal, newborn, and child health interventions in Countdown to 2015: a retrospective review of survey data from 54 countries. Lancet. 2012;379(9822):1225–33.

21. Abimbola S, Okoli U, Olubajo O, Abdullahi MJ, Pate MA. The midwives service scheme in Nigeria. PLoS Med. 2012;9(5):e1001211.

22. Witter S, Garshong B. Something old or something new? Social health insurance in Ghana. BMC Int Health Hum Rights. 2009;9(1):20.

23. Awoonor-Williams JK, Sory EK, Nyonator FK, Phillips JF, Wang C, Schmitt ML. Lessons learned from scaling up a community-based health program in the Upper East Region of northern Ghana. Glob Health Sci Pract. 2013;1(1):117–33.

24. keke E. The better obstetrics in rural nigeria (born) study: An impact evaluation of the nigerian midwives service scheme. Santa Monica: Rand Corporation; 2015.

25. Nyonator FK, Awoonor-Williams JK, Phillips JF, Jones TC, Miller RA. The Ghana community-based health planning and services initiative for scaling up service delivery innovation. Health Policy Plan. 2005;20(1):25–34.

26. Asante F, Chikwama C, Daniels A, Armar-Klemesu M. Evaluating the economic outcomes of the policy of fee exemption for maternal delivery care in ghana. Ghana Med J. 2007;41(3):110–7.

27. NHIA: MoH PPME Health Sector Indicator Database. 2012.

28. Ibiwoye A, Adeleke IA. Does National Health Insurance Promote Access to Quality Health Care? Evidence from Nigeria. The Geneva Papers on Risk and Insurance - Issues and Practice. 2008;33(2):219–33.

29. Africa Regional Report on the Sustainable Development Goals [https://www.uneca.org/publications/africa-regional-report-sustainable-development-goals]

30. Blanchet NJ, Fink G, Osei-Akoto I. The effect of Ghana's National Health Insurance Scheme on health care utilisation. Ghana Med J. 2012;46(2):76–84.

31. Odeyemi IA, Nixon J. Assessing equity in health care through the national health insurance schemes of Nigeria and Ghana: a review-based comparative analysis. Int J Equity Health. 2013;12(1):9.

32. Mensah J, Oppong JR, Schmidt CM. Ghana's National Health Insurance Scheme in the context of the health MDGs: an empirical evaluation using propensity score matching. Health economics. 2010;19 Suppl:95–106.

33. Ayanore MA, Pavlova M, Groot W. Unmet reproductive health needs among women in some West African countries: a systematic review of outcome measures and determinants. Reprod Health. 2016;13:5.

34. Dixon J, Tenkorang EY, Luginaah I. Ghana's National Health Insurance Scheme: a national level investigation of members' perceptions of service provision. BMC Int Health Hum Rights. 2013;13(1):35.

35. Do M, Soelaeman R, Hotchkiss DR. Explaining inequity in the use of institutional delivery services in selected countries. Maternal and child health journal. 2015;19(4):755–63.

36. Asamoah BO, Agardh A, Pettersson KO, Ostergren PO. Magnitude and trends of inequalities in antenatal care and delivery under skilled care among different socio-demographic groups in Ghana from 1988 - 2008. Bmc Pregnancy Childb. 2014;14:295.

37. Onwujekwe O, Onoka C, Uzochukwu B, Okoli C, Obikeze E, Eze S. Is community-based health insurance an equitable strategy for paying for healthcare? Experiences from southeast Nigeria. Health Policy. 2009; 92(1):96–102.

38. Fakunle B, Okunlola MA, Fajola A, Ottih U, Ilesanmi AO. Community health insurance as a catalyst for uptake of family planning and reproductive health services: the Obio Cottage Hospital experience. J Obstet Gynaecol. 2014;34(6):501–3.

39. Nigeria Midwives Service Scheme [http://www.who.int/workforcealliance/forum/2011/hrhawardscs26/en/]

40. DHS Methodology [https://dhsprogram.com/What-We-Do/Survey-Types/DHS-Methodology.cfm]

41. Reproductive health indicators: guidelines for their generation, interpretation and analysis for global monitoring [http://www.who.int/reproductivehealth/publications/monitoring/924156315x/en/]

42. Filmer D, Pritchett LH. Estimating wealth effects without expenditure data--or tears: an application to educational enrollments in states of India. Demography. 2001;38(1):115–32.

43. O'Donnell O, Van Doorslaer E, Wagstaff A, Lindelow M. Analyzing health equity using household survey data: a guide to techniques and their implementation. Washington: World Bank; 2008.

44. Wagstaff: On the measurement of Inequalitites in health. 1991.

45. O'Donnell O, O'Neill S, Van Ourti T, Walsh B. conindex: Estimation of concentration indices. Stata J. 2016;16(1):112–38.

46. Solar O, Irwin A. A conceptual framework for action on the social determinants of health. Social Determinants of Health Discussion Paper 2 (Policy and Practice); 2010.

47. Kwankye SO, Augustt E. Media exposure and reproductive health behaviour among young females in Ghana. African Population Studies. 2013;22(2).

48. Onwuzurike BK, Uzochukwu BS. Knowledge, attitude and practice of family planning amongst women in a high density low income urban of Enugu, Nigeria. Afr J Reprod Health. 2001;5(2):83–9.

49. Ajaero CK, Odimegwu C, Ajaero ID, Nwachukwu CA. Access to mass media messages, and use of family planning in Nigeria: a spatio-demographic analysis from the 2013 DHS. BMC Public Health. 2016;16:427.

50. Gupta N, Katende C, Bessinger R. Associations of mass media exposure with family planning attitudes and practices in Uganda. Stud Fam Plann. 2003; 34(1):19–31.

51. Onwuhafua PI, Kantiok C, Olafimihan O, Shittu OS. Knowledge, attitude and practice of family planning amongst community health extension workers in Kaduna State, Nigeria. J Obstet Gynaecol. 2005;25(5):494–9.

52. Omeje JC, Oshi SN, Oshi DC. Does possession of assets increase women's participation in reproductive decision-making? Perceptions of Nigerian women. J Biosoc Sci. 2011;43(1):101–11.

53. Crissman HP, Adanu RM, Harlow SD. Women's sexual empowerment and contraceptive use in Ghana. Stud Fam Plann. 2012;43(3):201–12.

54. Gakidou E, Vayena E. Use of modern contraception by the poor is falling behind. PLoS Med. 2007;4(2):e31.

55. Pell C, Menaca A, Were F, Afrah NA, Chatio S, Manda-Taylor L, Hamel MJ, Hodgson A, Tagbor H, Kalilani L, et al. Factors affecting antenatal care attendance: results from qualitative studies in Ghana, Kenya and Malawi.

PLoS One. 2013;8(1):e53747.

56. Onwujekwe O, Onoka C, Uzochukwu B, Hanson K. Constraints to universal coverage: inequities in health service use and expenditures for different health conditions and providers. Int J Equity Health. 2011;10:50.

57. Obiyan MO, Kumar A. Socioeconomic Inequalities in the Use of Maternal Health Care Services in Nigeria: Trends Between 1990 and 2008. Sage Open. 2015;5(4):2158244015614070.

58. Aremu O, Lawoko S, Dalal K. Neighborhood socioeconomic disadvantage, individual wealth status and patterns of delivery care utilization in Nigeria: a multilevel discrete choice analysis. Int J Womens Health. 2011;3:167–74.

59. Onah HE, Ikeako LC, Iloabachie GC. Factors associated with the use of maternity services in Enugu, southeastern Nigeria. Soc Sci Med. 2006;63(7):1870–8.

60. Ayanore MA, Pavlova M, Groot W. Focused maternity care in Ghana: results of a cluster analysis. BMC Health Serv Res. 2016;16(1):395.

61. Ochako R, Fotso JC, Ikamari L, Khasakhala A. Utilization of maternal health services among young women in Kenya: insights from the Kenya Demographic and Health Survey, 2003. Bmc Pregnancy Childb. 2011;11(1):1.

62. Fagbamigbe AF, Idemudia ES. Barriers to antenatal care use in Nigeria: evidences from non-users and implications for maternal health programming. Bmc Pregnancy Childb. 2015;15(1):95.

63. Arthur E. Wealth and antenatal care use: implications for maternal health care utilisation in Ghana. Health Econ Rev. 2012;2(1):14.

64. Mrisho M, Obrist B, Schellenberg JA, Haws RA, Mushi AK, Mshinda H, Tanner M, Schellenberg D. The use of antenatal and postnatal care: perspectives and experiences of women and health care providers in rural southern Tanzania. Bmc Pregnancy Childb. 2009;9:10.

65. Jallow IK, Chou YJ, Liu TL, Huang N. Women's perception of antenatal care services in public and private clinics in the Gambia. Int J Qual Health Care. 2012;24(6):595–600.

66. Fagbamigbe AF, Idemudia ES. Wealth and antenatal care utilization in Nigeria: Policy implications. Health Care Women Int. 2017;38(1):17–37.

67. Amoako Johnson F, Padmadas SS, Matthews Z. Are women deciding against home births in low and middle income countries? PLoS One. 2013;8(6):e65527.

68. Boerma JT, Bryce J, Kinfu Y, Axelson H, Victora CG. Mind the gap: equity and trends in coverage of maternal, newborn, and child health services in 54 Countdown countries. Lancet. 2008;371(9620):1259–67.

4

A comparison of misoprostol vaginal insert and misoprostol vaginal tablets for induction of labor in nulliparous women

Kjersti Engen Marsdal[1,2], Ingvil Krarup Sørbye[1], Lise C. Gaudernack[1] and Mirjam Lukasse[2*]

Abstract

Background: Since Misoprostol Vaginal Insert (MVI - Misodel ®) was approved for labor induction in Europe in 2013, to date, no study has been published comparing MVI to Misoprostol vaginal tablets (MVT). The aim of this study, performed as part of a quality improvement project, was to compare the efficacy and safety of 200 μg MVI versus 25 μg MVT for labor induction in nulliparous women.

Methods: This retrospective cohort study included 171 nulliparous singleton term deliveries induced with MVI ($n = 85$) versus MVT ($n = 86$) at Oslo University Hospital Rikshospitalet, Norway, from November 2014 to December 2015. Primary outcomes were time from drug administration to delivery in hours and minutes and the rate of cesarean section (CS). Results were adjusted for Bishop Score and pre-induction with balloon catheter.

Results: Median time from drug administration to delivery was shorter in the MVI group compared to the MVT group (15 h 43 min versus 19 h 37 min, $p = 0.011$). Adjusted for confounding factors, mean difference was 6 h 3 min ($p = 0.002$). The risk of CS was 67% lower in the MVI group compared to the MVT group (11.8% versus 23.3%, OR = 0.33; adjusted 95% CI 0.13–0.81). Adverse neonatal outcomes did not differ between the groups.

Conclusions: In a setting of routine obstetric care, MVI seems to be a more efficient labor induction agent than MVT, and with a lower CS rate and no increase in adverse infant outcomes.

Keywords: Labor induction, Cervical ripening, Misoprostol, Nulliparity, Cesarean section

Background

Induction of labor is one of the most frequently performed obstetrical interventions. The decision to induce labor is made if ending the pregnancy is considered more beneficial for the mother or the baby than awaiting spontaneous onset of labor. Induction of labor has increased over the last decades across Europe. In 2010, in 15 of 25 countries in Europe, more than 20% of the labors were induced [1]. In Norway, the induction rate increased from 12.5% in 2003 to 20.3% in 2013. The most common indications for induction of labor were pre-labor rupture of the membranes (PROM) and post-term pregnancy [2].

Whereas induction of multiparous women has a high success rate, the induction of nulliparous women poses a particular obstetrical problem. Inductions in nulliparous women with an unfavorable or unripe cervix carry an increased risk of dystocia and protracted labor [3, 4]. Conversely, induction of labor also poses a risk of uterine tachysystole and subsequent fetal distress [5]. Protracted labor and fetal distress are the two main indications for CS in Norway [6]. CS in the first delivery also has consequences for subsequent labors, as the repeat CS rate in Norway is 50% [6]. Thus it is of clinical importance to determine the safety and efficacy of new methods for induction of labor for nulliparous women in particular.

Misoprostol is a synthetic prostaglandin E1 analog and has been used off-label for cervical ripening and labor induction since the 1980s [7]. For labor induction in women with an

* Correspondence: mirjam.lukasse@hioa.no
[2]Oslo and Akershus University College, Faculty of Health Sciences, Department of Nursing and Health Promotion, P.O. Box 4, 0130 Oslo, Norway

unfavorable cervix, Misoprostol is more effective than other methods such as oxytocin, Dinoprostone and placebo, with no differences in adverse perinatal or maternal outcomes [7]. In Norway, Misoprostol 25 μg tablets administered vaginally every 4–6 h, has been the most commonly used method for inducing labor with an unfavorable cervix [2].

In 2013 a 200 μg Misoprostol vaginal insert (MVI – Misodel ®) received approval in Europe [8, 9]. In a phase III trial, MVI was compared to a Dinoprostone vaginal insert, a prostaglandin E2 analog. This trial reported significantly reduced times to delivery and no evidence of differences in maternal or neonatal safety outcomes [10]. Since the phase III trial, only three studies have compared MVI to other induction methods in terms of delivery outcomes [11–13]. Neither of these studies have presented data from nulliparous women exclusively, and no studies have compared MVI with MVT.

In a daily obstetric practice, individual care might lead to deviation from protocol. Thus, results from experimental studies are not always valid for obstetric care. The aim of the present study was to compare efficiency and safety of MVI versus MVT for labor induction in nulliparous women within a routine care setting. Our primary outcomes were time from drug administration to delivery and the rate of CS.

Methods

During 2014–2015 a national obstetric quality improvement project on CS was launched in Norway. One of the preselected focus areas was induction of labor in nulliparous women. During this period, our obstetrical unit improved our protocols for selecting women for induction of labor and improved adherence to the protocols for the induction procedures. As part of the project, MVI was introduced as an alternative to MVT in nulliparous women from November 2014 onwards.

In this study we included induced nulliparous women that delivered at Oslo University Hospital Rikshospitalet, Norway, from November 2014 through December 2015. The unit is a tertiary obstetrical unit with around 2800 deliveries annually. Women were included if their labors were induced with MVI or MVT, if they had no previous uterine surgery or other uterine abnormality and gave birth to a single fetus, in cephalic presentation, at gestational age of 37 weeks or more. This corresponds to Robson group 2a in the 10-group classification system [14]. As the study was a part of a quality improvement project conducted within a routine care setting, no randomization was performed. Both MVI and MVT were used for induction of labor during the whole study period and the choice of method was decided usually jointly by the obstetric consultant and the midwife on call. During the study period, 174 nulliparous women were initially included. Of these, three women, who received MVT after the MVI was accidentally removed, were excluded from the study.

In Norway, there is no standardized protocol for induction of labor. The department's protocol for induction of labor in nulliparous women during the study period is presented in Fig. 1.

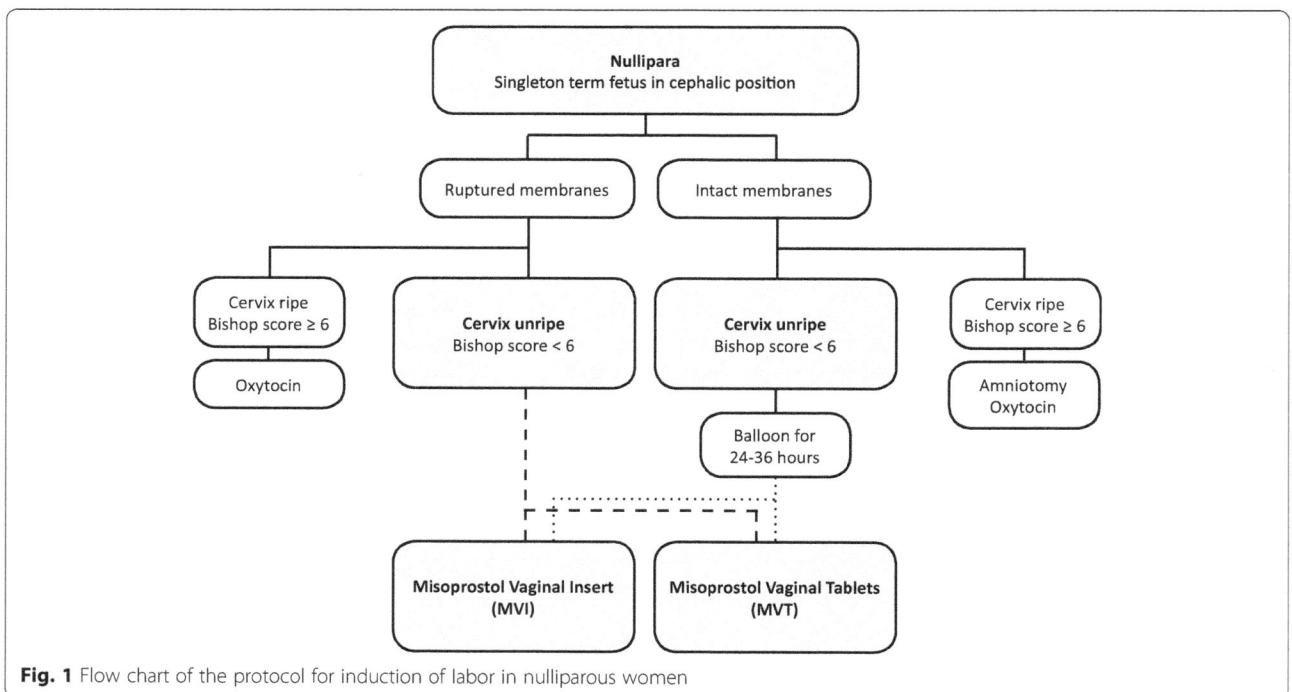

Fig. 1 Flow chart of the protocol for induction of labor in nulliparous women

MVI is a removable vaginal insert with a reservoir of 200 μg Misoprostol, released at a mean rate of approximately 7 μg per hour over a period of 24 h. MVI was inserted once, while the insertion of a 25 μg MVT was repeated every 4 h. After insertion of MVI or MVT, the women remained in bed with continuous cardiotocography (CTG) for one hour. A CTG was performed every 4–6 h; once regular contractions were established or according to the department's procedures. In women with a non-reassuring CTG during the induction process, the insert was withdrawn or tablet removal was attempted. The MVI was removed when the midwife considered that labor was established; if the CTG showed a non-reassuring pattern or if the 24-h dosing period was completed. For women not in labor after the dosing period, artificial rupture of membranes was performed, followed by oxytocin infusion. The oxytocin infusion was started at 5 mU/min and increased by 5 mU/min every 30 min until adequate uterine activity, defined as 4–5 contractions per 10 min. The maximum infusion rate was 30 mU/min. The oxytocin infusion was stopped or decreased if the woman had more than 5 contractions per 10 min. For inductions with MVT, artificial rupture of the membranes was performed when the Bishop Score reached 6 or more, followed by oxytocin infusion as described. At the end of day 3 or beginning of day 4, artificial rupture of the membranes was attempted even if the Bishop Score was below 6. The administration of MVT could be postponed if the woman was having regular contractions, if the woman needed to rest at night due to a long induction process and in rare cases due to logistic considerations. Inductions could be started any time during the day. No progress of labor and failed induction was according to the departments protocol defined as no progression after 6 h with the maximum dose of oxytocin. Individual assessments on labor progression were made by the obstetric consultant on call.

Our primary outcome regarding efficiency was time from drug administration to delivery. Secondary outcomes included time from drug administration to onset of the active phase of labor and labor duration. As to safety, our primary outcome was the rate of CS. Secondary outcomes included the proportion of operative and spontaneous vaginal deliveries, the use of oxytocin stimulation, the proportion of Apgar Score < 7 after 5 min and the rate of CS and operative vaginal deliveries due to fetal distress. All CTG-registrations from labors ending with operative delivery due to fetal distress were investigated for uterine tachysystole, defined as >5 contractions in 10 min.

Labor onset was defined as when the partogram was started by the attending midwife. Onset of active phase of labor was defined as regular, painful contractions that

led to a change in the cervix. PROM was defined as ruptured membranes without contractions. In this group, labor was induced after 24–48 h, and signs of infection were monitored until delivery. In women with PROM and meconium-stained amnion fluid, induction was started without delay.

Statistical analysis

Maternal characteristics and indications for labor induction were compared between the two groups using Student's t-test for continuous variables and chi-square test for dichotomous variables. For all outcomes, we identified potential confounding variables a priori according to previous knowledge of factors that could affect the likelihood of successful induction of labor using MVI or MVT [15–18]. Potential confounding factors included maternal age, body mass index, gestational age, birth weight, Bishop Score, PROM and pre-induction with balloon catheter. As a higher proportion of women in the MVI groups were induced due to hypertension/preeclampsia, the reason for induction was also considered a potential confounding factor. True confounders were defined as confounders that changed the results with more than 10%. For time outcomes, we used Student's t-test and Mann-Whitney U test to compare the two groups. Bishop Score and balloon catheter were identified as true confounding factors and were included in linear regression models with the forced entry method for the time outcomes. Due to skewed distributions, we also performed analyses with log transformed time variables in the model. To evaluate if labors interrupted by CS influenced the results, we also performed Cox regression with log rank test, censoring CS and with adjustment for Bishop Score and pre-induction with balloon catheter. In terms of delivery mode outcomes, we calculated crude and adjusted odds ratios (OR) with 95% confidence intervals (CI) in logistic regression models. In these analyses Bishop Score and balloon catheter were identified as true confounding factors and included in the models. To evaluate if fetal distress led to more operative deliveries in one of the groups, the proportion of CS and operative vaginal deliveries due to fetal distress were compared between the groups. Less than 2% of the data were missing. Missing data were excluded pairwise. A p-value of <0.05 was considered to indicate statistical significance. Statistical analyses were performed with IBM SPSS Statistics for Windows, Version 21 Armonk, NY: IBM Corp.

Ethical considerations

The study was approved by the Oslo University Hospital Data Protection Official for Research (2012/9668). The study was also evaluated by the Regional Committee for medical and health research ethics (REC South East in

Norway); however, as the study was limited to observations during standard clinical care, written informed consent was waivered.

Results

A total of 171 women were included in the study. Of these, 85 (49.7%) received MVI and 86 (50.3%) received MVT. Maternal and pregnancy characteristics were comparable in the two groups except for the mean Bishop Score, which was lower in the MVI group (Table 1).

As for the primary indication for induction, more women in the MVI group were induced due to preeclampsia/hypertension than in the MVT group, whereas other indications were similarly distributed.

The time interval from drug administration to delivery showed a skewed distribution with a right tail in both the MVI and the MVT groups (Fig. 2).

The average time from drug administration to delivery was significantly shorter in the MVI group compared to the MVT group (median time 15 h 43 min versus 19 h 37 min, $p = 0.011$), see Table 2. In regression models adjusting for Bishop Score and pre-induction with balloon catheter, the mean difference was 6 h 3 min ($p = 0.002$). The result did not change in models with log transformed outcomes ($p = 0.001$, data not shown). We conducted sensitivity analyses where we adjusted for additional potential confounders; however, the results did not change.

In the Cox model, where we censored deliveries interrupted by CS, the hazard ratio was increased by a factor of 2.1 in the MVI group compared to the MVT group, thus confirming the shorter time interval from drug administration to delivery in the former (see Fig. 3 and Table 3). In 9 women, the inductions were started in the evening and the 2nd dose of MVT was delayed so that the woman could rest at night. Excluding these women from the analyses did not change the results for the primary outcomes; time from drug administration to delivery and rate of CS.

As to delivery mode, women induced with MVI were less likely to be delivered by CS, compared to those induced with MVT (11.8% versus 23.3%), see Table 4. In models adjusting for Bishop Score and pre-induction with balloon catheter, there was a 67% reduced risk of CS in the MVI group compared to the MVT group (adjusted OR 0.33; 95% CI 0.13–0.81, $p = 0.016$). The results did not change in sensitivity analyses where we stratified for other potential confounders.

We found no difference in the rate of women delivered by CS due to fetal distress in the MVI versus the MVT groups; however, numbers were few ($n = 5$ (5.9%) versus $n = 8$ (9.3%)). Similarly we found no difference in the proportion of operative vaginal deliveries due to fetal distress in the two groups (MVI: n = 8 (9.4%) versus MVT: $n = 11$ (12.8%)). The number of labors diagnosed with uterine tachysystole and that ended with operative delivery due to fetal distress were few in both groups (MVI $n = 4$, MVT $n = 6$). Three neonates had an Apgar Score < 7 after 5 min; two in the MVI group and one in the MVT group. None of the neonates were diagnosed with metabolic acidosis (defined as umbilical artery pH

Table 1 Maternal characteristics and indications for labor induction in nulliparous women induced with Misoprostol Vaginal Insert (MVI) compared to Misoprostol Vaginal Tablets (MVT)

	MVI, $n = 85$		MVT, $n = 86$		
	mean or n	SD or %	mean or n	SD or %	p-value
Maternal age in years[a]	32.5	4.8	32.9	6.0	0.64
Body Mass Index[b]	24.6	5.5	24.4	4.8	0.807
Gestational age in days[a]	281	9.6	282	9.8	0.393
Bishop score[c]	3.1	1.2	3.6	1.5	0.016
Birthweight	3454	484	3485	520	0.692
Preinduction with balloon catheter	44	51.8	40	47.1	0.645
Primary indication for induction					
- Pre labor ruptures of membranes (PROM)	21	24.7	23	27.1	0.861
- Preeclampsia/hypertension	25	29.4	12	14.1	0.026
- Fetal concerns	16	18.8	18	21.2	0.848
- Postterm pregnancy[d]	8	9.4	13	15.3	0.351
- Maternal concerns	10	11.8	9	10.6	1.000
- Other	5	5.9	10	11.6	0.279

[a]At date of delivery
[b]From first prenatal visit
[c]At insertion of MVI or first MVT
[d]$\geq 42 + 0$ weeks, $\geq 41 + 2$ if maternal age ≥ 40 years

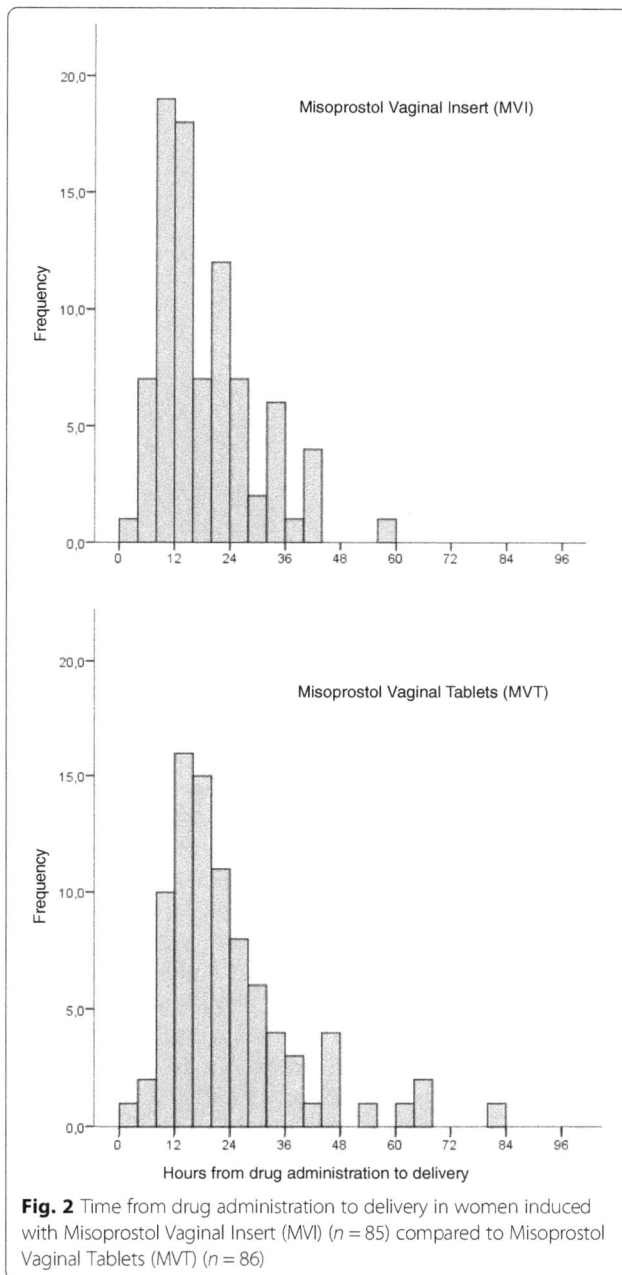

Fig. 2 Time from drug administration to delivery in women induced with Misoprostol Vaginal Insert (MVI) ($n = 85$) compared to Misoprostol Vaginal Tablets (MVT) ($n = 86$)

Table 2 Time outcomes in nulliparous women induced with Misoprostol Vaginal Insert (MVI) compared to Misoprostol Vaginal Tablets (MVT)

	MVI	MVT	Difference	p-value
Time intervals	$n = 85$	$n = 86$		
Time from drug administration to delivery				
Median (IQR)	15:43 (12:29)	19:37 (14:30)	3:54	0.011
Crude mean (SD)	18:39 (10:23)	23:42 (14:29)	5:03	0.010
Adjusted mean difference (CI; 95%)[a]			6:03 (2:20–9:46)	0.002
Time from drug administration to onset of active labor				
Median (IQR)	10:37 (10:42)	11:28 (12:13)	0:51	0.215
Crude mean (SD)	13:04 (8:32)	16:20 (13:27)	3:16	0.061
Adjusted mean difference (CI; 95%)[a]			4:16 (0:54–7:38)	0.013
Time from onset of active labor to delivery				
Median (IQR)	4:06 (6:54)	6:46 (5:50)	2:40	0.002
Crude mean (SD)	5:35 (4:36)	7:22 (4:09)	1:47	0.009
Adjusted mean difference (CI; 95%)[a]			1:47 (0:28–3:06)	0.008

Presented as hours:minutes
[a]Adjusted for Bishop Score and pre-induction with balloon catheter

with MVI had a lower risk of CS compared to women induced with MVT. There were no differences between the groups for the proportion of operative deliveries due to fetal distress or Apgar Score < 7 after 5 min.

To our knowledge, this is the first study comparing MVI to MVT. After the European approval on MVI, three studies comparing MVI other induction methods have been published [11–13]. Two studies comparing MVI to Dinoprostone insert [11, 13] did not find the same benefits for MVI over Dinoprostone insert as the phase III trial [10]. One study comparing MVI to Oral Misoprostol found shorter time from drug administration to delivery and a higher CS rate in the MVI group compared to Oral Misoprostol [12]. However, numbers for nulliparous women were not reported separately in any of the studies. Given the strong predictive value of parity on successful induction of labor, the results cannot directly be compared to our findings [15, 17].

We regard the mean adjusted difference in time from drug administration to delivery of 6 h 3 min as of clinical relevance, demonstrating MVI as the most effective induction agent. One contributory factor to the differences in efficiency could be deviation from the protocol in the MVT group, compared to the MVI group. Compliance with procedure is more likely with the MVI as

<7.00 and/or base deficit ≥12). Forty five (53%) women in the MVI group needed oxytocin during labor, compared to 63 (73%) in the MVT group ($p = 0.006$).

Discussion

In this study, in a setting of routine obstetric care, induction of labor with MVI was associated with a shorter time from drug administration to delivery compared to MVT. Both time from drug administration to onset of active labor and labor duration were shorter in the MVI group compared to the MVT group. Women induced

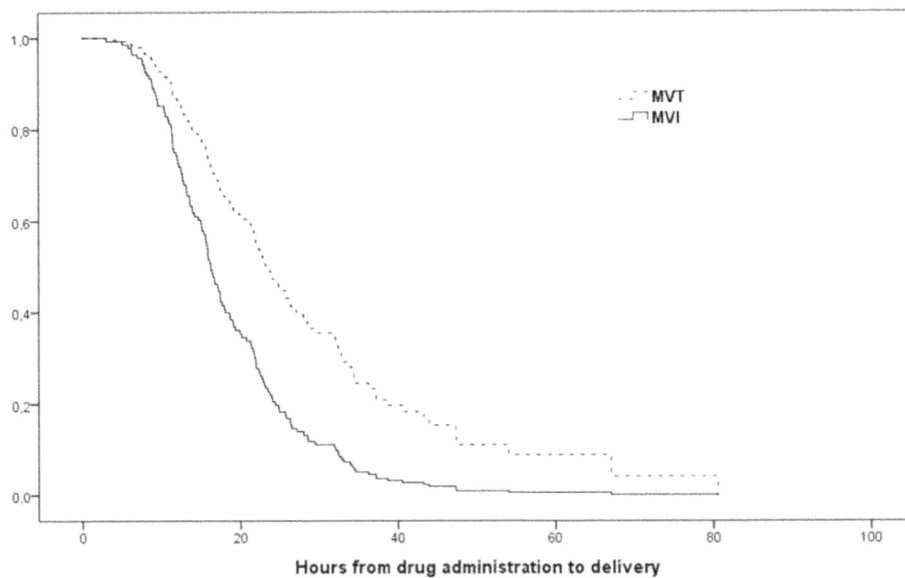

Fig. 3 Survival plot for time from drug administration to delivery in nulliparous women induced with Misoprostol vaginal insert (MVI) compared to Misoprostol vaginal tablets (MVT)

non-compliance would require removal of the insert, while non-compliance with the MVT is "just waiting a bit" with the next tablet. As prolonged latency and labor might lead to an increased risk of emergency CS and adverse maternal and neonatal outcome, an induction agent that is effective in the everyday routines of the department is preferable [6, 19, 20]. On the other hand, uterine tachysystole is a matter of considerable safety concern, especially for the fetus, when inducing labor [5]. The 5 min Apgar Score < 7 did not differ between the groups, neither did the proportion of operative deliveries due to fetal distress; however, cases were few. The lower rate of CS does however suggest that MVI is a safer alternative for the mother compared to MVT.

Compared to other studies, women in our study, both in the MVI and in the MVT groups, had more efficient induction processes and a lower CS rate. The median time from drug administration to delivery of 15.7 h in the MVI group is considerably shorter than the 25.9 h and 29.2 h reported on nulliparous women induced with

Table 3 Adjusted hazard ratio in relation to time from drug administration to delivery in nulliparous women induced with Misoprostol Vaginal Insert (MVI) compared to Misoprostol Vaginal Tablets (MVT)

	Adjusted Hazard ratio	95% CI	p-value*
Misoprostol vaginal insert (MVI)	2.11	1.48–3.02	0.001
Misoprostol vaginal tablets (MVT)	1	Reference	Reference

*From Log rank test

MVI in previous studies. However, in these studies MVI was compared to Dinoprostone [10, 21]. Previous studies of 25 μg MVT have also reported longer drug administration to delivery intervals compared to our findings, also in nulliparous women [22–24]. Median time has been reported to be 23.0 h [22], compared to 19.6 h in our study, and mean time 28.0 and 28.2 h [23, 24], compared to 23.7 h. In terms of CS, the rate found in our study is lower compared to previous studies on nulliparous women. In the MVI group, 11.8% underwent a CS in our study, compared to 32.9% and 34.5% in previous studies [10, 21]. For MVT, previous studies show more divergent results, from 20% to 42% [22, 25], compared to our result of 23.3%. These differences in efficiency and CS rate between the cited studies and our study may reflect provider-preference and a differential induction- and labor management policy. The overall CS rate in Norway and Scandinavia is low compared to other high income countries. In 2014, 16.6% were delivered by CS in Norway, compared to 32.2% in USA and 26.2% in UK [26–28]. A high proportion of pre-induction with balloon catheter (49.1%) and PROM (25.7%) might have contributed to increased efficiency and lower CS rate.

This study has several limitations. First, this retrospective cohort study was a part of a quality improvement project, focusing on induction in nulliparous women. Thus, there was no attempt of randomization. One could hypothesize that high risk pregnancies more often were induced using MVT, especially in the beginning of the study period, as the doctors and midwives were more familiar with this method. This might have

Table 4 Delivery mode in nulliparous women induced with Misoprostol Vaginal Insert (MVI) compared to Misoprostol Vaginal Tablets (MVT)

	MVI, n = 85		MVT, n = 86		Crude, n = 171			Adjusted[a], n=169[b]		
	n	%	n	%	OR	95% CI	p-value	OR	95% CI	p-value
Cesarean section	10	11.8	20	23.3	0.44	0.19–1.01	0.052	0.33	0.13–0.81	0.016
Operative vaginal delivery	19	22.4	18	20.9	1.09	0.53–2.25	0.821	1.14	0.54–2.39	0.733
Spontaneous vaginal delivery	56	65.9	48	55.8	1.45	0.78–2.69	0.236	1.60	0.84–3.04	0.150

[a]Adjusted for Bishop score and pre-induction with balloon catheter
[b]2 excluded due to missing data on Bishop score

contributed to a higher CS rate in the MVT group. However, as the maternal characteristics and the indications for induction of labor did not show major differences, this selection bias is unlikely to have had a major impact on our results. Conversely, the average Bishop Score was higher in the MVT group, which should correspond to more favorable cervix status. Furthermore fewer women had preeclampsia/hypertension in the MVT group which is a known risk factor for CS [29]. Although the lack of randomization could be considered a weakness, the results reflect what happened when MVI was introduced to a maternity department, without any adjustments in the treatment due to research considerations. Our results were robust across several different statistical models. Second, labor onset in this study was defined as when the midwife present defined active labor and started the partogram. This subjective assessment will differ between midwives. However, this is unlikely to represent a differential bias and is unlikely to influence the time from drug administration to delivery. Finally, the women in our study were not asked about their birth experience. As a negative birth experience is associated with an increased risk of postpartum depression, subsequent fear of childbirth and request for elective CS [6, 30], this would have added valuable information to the study.

Conclusions

In this study among nulliparous women in a routine care setting we found 200 μg MVI to be a more efficient and safe labor induction agent compared to 25 μg MVT. The time from drug administration to delivery was significantly shorter and the CS rate reduced in women induced with MVI, compared with MVT. Future studies comparing methods for labor induction should acknowledge the particular status of nulliparous women.

Abbreviations
CI: Confidence interval; CS: Cesarean section; CTG: Cardio-tocographic monitoring; MVI: Misoprostol vaginal insert; MVT: Misoprostol vaginal tablet; OR: Odds ratio; PROM: Pre-labor rupture of the membranes; SD: Standard deviation

Acknowledgements
Not applicable

Funding
Funder: Oslo and Akershus University College.

Authors' contributions
Kjersti Engen Marsdal (KEM), Ingvil Krarup Sørbye (IKS), Lise C Gaudernack (LCG) and Mirjam Lukasse (ML) conceived the idea of the study. KEM and LCG collected the data. KEM, IKS, LCG and ML were involved in developing the analyses strategy, the final analyses strategy was approved by all authors. KEM and IKS performed the analyses. KEM, IKS, LCG and ML were involved in interpreting the results and writing the manuscript, all authors approved the final draft.

Competing interests
Kjersti Engen Marsdal, Ingvil Krarup Sørbye, Lise C Gaudernack, Mirjam Lukasse. The authors declare that they have no competing interests.

Author details
[1]Department of Obstetrics, Oslo University Hospital Rikshospitalet, P.O. Box 4956 Nydalen, 0424 Oslo, Norway. [2]Oslo and Akershus University College, Faculty of Health Sciences, Department of Nursing and Health Promotion, P.O. Box 4, 0130 Oslo, Norway.

References
1. European perinatal health report: Health and Care of Pregnant Women and Babies in Europe in 2010. Euro-Peristat. http://www.europeristat.com/reports/european-perinatal-health-report-2010.html. Accessed 03 Sept 2016.
2. Dögl M, Vanky E, Heimstad R. Changes in induction methods have not influenced cesarean section rates among women with induced labor. Acta Obstet Gynecol Scand. 2016;95(1):112–5.
3. Yeast JD, Jones A, Poskin M. Induction of labor and the relationship to cesarean delivery: a review of 7001 consecutive inductions. Am J Obstet Gynecol. 1999;180(3 Pt 1):628–33.
4. Vahratian A, Zhang J, Troendle JF, Sciscione AC, Hoffman MK. Labor progression and risk of cesarean delivery in electively induced nulliparas. Obstet Gynecol. 2005;105(4):698–704.
5. Stewart RD, Bleich AT, Lo JY, Alexander JM, McIntire DD, Leveno KJ. Defining uterine tachysystole: how much is too much? Am J Obstet Gynecol. 2012;207(4):290–6.
6. Kolås T, Hofoss D, Daltveit AK, Nilsen ST, Henriksen T, Häger R, Ingemarsson I, Øian P. Indications for cesarean deliveries in Norway. Am J Obstet Gynecol. 2003;188(4):864–70.
7. Hofmeyr GJ, Gülmezoglu AM, Pileggi C. Vaginal misoprostol for cervical ripening and induction of labour. Cochrane Database Syst Rev. 2010;10
8. Misodel Summary of Product Characteristics. https://www.ferring.com/en/media/press-releases/2013/misodel-17oct13/. Accessed 01 Oct 2016.
9. Heads of Medicines Agencies. Misoprostol gynaecological indication PSUR SAR. 2015. http://www.hma.eu/search.html?id=6&q=misodel&L=0. Accessed 28 Sept 2016.
10. Wing DA, Brown R, Plante LA, Miller H, Rugarn O, Powers BL. Misoprostol vaginal insert and time to vaginal delivery: a randomized controlled trial. Obstet Gynecol. 2013;122(2 Pt 1):201–9.

11. Mayer RB, Oppelt P, Shebl O, Pömer J, Allerstorfer C, Weiss C. Initial clinical experience with a misoprostol vaginal insert in comparison with a dinoprostone insert for inducing labor. Eur J Obstet Gynecol Reprod Biol. 2016;200:89–93.

12. Dobert M, Brandstetter A, Henrich W, Rawnaq T, Hasselbeck H, Dobert TF, Hinkson L, Schwaerzler P. The misoprostol vaginal insert compared with oral misoprostol for labor induction in term pregnancies: a pair-matched case-control study. J of. Perinat Med. 2017;

13. Gornisiewicz T, Jaworowski A, Zembala-Szczerba M, Babczyk D, Huras H. Analysis of intravaginal misoprostol 0.2 mg versus intracervical dinoprostone 0.5 mg doses for labor induction at term pregnancies. Ginekologia pol. 2017;88(6):320–4.

14. Robson M, Murphy M, Byrne F. Quality assurance: the 10-group classification system (Robson classification), induction of labor, and cesarean delivery. Int J Gynaecol Obstet. 2015;131:23–7.

15. Pevzner L, Rayburn WF, Rumney P, Wing DA. Factors predicting successful labor induction with dinoprostone and misoprostol vaginal inserts. Obstet Gynecol. 2009;114(2 Pt 1):261–7.

16. Wing DA, Tran S, Paul RH. Factors affecting the likelihood of successful induction after intravaginal misoprostol application for cervical ripening and labor induction. Am J Obstet Gynecol. 2002;186(6):1237–40.

17. Crane JMG, Delaney T, Butt KD, Bennett KA, Hutchens D, Young DC. Predictors of successful labor induction with oral or vaginal misoprostol. J Matern Fetal Med. 2004;15(5):319–23.

18. Chen W, Xue J, Gaudet L, Walker M, Wen SW. Meta-analysis of Foley catheter plus misoprostol versus misoprostol alone for cervical ripening. Int J Gynaecol Obstet. 2015;129(3):193–8.

19. Laughon SK, Berghella V, Reddy UM, Sundaram R, Lu Z, Hoffman MK. Neonatal and maternal outcomes with prolonged second stage of labor. Obstet Gynecol. 2014;124(1):57–67.

20. Maghoma J, Buchmann EJ. Maternal and fetal risks associated with prolonged latent phase of labour. J Obstet Gynaecol. 2002;22(1):16–9.

21. Wing DA, Miller H, Parker L, Powers BL, Rayburn WF. Misoprostol vaginal insert for successful labor induction: a randomized controlled trial. Obstet Gynecol. 2011;117(3):533–41.

22. Gregson S, Waterstone M, Norman I, Murrells TA. Randomised controlled trial comparing low dose vaginal misoprostol and dinoprostone vaginal gel for inducing labour at term. BJOG. 2005;112(4):438–44.

23. Calder AA, Loughney AD, Weir CJ, Barber JW. Induction of labour in nulliparous and multiparous women: a UK, multicentre, open-label study of intravaginal misoprostol in comparison with dinoprostone. BJOG. 2008;115(10):1279–88.

24. Wing DA, Ham D, Paul RHA. Comparison of orally administered misoprostol with vaginally administered misoprostol for cervical ripening and labor induction. Am J Obstet Gynecol. 1999;180(5):1155–60.

25. van Gemund N, Scherjon S, LeCessie S, van Leeuwen JHS, van Roosmalen J, Kanhai HHH. A Randomised trial comparing low dose vaginal misoprostol and dinoprostone for labour induction. BJOG 2004; 111(1):42–49.

26. Norwegian Institute of Public Health. Medical Birth Registry of Norway. http://statistikk.fhi.no/mfr/. Accessed 18 Oct 2016.

27. European Medicines Agency. List of nationally authorised medical products Active substance: Misoprostol (gynaecological indication - labour induction). http://www.ema.europa.eu/docs/en_GB/document_library/Periodic_safety_update_single_assessment/2017/03/WC500223582.pdf. Accessed 02 Jan 2018.

28. NHS Digital. NHS Maternity Statistics - England, 2013–14. https://digital.nhs.uk/catalogue/PUB16725. Accessed 19 Oct 2016.

29. Kim LH, Cheng YW, Delaney S, Jelin AC, Caughey ABl. Preeclampsia associated with an increased risk of cesarean delivery if labor is induced? J Matern Fetal Med. 2010;23(5):383–8.

30. Righetti-Veltema M, Conne-Perréard E, Bousquet A, Manzano J. Risk factors and predictive signs of postpartum depression. J Affect Disord. 1998;49(3):167–80.

5

Unintended pregnancy is a risk factor for depressive symptoms among socio-economically disadvantaged women in rural Bangladesh

Pamela J. Surkan[1,2]* (iD), Donna M. Strobino[2], Sucheta Mehra[1], Abu Ahmed Shamim[3], Mahbubur Rashid[3], Lee Shu-Fune Wu[1], Hasmot Ali[3], Barkat Ullah[3], Alain B. Labrique[1], Rolf D. W. Klemm[1], Keith P. West Jr[1] and Parul Christian[1]

Abstract

Background: Little is known about the relation between unwanted pregnancy and intention discordance and maternal mental health in low-income countries. The study aim was to evaluate maternal and paternal pregnancy intentions (and intention discordance) in relation to perinatal depressive symptoms among rural Bangladeshi women.

Methods: Data come from a population-based, community trial of married rural Bangladeshi women aged 13–44. We examined pregnancy intentions among couples and pregnancy-intention discordance, as reported by women at enrollment soon after pregnancy ascertainment, in relation to depressive symptoms in the third trimester of pregnancy ($N = 14,629$) and six months postpartum ($N = 31,422$). We calculated crude and adjusted risk ratios for prenatal and postnatal depressive symptoms by pregnancy intentions.

Results: In multivariable analyses, women with unwanted pregnancies were at higher risk of prenatal (Adj. RR = 1.60, 95% CI: 1.37–1.87) and postnatal depressive symptoms (Adj. RR = 1.32, 95% CI: 1.21–1.44) than women with wanted pregnancies. Women who perceived their husbands did not want the pregnancy also were at higher risk for prenatal (Adj. RR = 1.42, 95% CI: 1.22–1.65) and postnatal depressive symptoms (Adj. RR = 1.30, 95% CI: 1.19–1.41). Both parents not wanting the pregnancy was associated with prenatal and postnatal depressive symptoms (Adj. RR = 1.34, 95% CI: 1.19–1.52; Adj. RR = 1.13, 95% CI: 1.06–1.21, respectively), compared to when both parents wanted it. Adjusting for socio-demographic and pregnancy intention variables simultaneously, maternal intentions and pregnancy discordance were significantly related to prenatal depressive symptoms, and perception of paternal pregnancy unwantedness and couple pregnancy discordance, with postnatal depressive symptoms.

Conclusions: Maternal, paternal and discordant couple pregnancy intentions, as perceived by rural Bangladeshi women, are important risk factors for perinatal maternal depressive symptoms.

Keywords: Unintended pregnancy, Pregnancy intention discordance, Perinatal depression, Depressive symptoms, Bangladesh

* Correspondence: psurkan@jhu.edu
[1]Center for Human Nutrition, Department of International Health, Johns Hopkins Bloomberg School of Public Health, 615 North Wolfe St., Room E2519, Baltimore, MD 21205-2179, USA
[2]Department of Population, Family and Reproductive Health, Johns Hopkins Bloomberg School of Public Health, Baltimore, MD 21205-2179, USA
Full list of author information is available at the end of the article

Background

Unintended pregnancies are a major problem worldwide, with 40% of pregnancies estimated to be unintended in less developed regions [1, 2]. Unintended pregnancies refer to pregnancies not wanted at the time (mistimed) or at any time (unwanted) [3]. Econometric analyses indicate that contraception is cost-effective relative to the consequences of unintended pregnancies [4]. As such, family planning initiatives have attempted to curb unwanted pregnancies; however, major socio-economic disparities in access to contraception still exist in developing countries [5]. In Bangladesh, a substantial number of unwanted pregnancies are terminated legally through 'menstrual regulation' for which manual vacuum aspiration is used to safely establish non-pregnancy up to 8–10 weeks after a women's missed period; yet, according to the 2007 Demographic and Health Survey about 30% of term live births are reported to be unintended [6].

A review of the literature suggested that, although findings are mixed, unwanted pregnancy is associated overall with adverse consequences, including limited antenatal care, short duration of breast feeding, adverse birth outcomes, and elevated infant and child mortality [7]. While there is a substantial literature on unintended pregnancy and mental health in developed countries, little is known about the relation between unwanted pregnancy and maternal mental health in lower- and middle-income countries [8]. Yet, high levels of common mental disorders, being predominantly maternal depressive symptoms, during pregnancy and postpartum (16 and 19%, respectively) have been estimated in lower- and middle-income countries [9]. In eastern Bangladesh, about one-third of women reported depressive symptoms between 34 and 35 weeks of pregnancy and 22% at 6–8 weeks postpartum [10, 11]. Furthermore, gendered inequalities related to reproductive decision-making and control exist within South Asia, with 48% of women in Bangladesh reporting that their husbands make decisions about their health and accessing healthcare services [12, 13]. Given this context, we were particularly interested in studying discordance of wantedness between couples in relation to depressive symptoms.

The principal aim of this study was to evaluate the relation between maternal and paternal pregnancy intentions and prenatal (in the 3rd trimester) and postnatal maternal depressive symptoms (at six months postpartum) among rural Bangladeshi women. In South Asia, women are often dependent on their husbands due to gaps in age, education, and control of financial resources [14]. Therefore, a second aim was to assess women's reports of the couple's discordance in intentions and unwantedness on the part of both parents in relation to women's perinatal depressive symptoms.

Methods

This study is a secondary analysis of data collected during the course of a cluster randomized, double-masked, placebo-controlled, community trial (JiViTA-1) of the effects of vitamin A or beta-carotene supplementation on all-cause, pregnancy-related mortality [15, 16]. The ClinicalTrials.gov identifier for that previous study was: NCT00198822, registered on 9/12/2005. JiViTA-1 was conducted between August 2001 and October 2007.

Study setting

This trial took place in 19 rural unions of Gaibandha and Rangpur Districts in northwestern Bangladesh, comprising an area of ~ 435 km^2. The site was selected to be typical of general living conditions in rural Bangladesh and eastern Gangetic region of South Asia. At the time of the study, about 40% of the married women of reproductive age in the area were literate, with < 5% having completed the 10th grade and < 40% were involved in income-generating work on their own. Husbands were mostly employed in subsistence agriculture, hired themselves out as daily wage laborers or ran a small business. Less than 15% of households had access to electricity, and households were mostly made of earth or tin.

Pregnancy ascertainment

Married women of reproductive age (13–44 years) who were neither sterilized nor menopausal and living with their husbands were recruited and placed under pregnancy surveillance [14]. All women were visited every five weeks to ask about their menstrual history during the past 30 days and offered a urine test if amenstrual to identify incident pregnancies. After obtaining verbal consent (due to illiteracy among many participants), pregnant women were enrolled in the trial, visited for an enrollment interview and began receiving supplements as per their allocation.

Data collection

Participants were interviewed by trained interviewers at inclusion (early pregnancy, median gestation age 9 weeks) to collect information on household socioeconomic factors (education, asset ownership, house construction), maternal nutritional status, diet, morbidity history, previous pregnancy history, wantedness of the incident pregnancy, hygiene, physical work history as well as tobacco and alcohol use [17]. Women were tracked through the course of their pregnancies and all women were interviewed again at 3 and 6 months post-partum and asked about labor and delivery, diet, morbidity history, work history and tobacco and alcohol use. In addition, from February 2004 to July 2017, a module of questions related to depression and suicide was introduced into the study and asked independently at two different times of eligibility, during the latter half of pregnancy (Median = 24.4 wks, Mean = 25.2 wks, SD = 2.1), and at ~ 6 months post-partum(Median 32.1 wks, Mean 32.4 wks, SD = 1.06 wks). All interviews were conducted one-on-one in women's homes and sufficient community counseling ensured that interviews were private and confidentiality could be maintained. If a woman could not be interviewed alone at a specific time, the interviewer rescheduled the visit until it could be conducted privately.

Data were collected at enrollment about unintended pregnancy from the woman for herself ("Did you want to become pregnant now?") and for her husband ("Did your husband want you to become pregnant now?"). Options included "wanted now", "mistimed" or "unwanted", asked approximately one week after a positive pregnancy test (Median = 1.0 wks; Mean = 11.6 wks, SD = 2.4). Pregnancy-intention discordance was defined from the mother's report of her intentions and those of her husband. For the purpose of the couple's discordance analysis, mistimed and unwanted pregnancies were combined and defined as "unwanted." Using 'wanted now' and the collapsed category of "unwanted" pregnancy (for the purpose of the discordance analyses), couples' discordance was defined as a non-match between the mother and her husband's intentions (not either both "wanted" or both "unwanted").

Because there was no validated depression scale in Bangladesh at the time of JiViTA-1, depressive symptom items were adapted from the nine-item Patient Health Questionnaire (PHQ-9) and the Center for Epidemiologic Studies Depression Scale (CES-D) [18, 19]. Selection of items (six prenatal and five postnatal) was based on pretesting in the study area. Questions were translated by a professional translator and an independent back-translation was done between Bangla and English to ensure that the meaning of the questions was retained. Women in the area struggled to grasp the meaning of some questions on the PHQ-9 and the CES-D, and so only questions that were clearly understood in focus group discussions were included. Two standard questions about suicidal ideation and suicide attempts were also included.

Maternal depressive symptoms during the latter half of pregnancy were measured using the following six symptoms reported in the last 30 days (yes/no): feeling sad all the time; becoming more forgetful; crying all the time; having thoughts of hurting yourself; sleeping more than before; and trying to hurt yourself. Postpartum maternal depressive symptoms were measured by asking women the first four items used in the prenatal period (listed above), along with a fifth symptom, not wanting to bathe or eat for several days in the last 60 days.

Socio-demographic and other covariates included: living standards index in quartiles (1st = low, 4th = high),

maternal education (none, 1–9, ≥10 years), maternal literacy (yes/no), maternal age at enrollment (≤19, 20–29, ≥30 years), maternal nutritional status during pregnancy (mid-upper arm circumference in the third trimester: < 21.5; ≥21.5 cm), anemia in the first trimester (symptoms of breathlessness at rest resulting in inability to work from the World Health Organization maternal screening questions), and infection in the first trimester (either urinary tract infection or pneumonia or both). [20] The living standards index was created using Principal Components Analysis, combining several household asset variables (toilet facilities, type of walls, kitchen, and roof, the number of clocks, living rooms, closets, beds, radios, irrigation pumps, televisions, rickshaws, and having electricity) [21]. Participants were classified in vitamin A, beta-carotene, and placebo groups representing their micronutrient supplementation assignment in the original trial.

The study protocol was reviewed and approved by the Johns Hopkins Bloomberg School of Public Health Institutional Review Board (IRB, #H.22.01.01.11.A1) and the Bangladesh Medical Research Council (BMRC, BMRC/ERC/1998–2001/2405). The informed consent process included, when so desired by the subjects, husbands, in-laws and sometimes community members. Individual consent was sought from the participating women and documented.

Data analysis

Descriptive demographic and pregnancy intention statistics were summarized for women in the subsample of the trial cohort who received prenatal and postnatal depressive symptoms assessments.

We restricted our analyses for prenatal depressive symptoms to women interviewed after the 23rd week and before the 37th week of gestation, in order to make sure that women were interviewed during a common time window, after a spontaneous loss (miscarriage) and before the very end of the pregnancy when hormonal changes related to pending delivery might affect their responses. Analyses were further restricted to women with singleton live births. The Cronbach alpha for prenatal symptoms with all items was 0.57 (unexplained variance = 0.67), and 0.63 (unexplained variance = 0.61) after removal of the item 'sleeping more than before.' The remaining five items were summed to achieve a total score of 0–5, with a score ≥ 3 considered our higher level of depressive symptoms. Only women with data on all five items were included in the analysis. Cronbach's alpha was 0.71 (unexplained variance = 0.49) for the five postpartum depressive symptoms. Items were summed and a cutoff of ≥3 was our basis for dichotomizing depressive symptoms based on the fact that this was the cutoff that conservatively optimized the number of women with symptoms (8% prenatally, 13% postnatally) that would be expected in rural Bangladesh.

Bivariate risk ratios (RRs) and 95% confidence intervals (CI) were calculated using a generalized linear model with binomial error structure and logarithmic link function. Unintended pregnancy included mothers' and their husbands' intentions separately (wanted and mistimed versus unwanted) and discordance between intentions (comparing unwanted by the mother/perceived as unwanted by the husband; unwanted by the mother/perceived as wanted by the husband; wanted by the mother/perceived as unwanted by the husband; wanted by the mother/perceived as wanted by the husband). Adjusted RRs were calculated for intentions and depressive symptoms at both time points including potential confounders and covariates of theoretical significance. We did not adjust for prenatal depressive symptoms in models for postpartum depressive symptoms due to the fact that we consider prenatal depressive symptoms potentially on the causal pathway, e.g. the negative effects of unintended pregnancy might first cause depressive symptoms during pregnancy which are sustained after the birth.

All models adjusted for geographic clustering sampled in the original study design and mothers' assigned vitamin supplementation group in the trial. All adjusted analyses at six months postpartum controlled for child sex. We were unable to include arm circumference, anemia and infection variables in all models simultaneously because of small numbers in some categories. Quasi-likelihood under the Independence Model Criterion Goodness of Fit tests indicated that arm circumference and anemia yielded the best fit; these two variables were included in our multivariable models.

Results

A total of 127,282 women were placed under 5-weekly pregnancy surveillance, of whom 59,666 became pregnant, of whom 16,792 were in the subsample that was eligible for assessment of depressive symptoms while pregnant during the eligible period that, for pregnant women, ran from February 2004 through November 2006. Excluding pregnancies in this subset who delivered, refused or died being assessed and mothers not meeting the gestational age window of eligibility, we assessed 14,629 3rd trimester gravida for depressive symptoms at a median gestational age of 32.1 weeks (IQR = 31.9–32.7 wks; mean = 32.4 wks, SD = 1.06 wks) (Fig. 1). Among all 59,666 pregnant women, 38,292 delivered a live, singleton birth such that they were eligible for the 6 month post-partum depressive symptom assessment during the active period of this study protocol, from February 2004 through July 2007. Among these,

36,851 mothers were assessed postpartum; however, because this assessment occurred across a wider postpartum interval, this analysis has been restricted to mothers whose depressive symptom interview occurred between 150 to 240 days (5–8 months), inclusive, leaving 31,422 women in the present analytical cohort (Fig. 1).

For the subsample for which prenatal depressive symptoms were reported, 59, 31 and 11% of mothers reported having a wanted, mistimed and unwanted pregnancy, respectively (Table 1). The respective proportions for mothers' perception of their husbands' pregnancy intentions were 67, 24 and 10% for wanted, mistimed and unwanted pregnancies (Table 1). In the postpartum sample, 57, 31 and 12% of mothers reported having a wanted, mistimed and unwanted pregnancy. The respective proportions based on the mother's perception of the fathers' pregnancy intentions were 63, 25 and 12% for wanted, mistimed and unwanted pregnancies (Table 1).

Finally, 8 and 13% of the mothers had ≥3 depressive symptoms during the prenatal and postnatal periods, respectively (Table 1). Mothers reporting a mistimed or unwanted pregnancy had a greater risk of prenatal depressive symptoms (RR 1.21, 95% CI 1.07, 1.37; RR 2.32, 95% CI 2.02, 2.66, respectively) than mothers with wanted pregnancies. Women reporting unwanted (RR 1.73, 95% CI 1.60, 1.87) but not mistimed pregnancies (RR 1.02, 95% CI 0.95, 1.10) were at greater risk for postnatal depressive symptoms (Table 1).

Women's mistimed (Adjusted RR 1.26, 95%CI 1.11, 1.43) and unwanted pregnancies (Adjusted RR 1.60, 95%OR 1.37, 1.87) had higher risk of prenatal depressive symptoms than women with wanted pregnancies after socio-demographic adjustment. Postpartum depressive symptoms were not related to mistimed pregnancies (Adjusted RR 1.05, 95% CI 0.98, 1.13), but women with unwanted pregnancies had an elevated risk of postpartum symptoms (Adjusted RR 1.32, 95% CI 1.21, 1.44) (Table 2).

Women with husbands who they perceived as not wanting the pregnancy were at higher risk for prenatal (Adjusted RR 1.42, 95% CI 1.22, 1.65) and postnatal depressive symptoms (Adjusted RR 1.30, 95% CI 1.19, 1.41), than women who perceived their husbands wanted the pregnancy (Table 3).

Perception of mistimed pregnancy for husbands was not related to prenatal or postnatal depressive symptoms. Maternal report of not wanting the pregnancy and also perceiving her husband to not want the pregnancy was associated with a 34% higher risk of prenatal depressive symptoms (Adjusted RR 1.34, 95%CI 1.19, 1.52) compared to when both parents wanted the pregnancy. Similarly, having the mother not want the pregnancy but perceive her husband want it was associated with a 51% higher risk of prenatal depressive symptoms (Adjusted

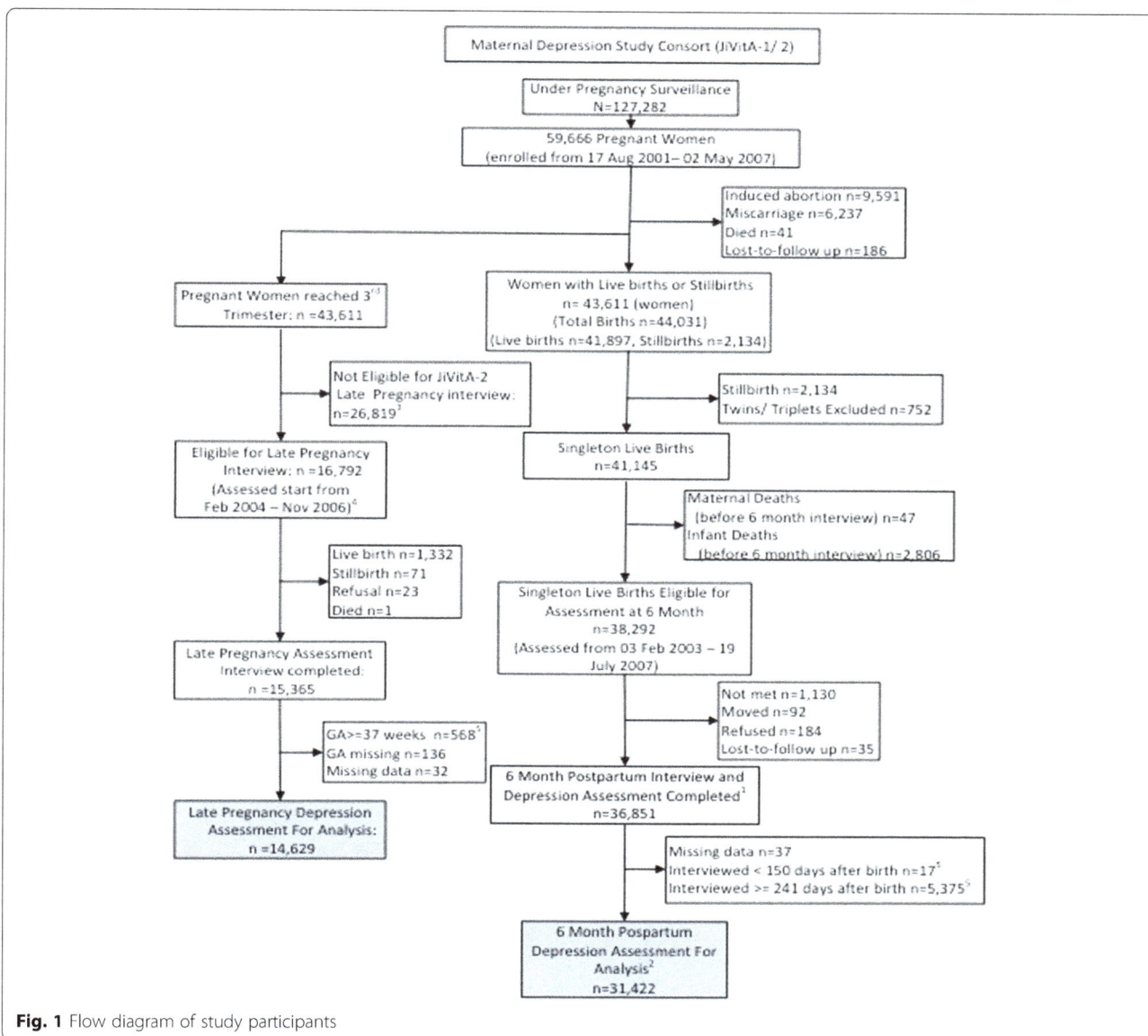

Fig. 1 Flow diagram of study participants

RR 1.51, 95% CI 1.29, 1.78), compared to cases in which both parents wanted the pregnancy. Finally, maternal report of wanting the pregnancy but perceiving that her husband did not want it was associated with a 30% higher risk of prenatal depressive symptoms (Adjusted RR 1.30, 95% CI 0.97, 1.74) compared to when both parents wanted the pregnancy (Table 3) compared to mothers who wanted the pregnancy and perceived that their husbands' also wanted it. A similar, but less pronounced, increase in the risk of depressive symptoms associated with unintended pregnancy was observed in the postpartum period, i.e. a 13% increased risk for mothers who did not want the pregnancy and perceived their husbands did not want it (Adjusted RR 1.13, 95% CI 1.06, 1.21), a 24% increased risk for mothers who did

not want the pregnancy but perceived their husbands wanted it (Adjusted RR 1.24, 95% CI 1.12, 1.37); and a 19% increased risk for mothers who wanted the pregnancy but perceived their husbands did not want it (Adjusted RR 1.19, 95% CI 0.99, 1.44).

Table 2 also shows multivariable results for the socio-demographic covariates and maternal depressive symptoms. Low maternal education was a risk factor for prenatal and postnatal depressive symptoms. Poor living standards showed an increased risk only for postnatal depressive symptoms. Older maternal age was associated with a higher risk of both prenatal and postnatal depressive symptoms. Anemia also was associated with greater risk of prenatal (Adjusted RR 2.08, 95% CI 1.85, 2.33) and postnatal (Adjusted RR 1.49, 95% CI 1.40, 1.58)

Table 1 Crude risk ratios of maternal wantedness of pregnancy and perceptions as risk factors for maternal depressive symptoms

	Prenatal depressive symptoms N = 1201 (8.2%)		Postnatal depressive symptoms N = 3965 (12.6%)	
	Total (%)/Cases (%)	RR [95% CI]	Total (%)/ Cases(%)	RR [95% CI]
PREGNANCY INTENTIONS				
Maternal pregnancy wantedness				
Wanted now	7835 (58.5)/563 (6.7)	Reference	15,647 (57.1)/2015 (11.4)	Reference
Mistimed	4091 (30.5)/372 (8.3)	1.21* [1.07, 1.37]	8352 (30.5)/1110 (11.7)	1.02 [0.95, 1.10]
Not wanted	1474 (11.0)/266 (15.3)	2.32* [2.02, 2.66]	3393 (12.4)/834 (19.7)	1.73* [1.60, 1.87]
Perceived paternal pregnancy wantedness				
Wanted now	8868 (66.8)/701 (7.3)	Reference	17,218 (63.3)/2285 (11.7)	Reference
Mistimed	3129 (23.6)/261 (7.7)	1.04 [0.91, 1.20]	6875 (25.3)/872 (11.3)	0.97 [0.90, 1.04]
Not wanted	1272 (9.6)/223 (14.9)	2.06* [1.80, 2.37]	3118 (11.5)/768 (19.8)	1.70* [1.57, 1.83]
Parental discordance of pregnancy wantedness				
Unwanted by mother/perceived as unwanted by husband	3975 (30.0)/440 (10.0)	1.52* [1.34, 1.72]	9325 (34.3)/1527 (14.1)	1.26* [1.18, 1.34]
Unwanted by mother/perceived as wanted by husband	1497 (11.3)/186 (11.1)	1.62* [1.38, 1.90]	2285 (8.4)/396 (14.8)	1.26* [1.13, 1.39]
Wanted by mother/perceived as unwanted by husband	425 (3.2)/44 (9.4)	1.36* [1.01, 1.83]	666 (2.4)/113 (14.5)	1.23* [1.03, 1.48]
Wanted by mother/perceived as wanted by husband	7363 (55.5)/515 (6.5)	Reference	14,925 (54.9)/1889 (11.2)	Reference
DEMOGRAPHIC CHARACTERISTICS				
Maternal education				
None	5175 (38.6)/620 (10.7)	2.87* [2.17, 3.81]	12,447 (45.4)/2154 (14.8)	1.83* [1.59, 2.10]
1–9	7143 (53.2)/538 (7.0)	1.82* [1.37, 2.40]	12,844 (46.8)/1620 (11.2)	1.36* [1.18, 1.57]
≥ 10	1102 (8.2)/42 (3.7)	Reference	2136 (7.8)/187 (8.1)	Reference
Living standard index				
1st quartile (poor)	2439 (18.2)/294 (10.8)	1.73* [1.48, 2.02]	6672 (24.3)/1179 (15.0)	1.47* [1.35, 1.61]

Table 1 Crude risk ratios of maternal wantedness of pregnancy and perceptions as risk factors for maternal depressive symptoms (*Continued*)

	Prenatal depressive symptoms N = 1201 (8.2%)		Postnatal depressive symptoms N = 3965 (12.6%)	
	Total (%)/Cases (%)	RR [95% CI]	Total (%)/ Cases(%)	RR [95% CI]
2nd	3276 (24.4)/333 (9.2)	1.52* [1.31, 1.77]	6831 (24.9)/1045 (13.3)	1.32* [1.20, 1.44]
3rd	3689 (27.5)/307 (7.7)	1.24* [1.06, 1.45]	6917 (25.2)/940 (12.0)	1.18* [1.09, 1.29]
4th quartile (rich)	4023 (30.0)/267 (6.2)	Reference	7016 (25.6)/797 (10.2)	Reference
Maternal age (yrs)				
≤ 19	5742 (42.8)/430 (7.0)	Reference	11,522 (42.0)/1340 (10.4)	Reference
20–29	6332 (47.2)/536 (7.8)	1.15* [1.03, 1.30]	13,097 (47.7)/1926 (12.8)	1.25* [1.17, 1.33]
≥ 30	1343 (10.0)/235 (14.9)	2.22* [1.90, 2.59]	2821 (10.3)/699 (19.9)	1.93* [1.78, 2.10]
Previous births				
Zero	6252 (46.6)/437 (6.5)	Reference	11,209 (40.9)/1245 (10.0)	Reference
≥ 1	7176 (53.4)/764 (9.6)	1.51* [1.35, 1.69]	16,226 (59.1)/2717 (14.3)	1.44* [1.35, 1.53]
Maternal literacy				
Yes	6969 (51.9)/435 (5.9)	Reference	12,994 (47.4)/1487 (10.3)	Reference
No	6458 (48.1)/766 (10.6)	1.82* [1.63, 2.05]	14,442 (52.6)/2474 (14.6)	1.43* [1.34, 1.51]
Maternal employment				
Yes	3008 (22.4)/240 (7.4)	0.90 [0.79, 1.02]	4428 (16.1)/661 (13.0)	1.00 [0.92, 1.08]
No	10,419 (77.6)/961 (8.4)	Reference	23,008 (83.9)/3300 (12.5)	Reference
Religion				
Non-Muslim	1145 (8.5)/90 (7.3)	Reference	2219 (8.1)/281 (11.2)	Reference
Muslim	12,281 (91.5)/1111 (8.3)	1.13 [0.91, 1.42]	25,217 (91.9)/3680 (12.7)	1.17* [1.02, 1.35]
HEALTH-RELATED INDICES				
Mid-upper arm circumference (cm)				
< 21.5	2705 (20.2)/264 (8.9)	1.13* [1.00, 1.28]	6517 (23.9)/1057 (14.0)	1.16* [1.09, 1.23]
≥ 21.5	10,700 (79.8)/934 (8.0)	Reference	20,796 (76.1)/2884 (12.2)	Reference
Anemia during pregnancy				
Yes	4081 (30.4)/629 (13.3)	2.28* [2.04, 2.56]	8648 (31.6)/1769 (17.0)	1.61* [1.51, 1.70]
No	9341 (69.6)/571 (5.8)	Reference	18,697 (68.4)/2177 (10.4)	Reference

Table 1 Crude risk ratios of maternal wantedness of pregnancy and perceptions as risk factors for maternal depressive symptoms *(Continued)*

	Prenatal depressive symptoms N = 1201 (8.2%)		Postnatal depressive symptoms N = 3965 (12.6%)	
	Total (%)/Cases (%)	RR [95% CI]	Total (%)/ Cases(%)	RR [95% CI]
Infections				
None	12,069 (89.9)/979 (7.5)	Reference	24,844 (90.8)/3323 (11.8)	Reference
At least one or both	1354 (10.1)/221 (14.0)	1.79* [1.55, 2.06]	2505 (9.2)/624 (19.9)	1.61* [1.49, 1.74]
Vitamin supplementation				
Vitamin A (Z)	4386 (32.7)/424 (8.8)	1.07 [0.86, 1.34]	9144 (33.3)/1332 (12.7)	1.00 [0.86, 1.17]
Beta-Carotene (X)	4532 (33.8)/378 (7.7)	0.94 [0.76, 1.16]	9168 (33.4)/1306 (12.5)	0.98 [0.85, 1.13]
Placebo (Y)	4510 (33.6)/399 (8.1)	Reference	9145 (33.3)/1327 (12.7)	Reference
Child sex				
Male	–	–	13,839 (50.4)/2010 (12.7)	1.01 [0.96, 1.06]
Female	–	–	13,618 (49.6)/1955 (12.6)	Reference

*indicates $P < 0.05$

Analyses at six months postpartum are restricted to mothers who had singleton births. All models are adjusted for geographic sector

The total sample size for the *prenatal depressive symptoms* analysis was 14,629. The number of missing observations were: maternal pregnancy wantedness = 28; perceived paternal pregnancy wantedness = 175; perception of couple pregnancy discordance = 184; maternal education = 9; assets index, maternal literacy and maternal employment were missing one observation each; maternal age = 11; religion = 2; MUAC = 26; anemia = 7; infection = 6; None were missing from the parity or vitamin supplementation group

The total sample size for *postnatal depressive symptoms* analysis was 31,422. The number of missing observations were: maternal pregnancy wantedness = 71; perceived paternal pregnancy wantedness = 286; perception of couple pregnancy discordance = 296; maternal education = 34; assets index = 25; maternal age = 17; parity, maternal literacy, maternal employment, and religion were missing 25; MUAC = 168; anemia = 131; infection = 126; None were missing from the vitamin supplementation group or child sex

Table 2 Adjusted risk ratios of maternal wantedness of pregnancy and demographic as risk factors for maternal depressive symptoms

	Maternal Depressive Symptoms	
	Prenatal RR [95% CI] N = 14,554	Postnatal RR [95% CI] N = 31,178
Maternal wantedness of pregnancy		
Wanted now	Reference	Reference
Mistimed	1.26* [1.11, 1.43]	1.05 [0.98, 1.13]
Not wanted	1.60* [1.37, 1.87]	1.32* [1.21, 1.44]
Maternal education		
None	1.50* [1.05, 2.15]	1.29* [1.07, 1.54]
1–9	1.45* [1.07, 1.98]	1.29* [1.11, 1.50]
≥ 10	Reference	Reference
Living standard index		
1st quartile (poor)	1.19 [1.00, 1.43]	1.15* [1.04, 1.27]
2nd	1.13 [0.95, 1.33]	1.08 [0.98, 1.19]
3rd	1.03 [0.88, 1.22]	1.04 [0.95, 1.14]
4th quartile (rich)	Reference	Reference
Maternal age (yrs)		
≤ 19	Reference	Reference
20–29	0.94 [0.80, 1.11]	1.09* [1.02, 1.20]
≥ 30	1.38* [1.12, 1.70]	1.44* [1.29, 1.61]
Previous births		
Zero	Reference	Reference
≥ 1	1.00 [0.85, 1.18]	1.03 [0.95, 1.12]
Maternal literacy		
Yes	Reference	Reference
No	1.39* [1.15, 1.67]	1.13* [1.02, 1.25]
Religion		
Muslim	1.01 [0.81, 1.25]	1.09 [0.95, 1.25]
Non-Muslim	Reference	Reference
Prenatal mid-upper arm circumference (cm)		
< 21.5	1.00 [0.89, 1.13]	1.06 [0.99, 1.13]
≥ 21.5	Reference	Reference
Anemia		
Yes	2.08* [1.85, 2.33]	1.49* [1.40, 1.58]
No	Reference	Reference
Vitamin Supplementation		
Vitamin A	1.11 [0.90, 1.37]	1.00 [0.86, 1.16]
Beta-Carotene	0.97 [0.79, 1.18]	1.02 [0.89, 1.18]
Placebo	Reference	Reference
Sex of resulting birth		
Male	–	1.01 [0.96, 1.07]
Female	–	Reference

*indicates P < 0.05

Analyses during pregnancy include only women interviewed between at or after 23 weeks or before 37 weeks of gestation. Analyses at six months postpartum are restricted to mothers who had singleton births. All models are adjusted for geographic sector

Table 3 Adjusted risk ratios of maternal perception of wantedness as risk factors for maternal depressive symptoms

	Maternal depressive symptoms	
	Prenatal RR [95% CI]	Postnatal RR [95% CI]
Paternal wantedness of pregnancy (n = 14,399; n = 30,964)		
Wanted now	Reference	Reference
Mistimed	1.10 [0.96, 1.26]	0.99 [0.92, 1.07]
Not wanted	1.42 [1.22, 1.65]*	1.30 [1.19, 1.41]*
Parental discordance of pregnancy wantedness (n = 14,399; n = 30,954)		
Unwanted by mother/perceived as unwanted by husband	1.34 [1.19, 1.52]*	1.13 [1.06, 1.21]*
Unwanted by mother/perceived as wanted by husband	1.51 [1.29, 1.78]*	1.24 [1.12, 1.37]*
Wanted by mother/perceived as unwanted by husband	1.30 [0.97, 1.74]	1.19 [0.99, 1.44]
Wanted by mother/perceived as wanted by husband	Reference	Reference

Analyses were conducted in the third trimester and at six months postpartum. All analyses were adjusted for maternal education (none, 1–9, ≥10 years); maternal age (≤19, 20–29, ≥ 30 years); parity (≥1, none); maternal literacy (no, yes); maternal employment (no, yes); religion (Muslim, non-Muslim); maternal mid-upper arm circumference in the first trimester (< 21.5, ≥21.5), anemia in first trimester (yes/no), vitamin supplementation group (vitamin A, beta-carotene, placebo) and geographic sector
Analyses for postnatal depressive symptoms were additionally adjusted for the sex of the child
In this table the "does not want" combines stating those who answered they did want the pregnancy and those who answered not wanting the pregnancy at this time
*indicates $P < 0.05$

symptoms. Religion, mid-upper arm circumference and child sex were not associated with depressive symptoms in any models (Table 2).

Discussion

Our results suggest pregnancy intentions, especially unwanted pregnancies, are related to maternal depressive symptoms during and after the pregnancy among impoverished rural Bangladeshi women. The likelihood of maternal prenatal depressive symptoms was 60 and 26% higher among women reporting unwanted or mistimed pregnancies, respectively, after adjustment. During the postpartum period, having an unwanted pregnancy was associated with 32% higher risk of maternal depressive symptoms. Mothers' perception that the pregnancy was unwanted by their husbands was also associated with a higher risk of prenatal and postnatal depressive symptoms. Finally, maternal perception of discordance between her own and her husband's pregnancy intentions conferred a higher risk especially of prenatal depressive symptoms, with over a 50% higher estimated risk occurring when the mother did not want the pregnancy but perceived her husband did want it. This elevated risk remained at 6 months postpartum, but was attenuated.

Our results are consistent with existing literature for South Asia. In Pakistan, women with higher levels of depressive symptoms between 20 and 26 weeks of pregnancy were also more likely to report unwanted pregnancies [17]. In an Indian study, unplanned pregnancy was associated with depression in women at 6–8 weeks postpartum [22]. A meta-analysis, including five

studies from lower- and middle-income countries, estimated 1.6 to 8.8 greater odds of maternal depressive symptoms associated with unwanted or unintended pregnancy [9]. In Bangladesh fathers' intentions appear to have more influence on a birth occurring than mothers' intentions [23]. Given these studies, it is possible that lack of control of fertility decisions in this context may contribute to women's depressive symptoms associated with unwanted pregnancy.

We found pregnancies unwanted by the husband, as reported by the mother, were associated with subsequent maternal depressive symptoms, a finding consistent with studies conducted in the United States and Japan [24–26]. As poor quality spousal relationships and interpersonal violence are linked to depression in Bangladeshi women, it is possible that a husband not wanting a pregnancy may reflect less family involvement or a poor quality relationship with the mother and child [27]. We found that the scenario in which mothers reported not wanting the pregnancy but perceived their husbands wanted it was the kind of pregnancy discordance most highly associated with the risk of maternal prenatal depressive symptoms. It is possible that this reporting pattern, i.e. the mother's perception that she did not want the pregnancy, but her husband did, may in some cases reflect sexual violence in which women are being forced to have sex in the context of their marital relationships.

We found an increased risk of prenatal and postnatal depressive symptoms for both discordant scenarios as well as for when the mother perceived that the child was unwanted by both parents, in comparison to when she perceived the pregnancy was desired by both husband and wife. To our knowledge only one study has examined this relation. In this US study of marital status and postpartum depressive symptoms, disagreement about pregnancy was significantly related to maternal depressive symptoms [28]. Perceived discordant pregnancy intentions may reflect conflict in the relationship or poorer relationship quality. Research from Bangladesh on pregnancy-intention discordance suggests fathers' desires may carry more weight; women have a higher likelihood of a birth if the father desires the pregnancy and the mother does not but a lower likelihood of a birth if the mother, but not the father, desires the pregnancy [23]. Thus, it is possible that pregnancy-intention discordance may partially reflect circumstances in which woman's desires are unfulfilled. When mothers did not want the pregnancy and perceived their husbands as not wanting the pregnancy may reflect circumstances in which the couple agreed that their condition was not ideal for having a child, either because of economic concerns or because they already had the number of children they desired.

The relation between unintended pregnancy and depressive symptoms can be viewed through a stressful life event lens [29]. Pregnancy and childbirth have been regarded as stressful life events and unintended pregnancy often exacerbates stress; for example, because of disruption of other life plans, being unprepared for parenthood, or lack of support [30]. Gender-based violence is pervasive in Bangladesh; over half of ever-married women age 15–49 report having experienced a form of physical or sexual violence from their husbands [31]. Of these women, 18% reporting his physically forcing her to have sex at some point, with 11% of those saying this occurred often or sometimes [31]. Spousal violence has been linked to suicidal ideation in Bangladesh and to poor mental health outcomes in India [32, 33]. Although we lacked data to examine the role of interpersonal violence, it is possible that sexual assault is a pathway to unintended pregnancy and is a root cause of the depressive symptoms we observed.

Maternal depressive symptoms and pregnancy intentions have been virtually unexplored among rural socio-economically disadvantaged women in developing countries, where unintended pregnancies are common and views toward childbearing and its cultural meaning may be different than in industrialized settings. The opportunity to follow a large cohort prior to pregnancy is rare in developing countries, with prospective data on pregnancy intentions gathered during the first trimester of pregnancy. Retrospective data on pregnancy intentions is thought to underestimate unwanted pregnancies. We also had data on perceived paternal pregnancy intentions, a topic with almost no published literature.

The fact that mothers reported on their husbands' pregnancy intentions is a limitation. However, mother's perception of her husband's attitude and perception of pregnancy-discordance between them may be, nevertheless particularly relevant to her mental health irrespective of his actual view. Another limitation was that there was no validated depression scale in Bangladesh at the time of our study, such that we used items drawn from several validated scales and suicide-related questions. As a result, we developed our own depressive symptom scales. The prenatal depressive symptom scale showed relatively low reliability based on Cronbach's alpha. This low alpha value may have been due to having relatively few items in these scales or may reflect poor interrelatedness of these items. The generalizability of our study is limited to women who are married, carried their baby throughout pregnancy, and had singleton births.

Conclusions

In summary, we found that maternal and paternal unwanted pregnancy, maternal report of mistimed pregnancy, and maternal report of couple pregnancy-intention discordance were risk factors for maternal depressive symptoms. Given that these symptoms may have important adverse consequences for mothers and children, knowledge that unwanted pregnancy is associated with an increased risk of depressive symptoms could be used to help identify women at risk. Especially in developing-country settings like rural Bangladesh where there is little funding and infrastructure for mental health, prevention efforts may take into account initiatives to prevent unwanted pregnancies and/or integrate family planning and mental health services. Future research is needed to understand the factors that determine whether pregnancies are unwanted or mistimed. Our results highlight an unmet need in Bangladesh, and likely other similar settings, for family planning services to target both wife and husband when offering pregnancy counseling to newly married couples in order to avoid unwanted pregnancies.

Acknowledgements
The authors wish to acknowledge Ellen Piwoz (The Bill & Melinda Gates Foundation), Maithilee Mitra and Allan Massie (Johns Hopkins University), and Richard Green and Margaret Neuse (US Agency for International Development).

Sources of funding
This work was supported by the National Institutes of Health, National Institute of Child Health and Development (NICHD) [1 RO3 HD069731-01A1]; the Bill and Melinda Gates Foundation, Seattle, WA (GH614, Global Control of Micronutrient Deficiency); the Office of Health, Infectious Diseases and Nutrition, US Agency for International Development (USAID, Micronutrients for Health Cooperative Agreement HRN-A-00-97-00015-00 and Global Research Activity GHS-A-00-03-00019-00), Washington DC, with additional support from the USAID Mission, Dhaka, Bangladesh; the Ministry of Health and Family Welfare, Government of Bangladesh, Dhaka; and the Sight and Life Global Nutrition Research Institute, Baltimore, Maryland.
The funders had no role in the design of the study and collection, analysis, and interpretation of data and in writing the manuscript.

Authors' contributions

PJS wrote the paper and conducted the statistical analyses; DMS edited the paper and contributed to the conceptualization of the study and interpretation of results; SM developed the assessment protocol and supervised implementation; AAS refined assessment protocol, trained field teams and implemented the study; MR supervised the epidemiological study, directed field investigation, and edited the manuscript; LW helped with data management and contributed to data analysis; HA refined assessment protocols, maintained study quality control, and assisted in study implementation; BU contributed to study implementation and training of field teams; AL was the project scientist of the parent trial, coordinated field operations, and edited the manuscript; RDWK contributed to study design and implementation of the study; KW was the PI of the parent trial, conceptualized study, and contributed to manuscript preparation; PC conceptualized the study, helped with procurement of funding and data interpretation and edited the manuscript. All authors read and approved the final manuscript.

Consent to participate

The informed consent process included, when so desired by the subjects, husbands, in-laws and sometimes community members. Individual consent was sought from the participating women and documented. Married women under 18 years of age who are living as a consensual couple starting to raise a family are formally considered to be emancipated minors. Their consent is considered acceptable without requiring parental consent, a facet of the protocol that was reviewed and approved by the IRB at Johns Hopkins University and the Bangladesh Medical Research Council.

Competing interests

The authors declare no competing interests.

Author details

[1]Center for Human Nutrition, Department of International Health, Johns Hopkins Bloomberg School of Public Health, 615 North Wolfe St., Room E2519, Baltimore, MD 21205-2179, USA. [2]Department of Population, Family and Reproductive Health, Johns Hopkins Bloomberg School of Public Health, Baltimore, MD 21205-2179, USA. [3]The JiVitA Project, Johns Hopkins University in Bangladesh, Gaibandha, Bangladesh.

References

1. Klima CS. Unintended pregnancy. Consequences and solutions for a worldwide problem. J Nurse Midwifery. 1998;43(6):483–91.
2. Singh S, Sedgh G, Hussain R. Unintended pregnancy: worldwide levels, trends, and outcomes. Stud Fam Plan. 2010;41(4):241–50.
3. Santelli J, Rochat R, Hatfield-Timajchy K, Gilbert BC, Curtis K, Cabral R, Hirsch JS, Schieve L. The measurement and meaning of unintended pregnancy. Perspect Sex Reprod Health. 2003;35(2):94–101.
4. Phillips CJ. Economics of family planning and birth control. Expert Rev Pharmacoecon Outcomes Res. 2002;2(1):23–8.
5. Ortayli N, Malarcher S. Equity analysis: identifying who benefits from family planning programs. Stud Fam Plan. 2010;41(2):101–8.
6. Demographic Health Surveys-Bangladesh. Final Report 2007. Calverton, Maryland: National Institute of Population Research and Training (NIPORT) Dhaka, Bangladesh, Mitra and Associates, Dhaka, Bangladesh and Macro International; 2007.
7. Gipson JD, Koenig MA, Hindin MJ. The effects of unintended pregnancy on infant, child, and parental health: a review of the literature. Stud Fam Plan. 2008;39(1):18–38.
8. Lancaster CA, Gold KJ, Flynn HA, Yoo H, Marcus SM, Davis MM. Risk factors for depressive symptoms during pregnancy: a systematic review. Am J Obstet Gynecol. 2010;202(1):5–14.
9. Fisher J, Cabral de Mello M, Patel V, Rahman A, Tran T, Holton S, Holmes W. Prevalence and determinants of common perinatal mental disorders in women in low- and lower-middle-income countries: a systematic review. Bull World Health Organ. 2012;90(2):139G–49G.
10. Gausia K, Fisher C, Ali M, Oosthuizen J. Antenatal depression and suicidal ideation among rural Bangladeshi women: a community-based study. Arch Womens Ment Health. 2009;12(5):351–8.
11. Gausia K, Fisher C, Ali M, Oosthuizen J. Magnitude and contributory factors of postnatal depression: a community-based cohort study from a rural subdistrict of Bangladesh. Psychol Med. 2009;39(6):999–1007.
12. van den Akker O. Reprod Health Psychology. West Sussex, UK: Wiley-Blackwell; 2012.
13. UNICEF. The state of the world's children 2008: Child survival, vol. 8. New York, NY: UNICEF; 2007.
14. Malhotra A, Vanneman R, Kishor S. Fertility, dimensions of patriarchy, and development in India. Popul Dev Rev. 1995;21(2):281–305.
15. West KP Jr, Christian P, Labrique AB, Rashid M, Shamim AA, Klemm RD, Massie AB, Mehra S, Schulze KJ, Ali H, et al. Effects of vitamin a or beta carotene supplementation on pregnancy-related mortality and infant mortality in rural Bangladesh: a cluster randomized trial. JAMA. 2011;305(19):1986–95.
16. Labrique AB, Christian P, Klemm RD, Rashid M, Shamim AA, Massie A, Schulze K, Hackman A, West KP Jr. A cluster-randomized, placebo-controlled, maternal vitamin a or beta-carotene supplementation trial in Bangladesh: design and methods. Trials. 2011;12:102.
17. Karmaliani R, Asad N, Bann CM, Moss N, McClure EM, Pasha O, Wright LL, Goldenberg RL. Prevalence of anxiety, depression and associated factors among pregnant women of Hyderabad, Pakistan. Int J Soc Psychiatry. 2009;55(5):414–24.
18. Kroenke K, Spitzer RL, Williams JB. The PHQ-9: validity of a brief depression severity measure. J Gen Intern Med. 2001;16(9):606–13.
19. Radloff LS. The CES-D scale: a self-report depression scale for research in the general population. Appl Psychol Meas. 1977;1:385–401.
20. World Health Organization. Reproductive health and research. Pregnancy, childbirth, postpartum, and newborn care: a guide for essential practice. Geneva. Switzerland: World Health Organization; 2003.
21. Gunnsteinsson S, Labrique AB, West KP, Christian P, Sucheta M, Shamim AA, Rashid M, Katz J, Klemm R. Constructing indices of rural living standards in Northwest Bangladesh. J Health Popul Nutr. 2010;28:509–19.
22. Patel V, Rodrigues M, DeSouza N. Gender, poverty, and postnatal depression: a study of mothers in Goa, India. Am J Psychiatry. 2002;159(1):43–7.
23. Razzaque A. Preference for children and subsequent fertility in Matlab: does wife-husband agreement matter? J Biosoc Sci. 1999;31(1):17–28.
24. Bronte-Tinkew J. Male pregnancy intendedness and children's mental proficiency and attachment security during toddlerhood. J Marriage Fam. 2009;71:1001–25.
25. Kitamura T, Shima S, Sugawara M, Toda MA. Psychological and social correlates of the onset of affective disorders among pregnant women. Psychol Med. 1993;23(4):967–75.
26. Leathers SJ, Kelley MA. Unintended pregnancy and depressive symptoms among first-time mothers and fathers. Am J Orthop. 2000;70(4):523–31.
27. Selim N. Cultural dimensions of depression in Bangladesh: a qualitative study in two villages of Matlab. J Health Popul Nutr. 2010;28(1):95–106.
28. Akincigil A, Munch S, Niemczyk KC. Predictors of maternal depression in the first year postpartum: marital status and mediating role of relationship quality. Soc Work Health Care. 2010;49(3):227–44.
29. Dohrenwend BS, Dohrenwend BP. Life stress and illness: formulation of the issues. New York: Prodist; 1981.
30. Geller PA. Pregnancy as a stressful life event. CNS Spectr. 2004;9(3):188–97.
31. National Institute of Population Research and Training (NIPORT), Mitra and Associates, and Macro International. Bangladesh Demographic and Health Survey. Chapter 14 domestic violence. Dhaka, Bangladesh and Calverton. USA: Maryland; 2007. p. 2009.
32. Kumar S, Jeyaseelan L, Suresh S, Ahuja RC. Domestic violence and its mental health correlates in Indian women. Br J Psychiatry. 2005;187:62–7.
33. Naved RT, Akhtar N. Spousal violence against women and suicidal ideation in Bangladesh. Womens Health Issues. 2008;18(6):442–52.

6

Prevalence of meconium stained amniotic fluid and its associated factors among women who gave birth at term in Felege Hiwot comprehensive specialized referral hospital, North West Ethiopia

Dagne Addisu[1]* , Azezu Asres[2], Getnet Gedefaw[3] and Simegnew Asmer[2]

Abstract

Background: Meconium stained amniotic fluid is one of the risk factors to increase the rate of perinatal morbidity and mortality both in developed and developing countries. Due to a multitude of factors associated with socioeconomic and quality of service, the ill effect of meconium stained amniotic fluid is even worse in developing countries. But very little information is known about the situation in Ethiopia, particularly the study area to design appropriate prevention strategies. Hence, this study aimed to determine the prevalence of meconium-stained amniotic fluid and its associated factors among women who gave birth at term in Felege Hiwot Referral Hospital, North West Ethiopia.

Methods: Institutional based cross-sectional study was conducted at Felege Hiwot Referral Hospital from March 02–May 27, 2018. A total of 495 mothers were included in the study. The study participants were selected by systematic random sampling technique. A combination of chart review and interview were used to collect the data. Data entry and analysis were made by using Epi-data version 3.1 and SPSS versions 23 respectively. Both descriptive & analytical statistics were computed. Statistical significance was considered at $P < 0.05$ and the strength of association was assessed by using adjusted odds ratio.

Result: The prevalence of meconium stained amniotic fluid was found to be 17.8%. Women whose age greater than 30 years [AOR =5.63, 95%CI =3.35–9.44], duration of labor greater than 24 h [AOR = 7.1, 95%CI =1.67–29.68], induced labor [AOR = 2.60, 95% CI =1.39–4.87], preeclampsia [AOR = 3.45, 95%CI =1.26–9.37] and obstructed labor [AOR =5.9, 95%CI =1.29–29.68] were found to be associated with meconium stained amniotic fluid.

Conclusions: The prevalence of meconium stained amniotic fluid was similar as compared to the international standard. Preeclampsia, maternal age, obstructed labor, induced labor and longer duration of labor were factors associated with an increased risk for meconium-stained amniotic fluid. Thus, early detection and timely intervention are mandatory to decrease prolonged and obstructed labor.

Keywords: Meconium, Amniotic fluid, Meconium stained amniotic fluid, Meconium aspiration syndrome, Felege Hiwot

* Correspondence: addisudagne7@gmail.com
[1]Department of midwifery, College of medicine and health science, Debre Tabor University, Debre Tabor, Ethiopia
Full list of author information is available at the end of the article

Background information

The occurrence of meconium-stained amniotic fluid (MSAF) during labor has been long considered the predictor of adverse fetal outcomes such as meconium aspiration syndrome and perinatal asphyxia, which leads to perinatal and neonatal morbidity and mortality [1, 2].

Meconium is a germ-free, thick, black-green, odorless material which is first recognized in the fetal intestine around 12 weeks of gestation and stores in the fetal colon throughout gestation [3, 4].

Passage of meconium in the newborn infants is a developmentally programmed incident; normally occurring within the first 24 to 48 h after birth. However, the fetus may pass meconium in the amniotic fluid during pregnancy due to different reasons. Meconium-stained amniotic fluid is uncommon before 37 weeks of gestation and the occurrence of a meconium-stained amniotic fluid increases with increasing gestational age [1, 5].

Meconium stained liquor (MSL) is the passage of meconium by a fetus in utero during the antenatal period or in labour. According to Royal College of Obstetricians and Gynecologists (RCOG) intrapartum care guideline, meconium stained amniotic fluid is classified as significant MSL and non-significant MSL. Non- significant MSL is defined as a thin yellow or greenish tinged fluid; containing non-particulate meconium whereas significant MSL is explained as dark green or black amniotic fluid that is thick and tenacious and consists lumps of meconium [6].

Meconium stained amniotic fluid contains masses of debris, desquamated cells from the intestine and skin, gastrointestinal mucin, lanugo hair, fatty material from the vernix caseosa and intestinal secretions [4].

The exact etiology of meconium stained amniotic fluid is not clear. However, previous studies suggested that obstetric factors such as (prolonged labour, post-term pregnancy, low-birth weight babies, oligohydramnios, intrauterine growth retardation and hypertensive disorders of pregnancy),medical factors (cholestasis of pregnancy and anemia) and socio-demographic and behavioral risk factors (higher maternal age, maternal drug abuse especially tobacco and cocaine use) are the major contributory factors for the passage of meconium into the amniotic fluid [7, 8].

Evidence showed that the incidence of meconium stained liquor is increasing as the gestational age increases. From 7 to 22% of term pregnancy were complicated by meconium stained liquor worldwide [9, 10].

Meconium-stained amniotic fluid has adverse long and short-term fetal outcomes; especially it increased rates of neonatal resuscitation, respiratory distress, lower Apgar score, neonatal nursery admissions, meconium aspiration syndrome, neonatal sepsis and pulmonary disease [2, 11, 12].

Meconium aspiration syndrome occurs all over the world about 5–10.5% of neonates with MSAF; which accounts around 12% of neonatal mortality (as much as 40% case fatality rate for the neonate and around 2% of perinatal mortality). Furthermore, the rates of severe mental retardation and cerebral palsy are significantly greater among infants born with MSAF [13, 14].

Meconium stained amniotic fluid significantly increase the rate of maternal complications such as meconium-laden amniotic fluid embolism, intrapartum chorioamnionitis, Puerperal endometritis, wound infection, increased risk of operative delivery and its complication [12, 15].

The perinatal morbidity and mortality related to MSAF can be decreased if major risk factors are recognized early and closely monitoring of the labor and careful decisions are made about the timing and mode of delivery [7].

Even though the magnitude and associated factors of meconium stained amniotic fluid were well studied in the developed countries, there is a paucity of locally generated evidence on the magnitude and associated factors of MSAF to design appropriate prevention strategies in the study area. Therefore, this study was aimed to determine the prevalence of meconium stained amniotic fluid and its associated factors among women who gave birth at term in Felege Hiwot comprehensive Specialized Referral Hospital.

Methods

Study settings and design

Hospital based cross-sectional study was conducted at felege Hiwot Comprehensive Specialized Referral Hospital Obstetrics and Gynecology department, Obstetrics ward from March 02–May 27, 2018 GC. This hospital is the only specialized hospital in Bahir Dar town and located in the Amhara region, Bahir Dar special zone, Bahir Dar City. It is located approximately 565 kms North West of Addis Ababa.

Felege Hiwot Comprehensive Specialized Referral Hospital is one of the top ten governmental hospitals in Ethiopia. This Hospital is having around 400 beds & 9 operating tables, serving over 7 million people within its catchment area. The labor ward gives services to around 612 deliveries per month. The Department of Obstetrics and Gynecology has a labor ward with seven beds in first stage room, two delivery couches in the second stage room, four beds in the recovery unit and sixty nine beds in the maternity ward along with two operating rooms. The ward is staffed with five obstetrics and gynecology specialists, thirty three midwives, seventeen clinical nurses, thirty five residents of different years (levels) of study and a varying number of interns.

Characteristics of participants

All women who gave birth at term in Felege Hiwot Referral hospital were the source population. This study included all women who gave birth at term throughout the day and night during the data collection period. Those mothers who presented with breech presentation and intrauterine fetal death before the onset of labor were excluded from the study.

Sample size determination

The sample size was determined by taking predictors for MSAF from previous studies and by using Epi info software version 7.2.0.1. After enrolling different significant factors in the previous studies, cord problem was one of the factors which had a maximum number for our sample size [16, 17]. Based on the previous finding, percent of outcome (MSAF) in women with cord problem (exposed group) were 25% and percent of outcome (MSAF) in women without cord problem (unexposed group) were 14.1% [16]. Based on the assumptions of one to one ratio of exposed to unexposed and 95% confidence interval of certainty to have a power of 80%, the sample size was 450. After 10% of non-response rate were added, the final sample size for this study was 495.

Sampling and sampling procedure

Systematic random sampling was applied to identify study participants from postnatal and maternity ward. To get study participants, first the average numbers of women who delivered during the data collection period was estimated based on the previous delivery, which was obtained by referring a two-month delivery registration book/record prior to data collection. Totally 1236 women were delivered in two months; on average 618 women were delivered per month. The data were collected within two-month duration. So as to find the sampling fraction, the total number of women who were delivered in two months (1236) was divided by the total number of sample size (495) and it was approximately 3. The first woman was selected by lottery method then every 3rd woman who gave birth was recruited for the study.

Meconium stained amniotic fluid was defined as the presence of meconium in the amniotic fluid which changes the color of the liquor from clear to various shades of green, yellow or brownish color depending on the degree of meconium stained liquor.

Data collection tools and procedures

Data were collected using a combination of interview and chart review by three BSc midwives who were trained for this purpose. Structured interviewer-administered data collection formats were adopted and modified from different kinds of literature. Questionnaires which guided chart review and interview were structured into four logical sections (socio -demographic characteristics, obstetric related factors; medical history and Behavioral related factors). Data on patient specific socio- demographic, obstetric,

medical and behavioral information were collected through interview of the mother and by reviewing her medical records.

Socio-demographic, obstetric, medical and behavioral variables

Socio-demographic, obstetric, medical and other factors were examined as a potential predictor in this analysis. Socio-demographic factors include age, ethnicity, residency, religion, educational status, marital status and occupation. Obstetric related factors include parity, Rh status, the onset of labor, late-term pregnancy, premature rupture of membrane, prolonged premature rupture of membrane, preeclampsia, oligohydramnios, IUGR, antepartum hemorrhage, cord problem, chorioamnionitis, duration of labor, mode of delivery, antenatal care follow up. Medically related factors include diabetes mellitus, gestational diabetes mellitus, anemia, hypothyroidism, hepatitis virus, chronic hypertension, asthma, jaundice, and cardiac disease. Behavioral factors include Cigarette smoking, Cocaine use, marijuana addict and chat chewing.

Data management and analysis

Data were entered into EPI data version 3.1 then exported to SPSS version 23 for analysis. Descriptive statistics like frequencies and cross tabulations were performed. Multiple logistic regressions were fitted for MSAF and odds ratio (OR) with their 95% confidence interval (95% CI) were calculated to identify associated factors of meconium stained amniotic fluid.

Variables with p-values ≤ 0.2 in bivariate analysis remained in the model as potential confounders for the next level analysis. The Hosmer -Lemeshow goodness-of-fit statistic was used to check if the necessary assumptions for multiple logistic regressions were fulfilled and the model had a p-value > 0.05 which proved the model was good.

Results

Socio-demographic characteristics

A total of four hundred ninety five women were enrolled in the study with a response rate of 100%. The mean age of the study participants was 28.05 years with standard deviation (SD) of ±5.1 years. Nearly two third, 344 (69.5%) of mothers were in the age group of > 30 years and 403 (81.4%) of them were from urban areas (Table 1).

Obstetrics related characteristics

The mean gestational age and duration of labor were 38.95 weeks and 11.45 h with SD of ±1.276 weeks and ± 5.7 h respectively. Half of, 251 (50.7%) mothers were Para I and 421 (85.1%) had spontaneous onset of labor. The majority (96.4%) mothers had a vertex presentation and the rest were face, brow and cord presentation with 2.63%, 0.61%, and 0.4% respectively. 22 (4.4%) of

Table 1 Socio-demographic characteristics of women who gave birth at term in Felege Hiwot Comprehensive Specialized Referral Hospital (n = 495)

Characteristics	Frequency	Percent (%)
Age		
≤ 30 years	344	69.5
> 30 years	151	30.5
Residence		
Urban	403	81.4
Rural	92	18.6
Ethnic group		
Amhara	473	95.6
Others	22	4.4
Religion		
Orthodox	458	92.5
Muslim	27	5.5
Protestant	10	2
Marital status		
Married/union	467	94.3
Others (Unmarried, single &divorced)	28	5.7
Educational status		
Non-formal education	175	35.4
Primary education	73	14.7
Secondary education	51	10.3
Tertiary education	196	39.6
Occupation		
Merchant	119	24
Governmental/private employee	100	20.2
House wife	249	50.3
Others(student, farmer, daily laborer)	27	5.5

Table 2 Obstetric characteristics of women who gave birth at term in Felege Hiwot Comprehensive Specialized Referral Hospital (n = 495)

Characteristics	Frequency	Percent (%)
Parity		
Primipara	251	50.7
Multipara	184	37.2
grand multipara	60	12.1
ANC follow up		
Yes	469	94.7
No	26	5.3
Gestational age		
37–40 weeks (term)	426	86.1
41 weeks (late term)	69	13.9
Rh status		
Positive	430	86.9
Negative	65	13.1
APH		
Yes	20	4
No	475	96
Obstructed labor		
Yes	11	2.2
No	484	97.8
IUGR		
Yes	19	3.8
No	476	96.2
Preeclampsia		
Yes	22	4.4
No	473	95.6
Oligohydramnios		
Yes	11	2.2
No	484	97.8
Onset of labor		
Spontaneous	421	85.1
Induced	74	14.9
Duration of labor		
≤ 24 h	485	98
> 24 h	10	2
Mode of delivery		
Spontaneous vaginal delivery	363	73.3
Cesarean section	120	24.2
Instrumental delivery	12	2.4
PROM		
Yes	63	12.7
No	432	87.3

mothers had preeclampsia and 9 (1.8%) mothers had obstructed labor (Table 2).

Medical and behavioral related characteristics
Concerning medical conditions of mothers, seven (1.4%) mothers had anemia, eight (1.6%) had gestational diabetes mellitus (GDM), four (0.8) had asthma and five (1%) of mothers had Hepatitis B virus. Almost all mothers, four hundred ninety five (100%) didn't use Cocaine, chat, Cigarette smoking and marijuana addict.

Prevalence of meconium stained amniotic fluid
The prevalence of meconium stained amniotic fluid was found to be 88 (17.8%) with [95% CI = 14.3–21.2]. Out of 88 cases delivered with MSAF, 35 (39.77%) were grade 3 MSAF, 42 (47.73%) were grade 2 MSAF and 11 (12.5%) were grade 1 MSAF.

Factors associated with meconium stained amniotic fluid

The association between socio-demographic, obstetrical, medical conditions of women, and MSAF were assessed. In the bivariate analysis; maternal age, marital status, Rh status, duration of labor, gestational age, the onset of labor, IUGR, preeclampsia and obstructed labor became significant at 0.2 level of significance. However, maternal age, the onset of labor, preeclampsia, duration of labor and obstructed labor were remained significantly and independently associated with MSAF in the multivariable analysis.

Mothers whose age greater than 30 years were 5.6 times more likely to develop meconium stained amniotic fluid during labor than those less than 30 years [AOR = 5.6, 95%C1 = 3.35–9.44].

Those women with duration of labor > 24 h had about 7.1 times higher odds of developing MSAF than those having less than 24 h [AOR =7.1, 95%Cl =1.67–29.68].

Women who had induced labor were 2.6 times more likely to develop MSAF as compared to the spontaneous onset of labor [AOR = 2.6, 95% CI =1.39–4.87].

Mothers who had preeclampsia were 3.4 times more likely to develop MSAF during labor as compared to those who didn't have [AOR = 3.4, 95%CI =1.26–9.37].

The chance of developing MSAF in obstructed labor was 5.9 times more likely than those without obstructed labor [AOR = 5.9, 95%CI =1.29–29.68] (Table 3).

Discussion

The prevalence of meconium stained amniotic fluid was 17.8% with [95% CI = 14.3–21.2]. This finding was in line with the finding from Jimma University specialized hospital (15.4%) [15]. This might be due to the similarity in socio-demography, health institution and quality of service they provided.

This finding was also in line with the finding from the Nigerian University Teaching Hospital (20.4%) [18]. This might be due to the similarity in accessibility and quality of services.

However, this finding was higher than the study finding in Southeastern Brazil (11.9%) [19] and Israel (10.9%) [20]. This discrepancy might be due to the difference between the accessibility and the quality of services in study settings. In addition to this, this study was done in a tertiary referral hospital which covers a wide catchment area and most of the patients referred to this hospital were already complicated and might have predisposing factors for MSAF.

On the other hand, this finding was lower than the study findings in IPGMER Hospital, India (30.6%) [21]. The difference could be attributed to the time gap between the studies. An additional explanation could be due to the emphasis is given by the Ethiopian government on maternal and child health services in the last years to improving maternal health services program. In addition to this, low behavioral risk factors for MSAF

Table 3 Bivariate and multivariable association of meconium stained amniotic fluid and independent factors among women who gave birth at term in Felege Hiwot Comprehensive Specialized Referral Hospital

Variables	MSAF		COR(95% CI)	AOR(95% CI)
	Yes	No		
Age				
≤ 30 years	34 (9.9%)	310 (90.1%)	1	1
> 30 years	54 (35.8%)	97 (64.2%)	5.0 (3.12–8.25)	5.6 (3.35–9.44)*
Marital status				
Married	79 (16.9%)	388 (83.1%)	1	1
Others	9 (32.1%)	19 (68.9%)	2.3 (1.015–5.33)	2.4 (0.96–6.18)
Rh status				
Positive	72 (16.7%)	358 (83.3%)	1	1
Negative	16 (24.6%)	49 (75.4%)	1.6 (0.87–3.01)	1.5 (0.73–3.07)
Onset of labor				
Spontaneous	64 (15.2%)	357 (84.8%)	1	1
Induced	24 (32.4%)	50 (67.6%)	2.6 (1.53–4.66)	2.6 (1.39–4.87)*
Duration of labor				
≤ 24 h	83 (17.1%)	402 (82.9%)	1	1
> 24 h	5 (50%)	5 (50%)	4.8 (1.37–17.10)	7.1 (1.67–29.68)*
IUGR				
Yes	7 (36.8%)	12 (63.2%)	2.8 (1.087–7.44)	2.4 (0.775–7.70)
No	81 (17.0%)	395 (83.0%)	1	1
Gestational age				
37-40wks	71 (16.7%)	355 (83.3%)	1	1
41wks	17 (24.6%)	52 (75.4%)	1.6 (0.894–2.99)	1.7 (0.896–3.46)
Preeclampsia				
Yes	9 (40.9%)	13 (59.1%)	3.4 (1.43–8.35)	3.4 (1.26–9.37)*
No	79 (16.7%)	394 (83.3%)	1	1
Obstructed labor				
Yes	6 (54.5%)	5 (45.5%)	5.8 (1.007–14.5)	5.9 (1.29–29.68)*
No	82 (16.9%)	402 (83.1%)	1	1

❖ Others mean (unmarried, windowed and divorce)
❖ * means $P < 0.05$

such as smoking, Cocaine use, and Marijuana addict were not found in this study area.

Age of the women was significantly associated with the development of MSAF. This finding was consistent with study findings in Indira Gandhi Medical College [22]. This could be explained as a woman gets older, she is more likely to have a gradual loss of compliance of the cardiovascular vessels that is mainly associated with aging of uterine blood vessels and arterial stiffness which may result in insufficient placental perfusion and in utero fetal hypoxia. This finally leads to passage of meconium into the amniotic fluid.

This study also indicated that a significant association was noted between induced labor and MSAF. This finding was in agreement with study findings in São Paulo, Southeastern Brazil [19]. This might be related to tetanic uterine contraction (uterine tachysystole) following oxytocin administration, which may result in intrauterine fetal hypoxia secondary to inadequate placental perfusion. When the fetus suffers from hypoxia or asphyxia, increased parasympathetic stimulation by vagus leads to passage of meconium.

In this study, longer duration of labor showed a statistically significant association with meconium-stained amniotic fluid. This finding was consistent with the study findings at SRM Medical College [17]. This could be due to a prolonged stressful environment for the fetus, which may result in increased peristalsis of a fetal gastrointestinal tract and relaxation of anal sphincter then the passage of meconium.

Preeclampsia had a statistically significant association with the development of MSAF. This finding was consistent with study findings in Kasturba Hospital Delhi and Somaiya Medical College Mumbai [23, 24]. The reason might be explained by the possibility of placental insufficiency in preeclampsia that leads to intrauterine fetal hypoxia or intestinal ischemia. This intrauterine hypoxia finally weakens the action of rectal sphincters and leading to the passage of meconium.

In this study, obstructed labor had a statistically significant association with the development of meconium-stained amniotic fluid. The finding was in agreement with the study conducted in the Nigerian University Teaching Hospital [18]. The reason might be due to the possibility of maternal dehydration, maternal distress and shock, which may result in intrauterine fetal hypoxia secondary to insufficient placental perfusion then the passage of meconium into the amniotic fluid.

This study shares the limitations of cross-sectional studies and hence may not be possible to establish a temporal relationship between MSAF and explanatory variables. Besides, as the study was conducted in a single referral hospital, the results might not be representative of other institutions and the community. Another limitation is possible to recall bias while determining the gestational age.

Conclusions

The prevalence of meconium stained amniotic fluid was similar compared to the international standard. Multifaceted factors such as preeclampsia, maternal age greater than 30 years, obstructed labor, induced labor and longer duration of labor were independently associated with an increased risk for meconium-stained amniotic fluid in term pregnancies. Hence, early detection by using a latent follow-up chart and partograph and timely intervention is recommended to decrease prolonged and obstructed labor. We also recommend using induction protocols strictly in a woman who is on induction to prevent uterine tachysystole.

Abbreviations
AOR: Adjusted Odd Ratio; APH: Ante Partum Hemorrhage; CI: Confidence Interval; COR: Crude Odd Ratio; IUGR: Intra-Uterine Growth Retardation; MAS: Meconium Aspiration Syndrome; MSAF: Meconium Stained Amniotic Fluid; MSL: Meconium Stained Liquor; PROM: Premature Rupture of Membrane; SD: Standard Deviation

Acknowledgments
The authors are indebted to the Bahir Dar University College of medicine and health science. Our gratitude also goes to the study participants and data collectors.

Funding
We are grateful to Bahir Dar University College of medicine and health science for their financial support. However, beyond finical support, the funders did not have any role in the design of the study and collection, analysis, and interpretation of data and in writing the manuscript.

Authors' contributions
DA wrote the proposal, gives training on data collection, analyzed the data and drafted the paper. AA, SA, and GG approved the proposal with some revisions, participated in data analysis and manuscript writing. All authors read and approved the final manuscript.

Competing interests
The authors declare that they have no competing interests.

Author details
[1]Department of midwifery, College of medicine and health science, Debre Tabor University, Debre Tabor, Ethiopia. [2]Department of midwifery, College of medicine and health science, Bahir Dar University, Bahir Dar, Ethiopia. [3]Department of midwifery, College of medicine and health science, Wolidia University, Wolidia, Ethiopia.

References
1. Khatun MHA, Arzu J, Haque E, Kamal M, Al Mamun MA, Khan MFH, et al. Fetal outcome in deliveries with meconium stained liquor. Bangladesh J Child Health. 2009;33(2):41–5.
2. Qadir S, Jan S, Chachoo JA, Parveen S. Perinatal and neonatal outcome in meconium stained amniotic fluid. Int J Reprod Contracept Obstet Gynecol. 2017;5(5):1400–5.
3. Jain PG, Sharma R, Bhargava M. Perinatal outcome of meconium stained liquor in pre-term, term and post-term pregnancy. Indian J Obstet Gynecol Res. 2017;4(2):146–50.
4. Parvin I, Khanam N, Alam A. Management Practices in Cases with Meconium Stained Amniotic Fluid (MSAF) Babies. 2008;6(12):102–5.
5. Begum N, Mahmood S, Munmun SA, Haque M, Nahar K, Chowdhury S. Perinatal outcome associated with meconium stained amniotic fluid in pregnancy. Journal of Paediatric Surgeons of Bangladesh. 2015;4(2):44–9.
6. Sarah M. In: SP SM, et al., editors. managments of meconium stained liquor. Cyprus: RCOG; 2016. p. 1–10.

7. Kumari R, Srichand P, Devrajani BR, Shah SZA, Devrajani T, Bibi I, et al. Foetal outcome in patients with meconium stained liquor. JPMA. 2012;62(474):474–6.

8. DR AK, Mahapatro A. obstetrics outcome at term in meconium stained amniotic fluid -A retrospective delivery. Inte J pharm bio sci. 2014;5(2):866–71.

9. Siriwachirachai T, Sangkomkamhang US, Lumbiganon P, Laopaiboon M. Antibiotics for meconium-stained amniotic fluid in labour for preventing maternal and neonatal infections. Cochrane Libr. 2014;6(11):CD007772.

10. Soni A, Vaishnav GD, Gohil J. Meconium stained amniotic fluid, its Significance and Obstetric Outcome. Med Sci. 2015;4(1):1861–68.

11. Shaikh EM, Mehmood S, Shaikh MA. Neonatal outcome in meconium stained amniotic fluid-one year experience. JPMA. 2010;60(9):711–4.

12. Desai D, Maitra N, Patel P. Fetal heart rate patterns in patients with thick meconium staining of amniotic fluid and its association with perinatal outcome. Int J Reprod Contracept Obstet Gynecol. 2017;6(3):1030–5.

13. Rajput U, Jain A. Impact of meconium stained amniotic fluid on early neonatal outcome. J Evol Med Dent Sci. 2013;2(45):8788–94.

14. Sharma U, Garg S, Tiwari K, Hans PS, Kumar B. Perinatal outcome in meconium stained amniotic fluid. J Evol Med Dent Sci. 2015;48:8319–27.

15. Sori D, Belete A, Wolde M. Meconium stained amniotic fluid: factors affecting maternal and perinatal outcomes at Jimma University specialized teaching hospital, south West Ethiopia. Gynecol Obstet (Sunnyvale). 2016;6(394):2161–0932.1000394.

16. Gupta V, Bhatia B, Mishra O. Meconium stained amniotic fluid: antenatal, intrapartum and neonatal attributes. Indian pediatrics. 1996;33:293–8.

17. Sundaram R, Murugesan A. Risk factors for meconium stained amniotic fluid and its implications. Int J Reprod Contracept Obstet Gynecol. 2017;5(8):2503–6.

18. David A, Njokanma O, Iroha E. Incidence of and factors associated with meconium staining of the amniotic fluid in a Nigerian University teaching hospital. J Obstet Gynaecol. 2006;26(6):518–20.

19. Osava R, Silva F, Oliveira S, Tuesta E, Amaral M. Meconium-stained amniotic fluid and maternal and neonatal factors associated. Revista de saude publica. 2012;46(6):1023–9.

20. Hiersch L, Krispin E, Aviram A, Wiznitzer A, Yogev Y, Ashwal E. Effect of meconium-stained amniotic fluid on perinatal complications in low-risk pregnancies at term. Am J Perinatol. 2016;33(04):378–84.

21. Chakraborty A, Mitra P, Seth S, Das A, Basak S, Paul J. Study on risk factors of meconium stained amniotic fluid and comparison of pregnancy outcome in clear and meconium stained amniotic fluid in a tertiary hospital, Kolkata. India Int J Biol Med Res. 2013;4(2):3084–7.

22. Naveen S, Kumar SV, Ritu S, Kushia P. Predictors of meconium stained amniotic fluid: a possible strategy to reduce neonatal morbidity and mortality. J Obstet Gynecol India. 2006;56(6):514–7.

23. Gupta P, Kaushik A, Chandra S, Mishra C. Amniotic fluid characteristics and their co-relates among females delivering in a tertiary care Hospital: a cross-sectional study. Indian J Prev Soc Med. 2014;45(1-2):106.

24. Bhatia P, Ela N. Fetal and neonatal outcome of babies in meconium stained amniotic fluid and meconium aspiration syndrome. J Obstet Gynecol India. 2007;57(6):501–4.

7

Increasing trend of exclusive breastfeeding over 12 years period (2002–2014) among women in Moshi, Tanzania

Ola Jahanpour[1*], Sia E. Msuya[1,2,3], Jim Todd[1,4], Babill Stray-Pedersen[5,6] and Melina Mgongo[1,3,6]

Abstract

Background: The World Health Organization has recommended that all infants under 6 months should be exclusively breastfed. An understanding of the trend of exclusive breastfeeding (EBF) over years and over smaller geographical areas is crucial to monitor the progress made in improving the proportions of infants' EBF.

Methods: Data on infant feeding practices on 2315 mother-infant pairs from 2002 to 2014 were extracted from cohorts of women who delivered in the Moshi Municipality. Descriptive statistics were used to establish the trend of EBF up to 1, 3 and 6 months across waves (2002/2004 = wave I, 2005/2012 = wave II and 2013/2014 = wave III), to relate EBF up to 6 months to wealth quintiles and to HIV status of mothers.

Results: The number of mothers in waves I, II and III were 1656 (71.5%), 256 (11.1%) and 403(17.4%) respectively. The percentages of EBF up to 6 months increased from 5.5, 13.7 to 16.9% from wave I to III. Overall, across the waves, the proportion of EBF up to 6 months among the mothers in the low wealth quintile was 4, 9 and 42%, and 7, 26 and 15% for the ones in the highest wealth quintile. The proportion of EBF up to 6 months has been increasing among HIV positive mothers while fluctuating among their counterparts across the waves.

Conclusion: The proportion of EBF up to 6 months has been increasing in the Moshi municipality but is below the national average. While establishing trends of EBF at the national level is commendable, research to establish trends over smaller geographical areas is needed to provide a true picture that may otherwise be masked.

Keywords: Trend, Exclusive breastfeeding, Regional level, Wealth quintile, HIV status, Tanzania

Introduction

There is ever growing evidence of the benefits of breastfeeding (BF) to the child and the mother [1]. The short term benefits to the child include the prevention of infections, such as acute respiratory infection and diarrhoea [1], which are among the leading causes of child mortality in low and middle income countries. Breastfeeding also provides long term benefits including the potential to prevent Type II diabetes and obesity [2]. Among all interventions that can reduce under-five mortality from preventable causes, optimal breastfeeding was found to lead, with a potential to prevent up to 13%

of this mortality [3]. The benefit was found to increase in proportion to the duration of breastfeeding.

The World Health Organization (WHO) recommends all children are exclusively breastfed (EBF). It has been recommended to have a target of 90% of infants being exclusively breastfed for the first six months of life [1, 3]. However, to date, only 43% are exclusively breastfed globally and no country has reached the target proportion of 90%, with Rwanda having the highest proportion (85%) of EBF [1]. It is important to be able to monitor the proportion of EBF and its changes over time towards meeting the set target.

The majority of countries, Tanzania included, have reported trends of EBF at the national level, but not at regional (smaller geographical) levels. However, national estimates may mask the true picture in the regions. With some studies reporting regional variability of EBF [4, 5],

* Correspondence: ola.jahanpour@gmail.com
[1]Institute of Public Health, Department of Epidemiology and Biostatistics, Kilimanjaro Christian Medical University College (KCMUCo), P.O. Box 2240, Moshi, Tanzania

the need to monitor the trend of EBF at the regional level cannot be overstated. The proportion of EBF is determined by socio-economic and demographic factors, which may vary considerably from one region to another. This study was carried out to determine the trend of EBF in the Moshi municipality in northern Tanzania from 2002 to 2014. The findings will give a picture of EBF at the regional level and of different sub-groups of mothers in the community. This understanding is crucial to enable health personnel at the national, regional, district and health facility level to develop interventions as per their scope.

Methods
Data source
The data for this study came from three open cohorts of women attending the Majengo and Pasua health centres in Moshi Municipality, Kilimanjaro region Tanzania [6–8]. To refer to these three distinct groups of women recruited in the parent study, the term "wave" will be used. Wave I for those who delivered between 2002 and 2004, wave II between 2005 and 2012 and wave III between 2013 and 2014, irrespective of when they were recruited into the cohort. Women were recruited between 2002 and 2004 and again in 2012–2014, primarily to evaluate the prevalence of HIV and sexually transmitted infections (STI) among pregnant women in the third trimester. Between 2005 and 2011, only HIV positive women were recruited. As some HIV negative women recruited up to 2004 may have delivered in 2005, their feeding practices are reported as wave II results. The same data collection and follow-up methods were used across all waves.

The women were followed up until delivery, during puerperium and afterwards, as long as they stayed in the cohort. After being seen at delivery, each mother-infant pair was seen at the centres at 1, 3 and 6 months and continued with visits until the child was 60 months old. Trained nurses carried out face to face interviews using questionnaires with structured and non-structured questions. During the visits, information on infant and young feeding practices, family planning use and growth monitoring data for children was collected. The information on infant and young child feeding that was collected included initiation of breastfeeding, colostrum giving, the practice of EBF, and complementary feeding. This paper analyses the data on EBF practices to give the trends of EBF. The practice of EBF was determined by asking at each visit whether the mother had fed her child anything other than breast milk since birth or the last clinic visit and, what she had introduced and how old the child was at the time. This information was then used to determine the age at which EBF ceased.

Study area
Data was from cohorts established in the Moshi Municipality in the Kilimanjaro region. In 2015–16, Kilimanjaro had a population of 1,560,354 with 285,263 being women of reproductive age (15–49 years) [9]. A large majority of pregnant women (98.3%) in Kilimanjaro region attend antenatal clinic care (ANC) at least once during their pregnancy and 87.6% have health facility deliveries [9]. This is very similar to the estimated national average for urban residents who attend ANC at least once of 98.4 and 81.6% who have health facility delivery [9].

Study design and population
Using the extracted data, a longitudinal study was carried out by following-up a mother and her infant from delivery up to when the infant was six months old. Any mother-infant pair with no information on initiation of breastfeeding or when other foods were introduced was excluded from the study. This is because the dependent variable was defined using these two variables.

Sample size
All eligible mothers in the cohort were included in this proposed study. Data from Demographic and Health Survey (DHS) reports over the study period (2002–2014) have shown an increase of 9% in the proportion of EBF among infants of 0–6 months at the national level from 41% in 2004/5 to 50% in 2014 [9]. Assuming a similar proportion in the studied area, and using a STATA (Stata Corporation, College Station, TX, USA) version 13 command;

Power two proportions p1 p2, n1() n2 () (p1 = 0.41, p2 = 0.5, n1 = 1656, n2 = 403).

With 1656 women in wave I, and 403 in wave III, the study has 90% power to show a difference of 9% in the proportion of women who exclusively breastfed infants under 6 months between the two groups, as significant at the 5% level.

Data analysis
Data was analysed using STATA Corporation, College Station, TX, USA version 13. Exclusive breastfeeding was categorized based on the World Health Organization (WHO) definition of EBF "The receipt of only breast milk (either directly from the breast or expressed); only oral rehydration solution, drops, and syrups (vitamins, minerals, or medicines) are permitted for the first 6 months of life" [10]. Infants who were exclusively breastfed up to 30 days or more were classified as exclusively breastfed up to 1 month. Infants who were exclusively breastfed up to 90 days or more, were classified as exclusively breastfed up to 3 months. And those who were exclusively breastfed up to 180 days were classified as exclusively breastfed up to 6 months. Breastfeeding

practices were analysed using the Chi-Square test to evaluate if there was a statistical difference in the proportion of those exclusively breastfed in each duration category (1, 3 and 6 months) across the waves. A Chi-square test for a linear trend in changes in exclusive breastfeeding up to 6 months across the three waves was carried out. All *p value* were derived from two-sided tests and a *p value* of less than 0.05 was considered statistically significant. Trends for wave I, wave II and wave III were established and compared. Also, separate proportions were made for HIV positive mothers and those that were negative, and for the ones in the highest and lowest wealth quintiles.

Wealth quintile was established using principle component analysis (PCA) [11]. The variables that were selected for Socioeconomic Status(SES) estimation were; employment status, level of education, travelling habits, income per month, house ownership, type of walls in a household, sanitation facility and source of water supply. The variables that had missing data was replaced by the mean. A total of 19 parameters were used to estimate the wealth quintile of the mothers. Wealth quintile was then categorized into 5 equal categories.

Ethical considerations

Ethical clearance certificate number 2020 was obtained from the College Research and Ethical Review Committee (CRERC) of Kilimanjaro Christian Medical University College. Permission to use the dataset was provided by the supervisor of the cohort. Mothers provided informed written consent and assented for their children to take part in the cohort. Mothers were informed that their information may be used for research purposes. Confidentiality and anonymity has been maintained whereby this study only accessed and used coded data without individual identifiers.

Results

Participants' flow

Information was available for 2802 mother-infant pairs. Out of these, 410 (14.6%) were excluded because the

mother-infant pair was not followed up to the age of six months and 77 (2.7%) missed information on when food or fluid were introduced. A total of 2315 (82.6%) mother-infant pairs met the inclusion criteria (Fig. 1).

A description of baseline characteristics of mothers and infants in the cohort

The median age of the mothers was 25 (Interquartile range (IQR) 21, 29) years. Most of the mothers (73.3%; $n = 1676$) had primary level education and 67.6% ($n = 1376$) had a parity of 2–4 children. The majority of women were HIV-negative $n = 1971$ (87.1%). A large proportion of the mothers $n = 1656$ (71.5%) came from wave I, while $n = 256$ (11.1%) were from wave II and $n = 403$ (17.4%) from wave III. The waves were different in the following characteristics; age of the mother, HIV status, parity and education of the mother (p *value* < 0.05), while similar in marital status and mode of delivery (p *value* > 0.05), (Table 1).

The majority (91.2%; $n = 2112$) were seen by the recruiter for only one pregnancy. There was almost an equal proportion of male (51.1%) and female (48.9%) infants. There were 26 (1.1%) twins, 32 (1.4%) preterm, and 646 (27.9%) born with a weight less than 2500 g i.e. low birth weight, (not shown).

Trend of exclusive breastfeeding over years

Overall, the proportion of infants who were exclusively breastfed up to 6 months increased from 5.5% in wave I to 13.7% in wave II to 16.9% in wave III. There was a statistically significant linear trend of EBF between the three waves with a χ2 = 63.4 and p *value* < 0.001, (Fig. 2).

A further analysis showed that the proportion of infants who were exclusively breastfed in all waves was higher at 1 month and continued to drop as an infant aged. The proportion of EBF at 1 month was the highest in wave II (94.9%). For EBF up to 3 months, the proportion ranged from 42 to 55.5% being again highest in wave II. The proportion of EBF up to 6 months was below 20% in all waves. There was a statistically

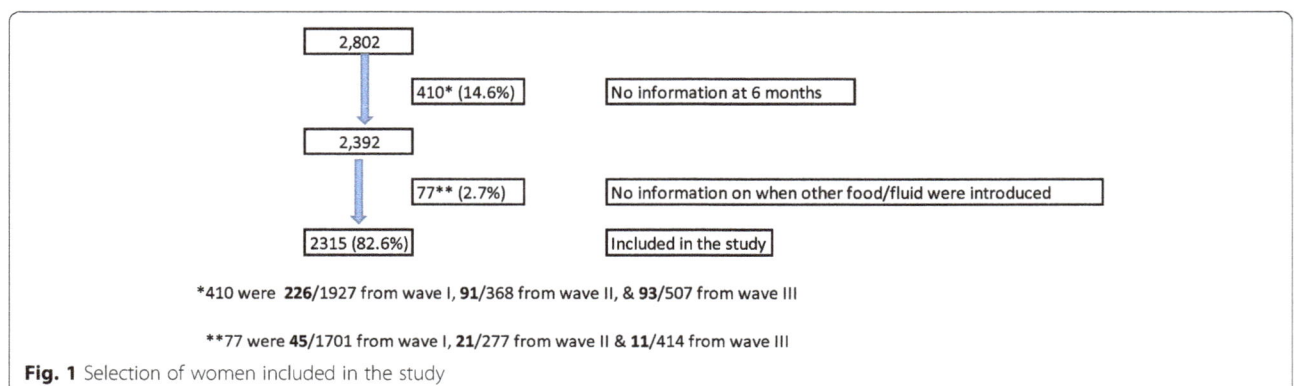

Fig. 1 Selection of women included in the study

Table 1 Baseline characteristics of mothers in the Moshi Municipality Cohort (N = 2315)

Characteristics	Total (N = 2315) n (%)	2002/4 (n = 1656, 71.5%) n (%)	2005/12 (n = 256, 11.1%) n (%)	2013/14 (n = 403, 17.4%) n (%)	χ2	P value
Age of the mother(years) (n = 2286)					97.971	< 0.001
≤ 24	1132 (49.5)	905 (55.1)	54 (22.4)	173 (43.0)		
> 24	1154 (50.5)	738 (44.9)	187 (77.6)	229 (57.0)		
HIV status (n = 2263)					668.41	< 0.001
Negative	1971 (87.1)	1535 (94.9)	87 (35.5)	349 (87.0)		
Positive	292 (12.9)	82 (5.1)	158 (64.5)	52 (13.0)		
Education of the mother (n = 2286)					1226.27	< 0.001
No formal education	87 (3.8)	82 (5.0)	4 (1.7)	1 (0.2)		
Primary education	1676 (73.3)	1419 (86.4)	215 (89.2)	42 (10.4)		
Secondary and higher	523 (22.9)	142 (8.6)	22 (9.1)	359 (89.3)		
Marital status(n = 2292)					4.0477	0.4
Married/cohabiting	2095 (91.4)	1508 (91.5)	228 (93.8)	359 (89.5)		
Single	173 (7.5)	122 (7.4)	13 (5.3)	38 (9.5)		
Once married	24 (1.1)	18 (1.1)	2 (0.8)	4 (1.0)		
Parity (n = 2160)					209.582	< 0.001
Multiparous [2–4]	1460 (67.6)	980 (59.7)	218 (89.7)	262 (94.9)		
Nulliparous	654 (30.3)	628 (38.3)	17 (7.0)	9 (3.3)		
Grand multipara (> 4)	46 (2.1)	33 (2)	8 (3.3)	5 (1.8)		
Mode of delivery (n = 2265)					2.752	0.252
Vaginal delivery	2126 (93.9)	1522 (94.1)	237 (95.2)	367 (92.2)		
Caesarean section	139 (6.1)	96 (5.9)	12 (4.8)	31 (7.8)		

significant association between the different waves and the proportion of exclusive breastfeeding at the different time durations (χ^2 = 13.2 p value = 0.001 up to 1 month, χ2 = 16.5, p value < 0.001 up to 3 months and χ2 = 65.2 p value < 0.001 up to 6 months), (Fig. 2).

Trend of exclusive breastfeeding by wealth quintile
The proportion of EBF among mothers of lowest wealth quintile increased across the waves at each time unit. Looking at the infants who were breastfed up to 6 months, the proportion of EBF among those of lowest wealth quintile increased from 4 to 9% to 42% across the three waves. Except for up to 1 month, there were significant differences in the proportion of EBF across waves among women with the lowest wealth quintile (χ^2 = 2.28 /p value = 0.319 up to 1 month, χ^2 = 7.56 p value = 0.023 up to 3 months and χ^2 = 29.76 p value < 0.001 up to 6 months), (Fig. 3).

Among women in the highest wealth quintile, those in wave II had the highest proportion of EBF at any time point. Looking at 6 months, the proportion changed from 7, to 26% to 15% from wave I to wave III. For mothers of the highest wealth quintile, except for the up

to 1 month observation, there were significant differences in the proportion of EBF across waves (χ^2 = 3.07 p value = 0.216 up to 1 month, χ^2 = 6.13 p value = 0.047 up to 3 months and χ^2 = 5.98 p value < 0.05 up to 6 months), (Fig. 3).

Trend of exclusive breastfeeding by HIV status
At 6 months, the proportion of EBF among HIV positive mothers increased from 6 to 11% to 27% across the waves. The significant difference in the proportion of EBF across the waves was only at 6 months (χ^2 = 3.10 p value = 0.212 up to 1 month, χ^2 = 4.14 p value = 0.126 up to-3 and χ^2 = 13.56 p value < 0.001 up to 6). On the other hand, among HIV negative mothers, the proportion of EBF up to 6 months increased from 6% in wave I to 17% in wave II, then dropped to 15% in wave III. Among HIV negative mothers, the great majority, these changes in the proportion were statistically different at 3 and 6 months (χ^2 = 4.19 p value = 0.123 up to1 month, χ^2 = 8.94 p value = 0.011 up to3 months and χ^2 = 47.49 p value < 0.001 up to 6 months). Except for wave II, at whatever time unit, the proportion of EBF among HIV positive mothers was higher. During wave I, the

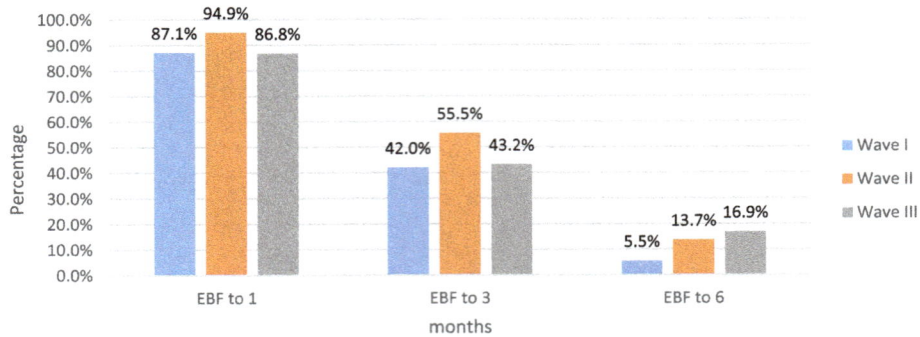

Fig. 2 Trend of exclusive breastfeeding over the three waves [N = 2315 wave I n = 1656, wave II n = 256, wave III n = 403]

proportion of EBF among HIV positive and negative mothers was the same at 6 months, (Fig. 4).

Discussion

This is the first study in Tanzania to establish the trend of EBF at a regional level over a period of 12 years. Although the proportion of EBF up to 6 months has been increasing overall across the years, it was not consistent across all the sub-groups of women. The proportion of EBF to 6 months showed the greatest increase among women of the lowest wealth quintile and those that are HIV positive, while there has been no significant increase among their counterparts. However, the general trend and that observed in all sub-groups of mothers is the decrease in EBF with an increase in infant age.

The overall trend of EBF up to 6 months in Moshi municipality has been observed to increase across the years. There has been a reported increase in the national average proportion of EBF in Tanzania [9] and Kenya [12],

while in the neighboring countries (e.g. Uganda) the proportion of EBF has been fluctuating [13–15]. Although it is encouraging to observe that the trend in Moshi municipality has been increasing across the years, the proportion of infants EBF up to 6 months is well below the recommended target of 90% [1]. Efforts to improve the proportion of EBF of infants under 6 months need to be emphasized in Tanzania and perhaps regional estimates taken as the guide to set targets.

The differences in proportions from the national average may be due to intrinsic differences between regions in a vast country like Tanzania. Other studies such as those conducted in Brazil [16], India [17], Nepal [5] and Nigeria [4] have reported regional variability. Kilimanjaro is one of the few regions in the country where the socio-demographic characteristics and the availability of well-being services are almost the same in rural and urban areas [9]. These characteristics are comparable to the national average for urban settings [9]. Other cross-sectional studies in other regions

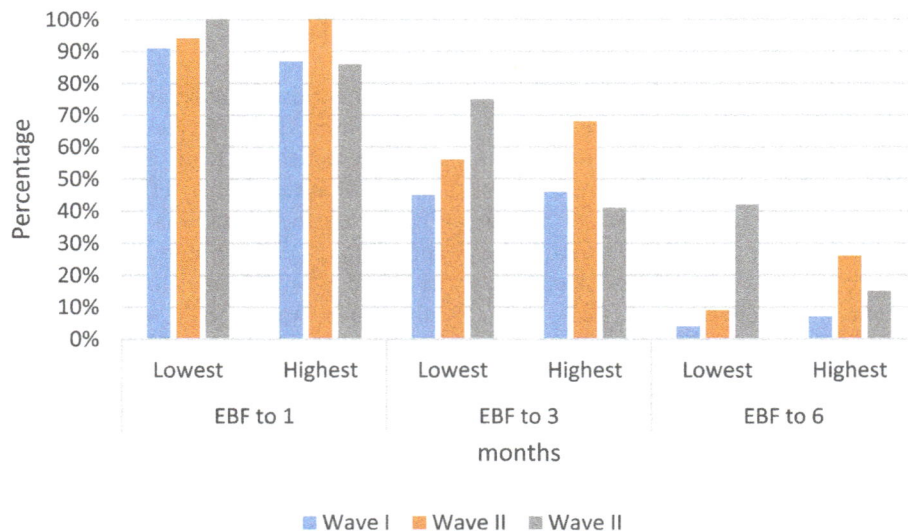

Fig. 3 Trend of exclusive breastfeeding practices between those with lowest and highest wealth quintile, 2002–2014. [N = 2315 lowest wealth quintile n = 473, highest wealth quintile n = 461]

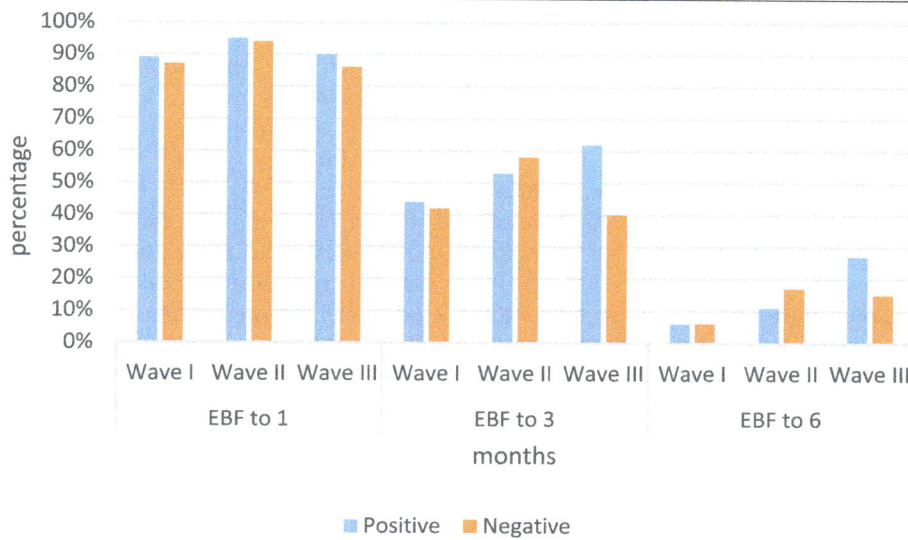

Fig. 4 Trend of exclusive breastfeeding practices based on HIV status of the mothers, 2002–2014. [N = 2315 HIV + ve *n* = 292, HIV –ve *n* = 1971]

have also shown the proportion of EBF of infants 0–6 months to be different from the national average [18, 19]. While providing national estimates of the proportion of EBF of infants 0–6 months is crucial [1], efforts to provide regional estimates may help to better understand the situation on the ground which may be different from the national status.

Another reason for the difference observed in the proportion of EBF of infants under 6 months may be due to differences in the study design [20] whereby this study used a cohort while estimates provided by DHS use a cross-sectional study design. Khanal et al. (2016) observed that cohort studies would provide lower proportions of EBF compared to cross-sectional studies although probably more 'realistic' proportions of EBF [20]. The proportions in this study are comparable to estimates in another cohort study in Nepal (8.9% EBF among infants up to 6 months, 2014) [20] and from the latest estimates made by DHS in the region (14.6% EBF among children 0–6 months 2015–16) [9].

A drop in EBF as infants age has been reported in global estimates [21], and in Brazil [16], India [17], Nepal [5], Nigeria [4] and Tanzania [9]. In this study, the proportion of EBF dropped by almost half from 1 month to 3 months. Understanding the point where there is a significant drop in EBF may guide the focus of interventions. For example, in Nepal the proportion of EBF among infants aged 0 up to 6 months increased mainly by increasing the proportion of those who were exclusively breastfed at 4 months [5]. The current vaccination schedule in Tanzania includes vaccines offered at six weeks after delivery. With an overall vaccination coverage of 75% in Tanzania and 93% in Kilimanjaro region [9], this contact with the health facility may be used as

an opportunity to strengthen interventions. The counselling that mothers receive during health facility visits has shown to improve EBF practices [4, 9, 22, 23] and particularly when provided after delivery [18].

We argue that Tanzania as a country has enough potential to do both make studies for trend of EBF at smaller geographical areas and establish satellite cohorts for EBF estimates. The latest DHS for the first time presented regional estimates of EBF [9], and showed regional variabilities. There are three schools of public health located in the northern, eastern and north-west areas of the country. Students at these institutions are required to conduct studies to graduate, and they have been doing this. This shows that there are enough resources (human, financial and time) and potential to conduct studies. A consideration may be made to make EBF related research a priority. Also, there are implementation partners (non-governmental organizations) all over the country. Taking the magnitude of the importance of EBF on the general well-being of the population, it may be important to give EBF a top priority for their interventions and explorations.

Making estimations at a global level, Victoria et al. (2016) found that the trend for EBF was increasing over years, the rate was higher among those with the highest wealth quintiles compared to those with the lowest [1]. With Sustainable Development Goal targeting equity [24], it is heartening to observe that, in the studied population, those of the lowest wealth quintile are doing well in this highly beneficial practice. However, caution has to be taken while looking at this. Studies have shown that the poor may tend to breastfeed for longer as they have nothing else to feed their infants, coined 'reverse causality' [25]. Ultimately, the infants do not benefit from the practice if they are EBF beyond 6 months. Other than that, it has been observed that ultimately the ones with the highest wealth quintile would adopt the recommended health beneficial practices. Efforts should be made to ensure that in Tanzania all women, despite their wealth quintiles, adopt and practice EBF.

Recommendations on EBF among HIV positive mothers have varied over the years [26] guided by research results, basically because of the fear of transmitting the infection through breast milk. In 2002–2004, the recommendation started with EBF for 3 months followed by abrupt cessation, but the current recommendation is using anti-retroviral treatment and breastfeeding the infants exclusively for the first six months of life followed by continued breastfeeding up to twelve months [27]. In this context, it is encouraging that the proportion of EBF among HIV positive mothers is higher than their negative counterparts. However, this is not surprising given that in the current PMTCT program, HIV-positive pregnancy women and postpartum women are seen monthly for counselling and care, including counselling on breastfeeding and infant feeding practices. Nevertheless, the proportion of HIV-positive mothers EBF in wave III were still lower than the recommended proportions. The proportion of EBF reported in this study among HIV positive mothers are similar to the proportion of a study carried out in the eastern part of the country (proportion of EBF up to 6 months 13.3%) in 2010 [28], but lower than that reported in a recent study carried out also in the same area (proportion of EBF among children 0–6 months 77%) in 2016 [22]. The differences in the proportion of EBF with those observed in the recent study may have resulted from using different study designs. The differences may also have been because of different settings. With the change in EBF policy among HIV positive mothers, the adoption may be faster in the sites used in the recent study. Authors in the article observed that providers in one of the facility were probably exposed to more trainings [22] which might have made providers more aware of recommendations. However, this referred study [22] shows that it is possible to increase the proportion of EBF among HIV positive mothers and strategies to meet this are to be strengthened.

The limitations for this study include being a hospital based study of a cohort with a loss to follow-up of about 20%. This may introduce selection bias, whereby those who stayed with the cohort for at least 6 months after delivery may be different from those that were lost. Information bias was limited by using a standardized questionnaire and training the research assistants. Establishing EBF by making a follow-up of feeding practices from delivery until the child was six months of age, rather than a 24-h recall, is among the strength of this study [20].The findings are to be

interpreted with caution; wave II contains more HIV positive mothers as the cohort recruitment focused on them and hence over representation of HIV positives in the whole cohort.

Conclusion

While establishing trends of EBF at a national level is commendable, efforts to establish the trend in the smaller geographical areas are needed to provide a true picture that may otherwise be masked and which is necessary to guide localized interventions. The trend may also need to be explored for women of different socio-economic and health status. Interventions such as counselling should focus on mothers with infants of one month of age.

Abbreviations

ANC: Antenatal clinic care; CRERC: College Research and Ethical Review Committee; DHS: Demographic Health Survey; EBF: Exclusive breastfeeding; IQR: Interquartile range; PCA: Principle Component Analysis; STI: Sexually Transmitted Infections

Acknowledgments

We would like to thank the Catholic University of Health and Allied Sciences, the Letten Foundation and Sub-Saharan Africa Consortium for Advanced Biostatistics Training programme for making it possible to carry out this study. We would like to also thank the Better Health for African Mother and Child faculty for their tireless support in seeing this work through to publication. Authors are grateful to Dr. Michael Mahande, the staff and colleagues at the department of Epidemiology and Applied Biostatistics at Kilimanjaro Christian Medical University College for their continuous mentorship and support. We graciously appreciate and acknowledge Mr. Edward (Ned) Cundal and Chandra Almony for their help in editing this manuscript.

Funding

This study was supported through the DELTAS Africa Initiative SSACAB (Grant No. 107754/Z/15/Z). The DELTAS Africa Initiative is an independent funding scheme of the African Academy of Sciences (AAS) Alliance for Accelerating Excellence in Science in Africa (AESA) and is supported by the New Partnership for Africa's Development Planning and Coordinating Agency (NEPAD Agency) with funding from the Wellcome Trust (Grant No. 107754/Z/15/Z) and the UK government. The views expressed in this publication are those of the authors and not necessarily those of the AAS, NEPAD Agency, Wellcome Trust or the UK government. Data collection for the period of 12 years was funded by the Letten Foundation Oslo, Norway.

Author's contribution

OJ, SM, MM, BP, contributed in the study design. OJ analysed the data under the guidance of JT. OJ and JT interpreted the results. OJ prepared the manuscript and all the other authors reviewed the manuscript before submission. All authors read and approved the final manuscript.

Competing interests

The authors declare that they have no competing interests.

Author details

[1]Institute of Public Health, Department of Epidemiology and Biostatistics, Kilimanjaro Christian Medical University College (KCMUCo), P.O. Box 2240, Moshi, Tanzania. [2]Department of Community Medicine, Kilimanjaro Christian Medical Centre (KCMC), Moshi, Tanzania. [3]Better Health for African Mother and Child (BHAMC), Moshi, Tanzania. [4]London School of Hygiene and Tropical Medicine, bloomsbury, UK. [5]Division of Women, Oslo University

Hospital, University of Oslo, Oslo, Norway. [6]Institute of Clinical Medicine, University of Oslo, Oslo, Norway.

References

1. Victora CG, Bahl R, Barros AJD, Franca GVA, Horton S, Krasevec J, et al. Breastfeeding in the 21st century: epidemiology, mechanisms, and lifelong effect. Lancet [Internet]. 2016;387(10017):475–90. Available from:. https://doi.org/10.1016/S0140-6736(15)01024-7.
2. Horta BL, Loret de Mola C, Victora CG. Long-term consequences of breastfeeding on cholesterol, obesity, systolic blood pressure and type 2 diabetes: a systematic review and meta-analysis. ActaPaediatr [Internet]. 2015;104:30–7. Available from: https://doi.org/10.1111/apa.13133
3. Jones G, Steketee RW, Black RE, Bhutta ZA, Morris SS. How many child deaths can we prevent this year? Lancet. 2003;362(9377):65–71.
4. Agho KE, Dibley MJ, Odiase JI, Ogbonmwan SM. Determinants of exclusive breastfeeding in Nigeria. BMC Pregnancy Childbirth. 2011;11(2):2–9.
5. Khanal V, Sauer K, Zhao Y. Exclusive breastfeeding practices in relation to social and health determinants : a comparison of the 2006 and 2011 Nepal demographic and health surveys. BMC Public Health. 2013;13(958):13.
6. Msuya SE, Mbizvo E, Hussain A, Uriyo J, Sam NE, Stray-Pedersen B. HIV among pregnant women in Moshi Tanzania: the role of sexual behavior, male partner characteristics and sexually transmitted infections. AIDS Res Ther. 2006;3(27):1–10.
7. Katanga J, Mgongo M, Hashim TH, Stray-pedersen B, Msuya SE. Screening for syphilis, HIV, and hemoglobin during pregnancy in Moshi municipality, Tanzania: how is the health system performing (short communication). Sci J Public Heal [Internet]. 2015;3(1):93–6 Available from: http://www.sciencepublishinggroup.com/journal/paperinfo.aspx?journalid=251&doi=10.11648/j.sjph.20150301.26.
8. Hussein TH, Mgongo M, Uriyo JG, Damian DJ, Stray-pedersen B, Msuya SE. Exclusive breastfeeding up to six months is very rare in Tanzania : a cohort study of infant feeding practices in Kilimanjaro area. Sci J Public Heal. 2015; 3(2):251–8.
9. Ministry of Health Community Development Gender Elderly and Children D es S, Ministry of Health Z, Statistics TNB of, Zanzibar O of CGS. Tanzania Demographic and Health Survey and Malaria Indicator Survey, 2015–16. 2016.
10. UNICEF and World Health Organization. Indicators for Assessing Infant and Young Child Feeding Practices [Internet]. Vol. 2007. 2008. Available from: http://www.who.int/nutrition/publications/infantfeeding/9789241596664/en/
11. Seema V, Kumaranayake L. Constructing socio-economic status indices : how to use principal components analysis. Oxford University Press. 2006.
12. National Bureau of Statistics (NBS)[Kenya]. Kenya Demographic and Health Survey. 2014:2014.
13. National Bureau of Statistics (NBS)[Rwanda]. Rwanda Demographic and Health Survey 2014–15. 2014.
14. National Bureau of Statistics (NBS) [Uganda]. Uganda Demographic and Health Survey. 2015/16:2017.
15. National Bureau of Statistics (NBS) [Burundi]. Burundi Demographic and Health Survey. 2016/17:2017.
16. Parizoto GM, Parada CMGDL, Venâncio SI, Carvalhaes MADBL. Trends and patterns of exclusive breastfeeding for under-6-month-old children. J Pediatr. 2009;85(3):201–8.
17. Chandhiok N, Singh KJ, Sahu D, Singh L, Pandey A. Changes in exclusive breastfeeding practices and its determinants in India , 1992–2006 : analysis of national survey data. Int Breastfeed J. 2015;10(34):1–13. Available from: https://doi.org/10.1186/s13006-015-0059-0
18. Mgongo M, Mosha MV, Uriyo JG, Msuya SE, Stray-pedersen B. Prevalence and predictors of exclusive breastfeeding among women in Kilimanjaro region , Northern Tanzania : a population based cross-sectional study. Int Breastfeed J. 2013;8(12):1–8.
19. Kazaura M. Exclusive breastfeeding practices in the coast region. Tanzania Afr Health Sci. 2016;16(1):44–50.
20. Khanal V, Lee AH, Scott JA, Karkee R, Binns CW. Implications of methodological differences in measuring the rates of exclusive breastfeeding in Nepal : findings from literature review and cohort study. BMC Pregnancy Childbirth. 2016:1–9. Available from:. https://doi.org/10.1186/s12884-016-1180-9.
21. Cai X, Wardlaw T, Brown DW. Global trends in exclusive breastfeeding. Int Breastfeed J. 2012;7(12):2–6.
22. Williams AM, Chantry C, Geubbels EL, Ramaiya AK, Shemdoe AI, Tancredi DJ, et al. Breastfeeding and complementary feeding practices among HIV-exposed infants in coastal Tanzania. J Hum Lact. 2016;32(1):112–20.
23. Yalcin S, Berde a, Suzan Y. determinants of exclusive breast feeding in sub-Saharan Africa : a multilevel approach. Paediatr Perinat Epidemiol. 2016; 30(5):433–9.
24. United Nations. Global indicator framework for the Sustainable Development Goals and targets of the 2030 Agenda for Sustainable Development 2015. Available from: https://unstats.un.org/sdgs/indicators/Global%20Indicator%20Framework_A.RES.71.313%20Annex.pdf
25. Kramer MS, Moodie EEM, Dahhou M, Platt RW. Breastfeeding and infant size: evidence of reverse causality. Am J Epidemiol. 2011;173(9):978–83.
26. Young SL, Mbuya MNN, Chantry CJ, Geubbels EP, Israel-ballard K, Cohan D, et al. Current Knowledge and Future Research on Infant Feeding in the Context of HIV : Basic , Clinical , Behavioral, and Programmatic Perspectives. Adv Nutr 2011;2(6):225–243.
27. World Health Organization. Use of antiretroviral drugs for treating pregnant women and preventing HIV infection in infants. Executive summary. 2012. Available from: http://apps.who.int/iris/bitstream/10665/70892/2/WHO_HIV_2012.6_eng.pdf
28. Young SL, Israel-ballard KA, Dantzer EA, Ngonyani MM, Nyambo MT, Ash DM, et al. Infant feeding practices among HIV-positive women in Dar es Salaam , Tanzania , indicate a need for more intensive infant feeding counselling. Public Health 2010;13(12):2027–2033.

Knowledge of danger signs during pregnancy and subsequent healthcare seeking actions among women in Urban Tanzania

Beatrice Mwilike[1,5]* , Gorrette Nalwadda[2], Mike Kagawa[3], Khadija Malima[4], Lilian Mselle[1] and Shigeko Horiuchi[5]

Abstract

Background: Tanzania is among the countries with a high maternal mortality ratio. However, it remains unclear how information and education on danger signs of pregnancy translate into appropriate actions when a woman recognizes danger signs. This study aimed to determine women's knowledge of obstetric danger signs during pregnancy and their subsequent healthcare seeking actions.

Methods: The study design was a health facility-based cross-sectional study. Quantitative data were collected through interviewer-administered questionnaires. Descriptive and inferential statistics were used to analyze the data. The study enrolled 384 women from two health centers in Kinondoni Municipality, Dar es Salaam, Tanzania. A woman who had not mentioned any danger sign was categorized as *having no knowledge*, mentioned one to three danger signs as *having low knowledge*, and mentioned four or more danger signs as *having sufficient knowledge*.

Results: Among the 384 participants, 67 (17.4%) had experienced danger signs during their pregnancy and reported their healthcare seeking actions after recognizing the danger signs. Among those who recognized danger signs, 61 (91%) visited a healthcare facility. Among the 384 participants, five (1.3%) had no education, 175 (45.6%) had primary education, 172 (44.8%) had secondary education, and 32 (8.3%) had post-secondary education as their highest educational levels. When asked to spontaneously mention the danger signs, more than half of the participants ($n = 222$, 57.8%) were able to mention only one to three danger signs. Only 104 (31%) had correct knowledge of at least four danger signs and nine (2.7%) were not able to mention any item. The most commonly known pregnancy danger signs were vaginal bleeding (81%); swelling of the fingers, face, and legs (46%); and severe headache (44%). Older women were 1.6 times more likely to have knowledge of danger signs than young women (OR 1.61; 95% CI 1.05-2.46)".

Conclusion: Women took appropriate healthcare seeking action after recognizing danger signs during pregnancy. However, the majority had low knowledge of pregnancy danger signs. Additional studies are warranted to address the knowledge gap and to plan interventions for improving health education under limited resource settings.

Keywords: Knowledge, Danger signs, Pregnancy, Healthcare seeking action

* Correspondence: beatricemwilike@yahoo.com; 15dn013@slcn.ac.jp
[1]Muhimbili University of Health and Allied Sciences, School of Nursing, P.O. Box 65004, Dar es salaam, Tanzania
[5]St. Luke's International University, 10-1 Akashi-cho, Chuo-ku, Tokyo 104-0044, Japan
Full list of author information is available at the end of the article

Background

In 2013, about 289,000 women across the world were reported to have died from pregnancy and childbirth-related complications [1]. It is estimated that the majority (62%) of global maternal deaths occur in Sub-Saharan Africa [1]. A high maternal mortality ratio usually characterizes most countries within the Sub-Saharan region, one of which is Tanzania at 556 deaths per 100,000 live births [2]. Other countries in the East African region with a high maternal mortality ratio include Kenya (510/100,000 live births) and Uganda (343/100,000 live births) [3]. The major complications that account for 80% of all maternal deaths are severe bleeding, infections, high blood pressure during pregnancy, obstructed labor, and unsafe abortion. However, many maternal deaths can be prevented if appropriate action is taken early and promptly.

Tanzania's ongoing efforts to improve maternity care has resulted in the adoption of the World Health Organization's focused antenatal care (FANC) program consisting of only four visits for low-risk pregnancy without complications. This version of an antenatal care (ANC) program included health promotion, prevention, detection, and treatment of existing diseases. It contained critical information for birth preparedness including the seven danger signs of pregnancy [4].

Every woman needs to be aware of the danger signs that occur during pregnancy, as complications can be unpredictable. These danger signs include vaginal bleeding, severe headache, vision problems, high fever, swollen hands/face, and reduced fetal movement [4]. These danger signs usually indicate the presence of an obstetric complication that may arise during pregnancy, delivery or postdelivery. Knowledge of these danger signs will help women to make the right decisions and take appropriate healthcare seeking actions [5]. Eventually, taking the right healthcare seeking action means receiving immediate and appropriate care, which reduces maternal mortality and morbidity. Therefore, women should receive health education about pregnancy including outcomes, danger signs during pregnancy, nutrition and family planning, as well as other services when they visit an ANC clinic [2].

The 2011 demographic health survey report of Tanzania [2] showed that only 53% of pregnant women were informed about the danger signs of pregnancy during their ANC visits. Other studies have also identified women's lack of knowledge of these danger signs [5–12]. However, the healthcare seeking actions of women after recognizing a danger sign during pregnancy have not yet been investigated. As all pregnant women are at risk of developing pregnancy-related complications, education on danger signs of pregnancy should be provided to all women who are attending an ANC clinic [3].

During a visit to a clinic, women receive an antenatal card wherein all the services provided during each visit are recorded [4]. However, the antenatal card does not usually include information on danger signs, thus such information may be missed during a visit [11, 12]. Women are advised to go to a nearby health facility and seek care in case they experience any pregnancy danger signs; however, visiting traditional healers, friends, or relatives before going to a health facility is also apparent [13]. In addition, women in South Africa [14] weighed the expected benefits against the anticipated costs before making a decision to avail of healthcare. Thus, travel time and perceptions of staff receptivity were also influential in their decision-making.

However, there are apparently no studies that have found a link between women's knowledge of danger signs during pregnancy and their subsequent healthcare seeking action if they recognize a danger sign. In this study, we assessed the knowledge of danger signs of pregnant women in Tanzania and their subsequent healthcare seeking action after recognizing the danger signs.

Methods

Study design

The study design was a health facility-based cross-sectional study whereby data were gathered at one point in time in a clinical setting. The researcher interviewed the participants using a Swahili questionnaire.

Study setting

The study was performed in two health centers in Kinondoni municipality, an urban district located in the Dar es Salaam region, Tanzania. The total population of this municipality is 1,775,049 (914,247 women and 860,802 men) according to the 2012 national census report [15]. The maternal mortality ratio of this municipality was 529/100,000 live births [16]. At the time of data collection, there were two health centers available, and data were collected at the Reproductive and Child Health Clinic (RCHC) of these health centers from May 2013 to June 2013. These health centers provide reproductive and child health services as well as maternity services for women who attend the clinic. Normally, antenatal education is provided in the form of a group session with women who have attended the clinic on a particular day. The total number of women who receive care at the RCHC ranged from 60 to 100 women per day. Nurse-midwives provide information about nutrition, birth preparations, obstetric danger signs, and vaccinations following uniform guidelines for providing information according to the available FANC guidelines in the country. Women are advised to visit a nearby health facility for care when they recognize a danger sign during their pregnancy.

Study participants

Potential participants were 392 postpartum women who were seeking immunization services for their children in

May and June 2013. The participants were selected by proportionate systematic random sampling. A woman who had given birth within the past 6 weeks from the day of data collection was eligible for the study.

Instrument

We developed a questionnaire based on a previous questionnaire about awareness of danger signs among rural women in a study conducted in Tanzania [5]. The questionnaire was translated from English to Swahili, which is a language most familiar to Tanzanians, by a trained research assistant and an experienced midwife. The questionnaire is composed of four sections: socio-demographic characteristics, experiences in the last pregnancy, knowledge of pregnancy danger signs, and healthcare seeking actions.

The section for knowledge of danger signs was adopted from a tool by Pembe et al. [5] and is composed of five open-ended questions regarding general knowledge about danger signs during pregnancy, recognition of danger signs, and source of information. Based on the danger signs that a woman can recognize, a list of nine danger signs stated in the WHO guide for essential practice (Childbirth, Postpartum and Newborn Care) [17] was used. These danger signs included the following: (1) severe vaginal bleeding, (2) convulsions, (3) severe headache with blurred vision, (4) severe abdominal pain, (5) too weak to get out of bed, (6) fast or difficulty in breathing, (7) reduced fetal movement, (8) fever, and (9) swelling of the fingers, face, and legs [5]. A woman was considered to *have sufficient knowledge* if she was able to spontaneously mention at least four of the nine danger signs [12]. On the other hand, a woman was considered to *have low knowledge* if she was able to spontaneously mention one to three danger signs, and to *have no knowledge* if she was not able to spontaneously mention any danger sign.

The section for healthcare seeking actions included six questions (forced choice and open-ended) about the recognized danger signs and health actions women had taken for each danger sign. An example of an open-ended question was to explain further why the woman decided to take a particular action after recognizing a danger sign. Visiting a health facility for care was considered as appropriate healthcare seeking action, whereas not doing anything, visiting a traditional healer, self-medication, and going to a traditional birth attendant were considered as inappropriate healthcare seeking actions.

The ANC experience during their last pregnancy involved answering a questionnaire consisting of nine questions (forced choice and open-ended) that queried about the type of care women received during their clinic visits including education and advice.

The tool was pretested in another health center within the municipality to check for clarity. Twenty women of similar status were interviewed and appropriate modifications were made to the questionnaire.

Data collection

All the women enrolled in this study provided informed consent before participating. Using the questionnaire, the lead researcher and five trained research assistants interviewed women in Swahili at the health facilities. After the interview, the lead researcher collected the questionnaires for data entry and cleaning. There were 384 pregnant women who agreed to participate in the study.

Data analysis

Descriptive and inferential statistics were used. The participants' characteristics were evaluated in terms of frequencies. The F-test was used to compare knowledge scores, demographic characteristics, and healthcare seeking actions. The confounding variables that were controlled included educational level, marital status, occupation, parity, gravidity, and ANC visit. A P-value <0.05 was considered to indicate a statistically significant difference. Data were analyzed using an SPSS statistical package.

Results

Of the 392 pregnant women who were eligible, 384 (98%) consented to participate in the study. The participating women responded to all the questions in the questionnaire. Among these 384 women, 67 (17.4%) had experienced danger signs during their pregnancy and reported their healthcare seeking actions after recognizing the danger signs.

Characteristics of participating women

More than half of the participants (68.8%) were aged 21 to 30 years, and 329 (85.7%) were living with their partners. Among the participants, five (1.3%) had no education, 175 (45.6%) had primary education, 172 (44.8%) had secondary education, and 32 (8.3%) had post-secondary education as their highest educational levels. About half (54.4%; $n = 209$) were either employed or engaged in business which was conducted outside of their home. A total of 374 (97.4%) participants had attended ANC at least once during their last pregnancy, and among these, 271 (70.6%) had visited an antenatal clinic more than four times (Table 1). The gestational age at the first ANC visit was 4 months or more for 204 women (54.4%). Furthermore, 34.9% ($n = 134$) of the respondents were primiparas. About 99% of the participants delivered at a health facility (i.e., hospital, healthcare center, or dispensary). The mean distance to the health facility was 2.4 km (SD = 3.1).

Table 1 Characteristics of women and relationship with knowledge about danger signs (N = 384)

Variable	Categories	n (%)	Knowledge Mean score	F	P
Age	<20	30 (7.8)	1.77	4.05	**0.018**
	21-30	264 (68.8)	2.64		
	>30	90 (23.4)	2.83		
Education level	No education	5 (1.3)	1.40	2.42	0.066
	Primary	175 (45.6)	2.41		
	Secondary	172 (44.8)	2.80		
	Post-secondary	32 (8.3)	2.91		
Marital status	Living with partner	329 (85.7)	2.42	0.759	0.384
	Not living with partner	55 (14.3)	2.65		
Occupation	With occupation	209 (54.4)	2.59	0.419	0.658
	No occupation	163 (42.4)	2.61		
	Student	12 (3.2)	3.08		
Parity	1	160 (41.7)	2.64	0.425	0.654
	2-4	214 (55.7)	2.57		
	≥5	10 (2.6)	3.10		
Gravidity	1	134 (34.9)	2.50	1.032	0.357
	2-4	229 (59.6)	2.64		
	≥5	21 (5.5)	3.10		
ANC visit	<4 visits	113 (29.4)	2.05	1.747	0.187
	≥4 visits	271 (70.6)	2.15		

Knowledge of danger signs during pregnancy

A total of 335 (87.2%) women reported that they had heard about danger signs during pregnancy. The source of information about the danger signs during pregnancy was from the RCHC for 274 women (81.8%), social gatherings for 58 women (17.4%), and the radio for three women (0.8%).

When asked to spontaneously mention the danger signs, more than half of the participants (n = 222, 57.8%) were able to mention only one to three danger signs.

Only 104 (31%) had correct knowledge of at least four danger signs and nine (2.7%) were not able to mention any item. The mean score for knowledge of danger signs was 3.0 (SD = 1.609). Figure 1 shows the danger signs in ascending frequency. The most commonly known danger signs were vaginal bleeding (81.2%), edema (46.3%), and headache (43.6%).

The rest of the participants (n = 49, 12.8%) were not able to spontaneously mention the danger signs. These participants were thus provided with a list of danger

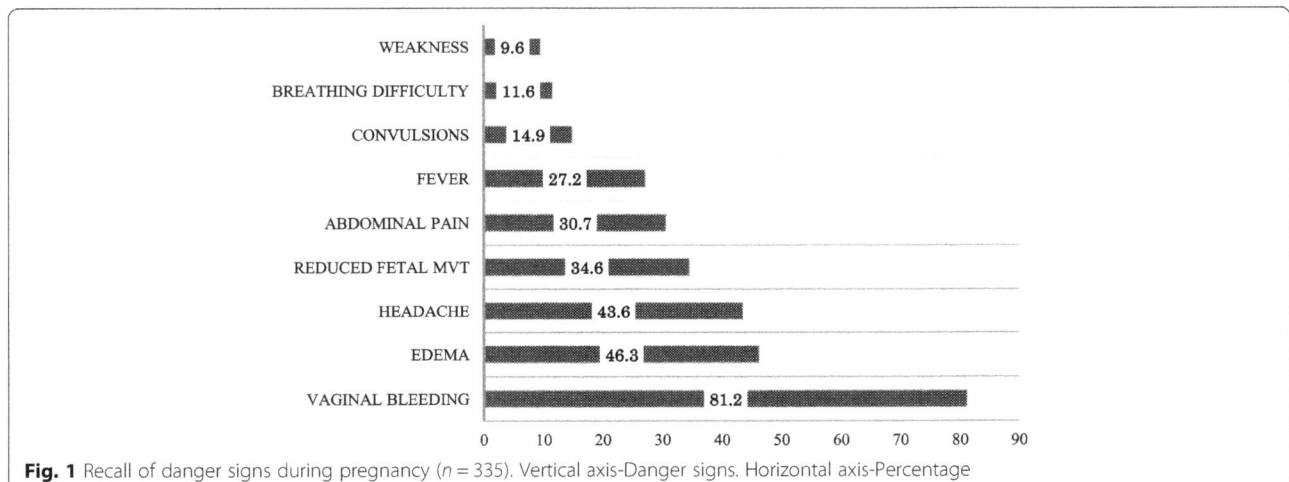

Fig. 1 Recall of danger signs during pregnancy (n = 335). Vertical axis-Danger signs. Horizontal axis-Percentage

signs to help them recall the signs. The most commonly known danger signs in this group were vaginal bleeding (65.3%) and abdominal pain (65.3%).

Knowledge scores and characteristics of women

There was a significant relationship between age and knowledge of danger signs ($P = 0.018$). The women were classified into three age groups; young age: < 20 years; middle age: 21-30 years; old age: > 31 years. Participants who were older had higher scores than those who were younger (Table 1). The mean score for knowledge of danger signs among women aged 30 years and above was 2.83, whereas that among women aged 20 years and below was 1.77. The other variables, namely, educational level, marital status, occupation, parity, gravidity, and ANC visit were not significantly related to knowledge of danger signs during pregnancy. After performing further analysis and controlling for confounding variables using logistic regression, it was determined that older women were 1.6 times more likely to have knowledge of danger signs than younger women (OR 1.61; 95% CI 1.05-2.46).

Healthcare seeking actions after recognition of danger signs

The healthcare seeking actions were categorized as either appropriate (visiting a health facility) or inappropriate (taking no action; consulting a friend/relative, or self-medication). A total of 67 (17.4%) participants had recognized danger signs during their last pregnancy. The majority of the women who recognized danger signs ($n = 61$, 91%) went to a health facility for care after experiencing the danger signs. The actions taken for each danger sign experienced are shown in Table 2. All the women who experienced danger signs such as edema and reduced fetal movement went to a health facility for care. The mean score for knowledge of danger signs for those who experienced danger signs was 3.17 (SD = 2.196). For crucial and vivid danger signs such as vaginal bleeding (n

= 1), convulsions ($n = 1$), and abdominal pain ($n = 2$), some of the women did not visit a health facility for care.

Other danger signs such as fever, headache, and being too weak to get out of bed were dealt with inappropriately because the participants considered these signs as normal events during pregnancy and therefore they decided to either not take any action or buy over-the-counter medicines. Women were asked to further explain why they decided to take the actions they took, and the majority of the participants ($n = 53$, 79.1%) who experienced danger signs explained that they preferred to be treated at the hospital because they believed that their problem would be solved in health facilities. Moreover, seven (10.5%) participants explained that they were educated about the danger signs so they knew that they were supposed to go to the hospital; five women (7.5%) responded that their condition worsened and therefore they had to rush to the hospital to save their lives and their babies. However, two women (3%) explained that the danger signs were normal events during pregnancy and therefore they decided to stay at home.

Discussion
Knowledge of danger signs during pregnancy

Our findings indicate that knowledge of danger signs during pregnancy was low among the pregnant women in Tanzania who participated in this study. Slightly less than one-third of the participants were spontaneously able to mention four or more danger signs. Notably, this finding is similar to those of other studies in Africa regarding knowledge of danger signs among pregnant women. In fact, only 26% of women in rural areas in Tanzania were reported to be aware of danger signs during pregnancy [5]. The same trend was also found in a study conducted in Aleta Wondo in Ethiopia, where only 30.4% of the women were aware of at least two danger signs [8].

The most common spontaneously mentioned danger sign of pregnancy was vaginal bleeding (81.2%), possibly

Table 2 Healthcare seeking actions for danger signs during pregnancy

Danger signs	Experienced (n = 67)		Total
	Appropriate Action	Inappropriate action	
Vaginal bleeding	34	1	35
Edema	25	0	25
Headache	37	3	40
Reduced fetal movement	24	0	24
Abdominal pain	32	2	34
Fever	26	3	29
Convulsions	23	1	24
Difficulty Breathing	30	1	31
Weakness	34	2	36

Multiple response table. The values are over a total of participants who experienced a particular danger sign

because it is the most visible sign compared with other signs such as reduced fetal movement. This finding is similar to that of studies in Ethiopia [8] and Uganda [9] whereby most respondents spontaneously identified vaginal bleeding as a danger sign more than others. However, some previous studies showed a contrasting finding whereby in rural Tanzania only 9.6% and Uganda 49% women were aware of vaginal bleeding as a danger sign during pregnancy [5, 9].

This difference might be due to the study design and location differences as they were all community surveys. Nevertheless, emphasis should also be placed on other danger signs that were not commonly mentioned such as abdominal pain and convulsions. A study by Hailu et al. in Ethiopia revealed that these danger signs were not spontaneously mentioned even though they indicated the presence of (pre-)eclampsia [8]. Only 7% of the participants mentioned abdominal pain and 4.7% convulsion as danger signs.

A significant relationship was found between having knowledge about danger signs and age of the participants. Similar findings were reported from studies in rural Tanzania and South Africa, which found increased awareness among older and multiparous women [5, 10]. Thus, older women have more experience with pregnancy issues. The total fertility rate in Tanzania is 5.4 births per woman. The total fertility rate among rural women on the mainland (6.1 births) is higher than that among urban women (3.7 births) [2]. Therefore, it was likely that they were more aware of danger signs either from their own experience or from events in their society. This implies a need for special consideration among young women, particularly adolescents, when providing health counseling and education at antenatal clinics.

Being young and immature may likely affect the reception of antenatal education and the recognition of signs of obstetric complications. WHO reported that adolescent pregnancy remains a major contributor to maternal mortality and that obstetric complications are the second cause of death among 15 to 19 year olds globally [18]. Most pregnant adolescents lacked social support, experienced community stigmatization, and were treated improperly by health workers [19]. There is therefore a need to introduce and implement special adolescent friendly interventions to empower pregnant adolescents by providing them health information on pregnancy as well as delivery and early childhood care [20]. Pregnant adolescents need to know and be assured that healthcare workers care about them and that they can receive assistance in using the available health facility services. Moreover, techniques such as producing pictorial gifts with health messages that can remind pregnant adolescents of the danger signs during pregnancy and what appropriate actions to take when they recognize a danger

sign should be used. Although this study was conducted in an urban district where 97% of women visited an ANC clinic at least once, the present findings suggest that the quality of antenatal health education was poor.

During antenatal health education, a large group of more than 40 women usually gather, with only one or two nurse-midwives handling the hour-long session. The likelihood of some women missing or misinterpreting the educational information provided is higher in a large group than in a small group. A previous study on the quality of antenatal care in rural Tanzania showed that two out of every five women were not counselled on pregnancy danger signs [21]. Regarding the amount of time spent for antenatal care consultation in Tanzania, the mean total duration for the initial ANC consultation was reported to be only about 20 min [22], which is not sufficiently long for proper counselling [11]. These findings imply a poor quality of counselling regarding the danger signs during pregnancy for women who had attended the antenatal clinic. Furthermore, there was an apparent imbalance between demand and supply owing to the overwhelming numbers of women attending the clinics, inadequately skilled staff, and indifferent attitudes of healthcare workers. Nyamtema et al. [11] found substandard ANC in rural Tanzania owing to the lack of staff, equipment, and supplies. The lack of simplicity in the information delivery system for pregnant KwaZulu-Natal women in South Africa [10]. Therefore, considerable and sustained efforts are needed to improve the quality of health education provided at health facilities in Tanzania, aiming at increasing knowledge of danger signs during pregnancy.

Healthcare seeking action

The present findings revealed that the majority of women who had recognized signs of complications during their pregnancy visited a health facility for care and management. They likely feared for the life of their infant. Also, the majority were living less than five kilometers from the hospital, hence they could easily access the services. They believed that being in a hospital environment could solve most of their health-related concerns.

What was surprising was the decision of some women who experienced danger signs not to take any action. The results showed that those who experienced fever and headache decided to either do nothing or take over-the-counter medicine. These findings in some respects resemble those of a study conducted in Ghana reporting on obstetric danger signs and factors affecting the healthcare seeking behavior which identified a traditional hierarchy of seeking care [23]. For symptoms such as vaginal bleeding, headache, and fever, women usually started with home remedies, progressed to consulting traditional healers, and ended up at a health facility.

Furthermore, Kilewo et al. identified perceived delay in healthcare seeking in a study from Bangladesh [24]. They reported that only 33% of the patients sought treatment from a qualified health provider during their pregnancy. More than 75% of the women with time-sensitive complications of convulsions or vaginal bleeding had either failed to seek any treatment or sought treatment from an unqualified provider.

Therefore, factors that affect women's healthcare seeking should be thoroughly clarified and addressed in the community. Studies have shown that women's decision to seek care could be greatly influenced by the perceived severity of the condition, distance to the health facility, and financial status to cover hospital bills in case payment was necessary [12, 24]. Furthermore, consideration must be given to the limited decision-making capability of women within marriage and family [4]. Women need to be empowered with knowledge and birth preparedness during the antenatal clinic visit.

Implications for practice
The present results imply that having knowledge of danger signs is not enough; additional changes in attitude and empowerment to take appropriate action are also required. A lack of educational opportunities and poor understanding of both danger signs and possible complications indicate that many women may not be familiar with the presentation of complications and consider them normal appearances in pregnancy. Delay in seeking appropriate healthcare owing to lack of knowledge of danger signs can be reduced by improving access to health information and education through the development of community outreach projects that specifically provide information on childbearing issues particularly danger signs for obstetric complications. Such information should be given to individual women and their families to facilitate their collaboration when care is needed. The establishment of community-based programs is also of particular importance to assist women with limited ability to visit health facilities. It will also be beneficial if other members of the community receive education and eventually provide a community support group that will offer help when a complication occurs. Importantly, the quality of health education at the health facility should be carefully checked for relevance and usability.

Limitations and further research
One main limitation of the present study was that the structured interview format limited the ability to explore extensively the reasons for the subsequent actions the women took after recognizing the danger signs and how long it took them to decide to seek care. Future exploratory studies on healthcare seeking behavior will provide insights into the association between having knowledge

and subsequent healthcare seeking actions. In addition, the small number of those who recognized danger signs and the use of only two health facilities limit the generalization of our findings. Also, other factors standing in between knowledge and action have not been clearly stated and assessed systematically in the data collection tool. As these other factors were not considered in this study, additional studies are recommended to further assess these factors. Our study was conducted in a clinical setting and in facilities located in an urban district. Therefore, the findings cannot be generalized to women who have failed to attend a clinic soon after delivery and to those living in rural areas. Our sample was biased by the fact that we did not include women who delivered at home as well as women who experienced perinatal deaths, because we sampled after delivery in a clinic where women brought their newborns for immunization.

Conclusion
This is apparently the first study that assessed the knowledge of danger signs during pregnancy and subsequent healthcare seeking actions of women in urban Tanzania. The findings indicate their low knowledge of danger signs during pregnancy and provide important insights into the possible underlying factors. Older participants had higher scores for knowledge of danger signs than younger participants. Women's knowledge of danger signs during pregnancy positively influenced their decisions regarding when to seek medical care and when to take appropriate action. Further studies are recommended to address the knowledge gap and to plan more effective interventions for improving antenatal care in limited resource settings.

Abbreviations
ANC: Antenatal Care; FANC: Focused Antenatal Care; IRB: Institutional Review Board; MUHAS: Muhimbili University of Health and Allied Sciences; RCHC: Reproductive and Child Health Clinic; WHO: World Health Organization

Acknowledgements
We express our special thanks to the research assistants and midwives of the health facilities for their cooperation with the data collection.
We gratefully thank NORAD's Program for Master Studies (NOMA) from Bergen Norway for funding this study.
We appreciate Dr. Sarah E. Porter for the English editorial support and critique on behalf of St. Luke's International University, Tokyo Japan.
We sincerely thank Dr. Edward Barroga (http://orcid.org/0000-0002-8920-2607) for the comprehensive editorial review and detailed guidance in writing the manuscript.

Funding
This research study was funded by NORAD's Program for Master Studies (NOMA) from Bergen Norway and the Japan Society for the Promotion of Science (JSPS) Core-to-core program, Asia-Africa Science Platforms (2015-2018).

Authors' contributions

BM conceptualized the study design, collected the data, performed statistical analysis, and prepared the first draft of the manuscript. GN, MK, KYM, and LM participated in conceptualizing the study design and data analysis. SH co-conceptualized and supervised the whole study, crosschecked all data analysis, and provided important content revisions in the drafting of the manuscript. All authors read and approved the final manuscript.

Competing interests

The authors declare that they have no competing interests.

Author details

[1]Muhimbili University of Health and Allied Sciences, School of Nursing, P.O. Box 65004, Dar es salaam, Tanzania. [2]Department of Nursing, Makerere University, P.O. Box 7072, Kampala, Uganda. [3]Department of Obstetrics and Gynecology, Makerere University, P.O. Box 7072, Kampala, Uganda. [4]Tanzania Commission for Science and Technology, Dar es Salaam, Tanzania. [5]St. Luke's International University, 10-1 Akashi-cho, Chuo-ku, Tokyo 104-0044, Japan.

References

1. WHO, UNICEF, UNFPA, The World Bank and the United Nations Population Division 2013. Trends in Maternal Mortality: 1990 to 2013. http://www.who.int/reproductivehealth/publications/monitoring/maternal-mortality-2013/en/. Accessed 15 Aug 2017.

2. Ministry of Health, Community Development, Gender, Elderly and Children - MoHCDGEC/Tanzania Mainland, Ministry of Health - MoH/Zanzibar, National Bureau of Statistics - NBS/Tanzania, Office of Chief Government Statistician - OCGS/Zanzibar, and ICF. 2016. Tanzania demographic and health survey and malaria indicator survey (TDHS-MIS) 2015-16. Dar es salaam/Tanzania: MoHCDGEC, MoH, NBS, OCGS, and ICF. http://dhsprogram.com/publications/publication-FR321-DHS-Final-Reports.cfm. Accessed 15 Aug 2017.

3. WHO, UNICEF, UNFPA, World Bank Group and the United Nations Population Division. Trends in Maternal Mortality 1990-2015. WHO publication. http://www.who.int/reproductivehealth/publications/monitoring/maternal-mortality-2015/en/.

4. Kearns A, Hurst T, Caglia J, Langer A. Focused antenatal Care in Tanzania. Women and health initiative, maternal health task force, Harvard School of Public Health. 2014. https://cdn2.sph.harvard.edu/wp-content/uploads/sites/32/2014/09/HSPH-Tanzania5.pdf. Accessed 8 Apr 2016.

5. Pembe AB, Urassa DP, Carlstedt A, Lindmark G, Nyström L, Darj E. Rural Tanzanian women's awareness of danger signs of obstetric complications. BMC Pregnancy Childbirth. 2009; https://doi.org/10.1186/1471-2393-9-12.

6. Gross K, Armstrong-Schellenberg J, Kessy F, Pfeiffer C, Obrist B. Antenatal care in practice: an exploratory study in antenatal care clinics in the Kilombero Valley, south-eastern Tanzania. BMC Pregnancy Childbirth. 2011; https://doi.org/10.1186/1471-2393-11-36.

7. Gupta S, Yamada G, Mpembeni R, Frumence G, Callaghan-Koru JA, Stevenson R, Brandes R, Baqui AH. Factors associated with four or more antenatal care visits and its decline among pregnant women in Tanzania between 1999 and 2010. PLoS One. 2014; https://doi.org/10.1371/journal.pone.0101893.

8. Hailu M, Gebremariam A, Alemseged F. Knowledge about obstetric danger signs among pregnant women in Aleta Wondo District, Sidama Zone, Southern Ethiopia. Ethiopian J Health Sci. 2010; https://doi.org/10.4314/ejhs.v20i1.69428.

9. Kabakyenga JK, Östergren PO, Turyakira E, Pettersson KO. Knowledge of obstetric danger signs and birth preparedness practices among women in rural Uganda. Repro Health. 2011; https://doi.org/10.1186/1742-4755-8-33.

10. Hoque M, Hoque ME. Knowledge of danger signs for major obstetric complications among pregnant KwaZulu-Natal women implications for health education. Asia-Pacific J Publ Health. 2011;23(6):946–56.

11. Nyamtema AS, Bartsch-de Jong A, Urassa DP, Hagen JP, van Roosmalen J. The quality of antenatal care in rural Tanzania: what is behind the number of visits? BMC Pregnancy Childbirth. 2012;12:70.

12. Okour A, Alkhateeb M, Amarin Z. Awareness of danger signs and symptoms of pregnancy complication among women in Jordan. Int J Gynecol Obstet. 2012;118(1):11–4.

13. Dako-Gyeke P, Aikins M, Aryeetey R, Mccough L, Adongo PB. The influence of socio-cultural interpretations of pregnancy threats on health-seeking behavior among pregnant women in urban Accra, Ghana. BMC Pregnancy Childbirth. 2013; https://doi.org/10.1186/1471-2393-13-211.

14. Abrahams N, Jewkes R, Mvo Z. Health care–seeking practices of pregnant women and the role of the midwife in Cape Town, South Africa. J Midwifery Women's Health. 2001; https://doi.org/10.1016/S1526-9523(01)00138-6.

15. United Republic of Tanzania. 2012 population and housing census. Population distribution by administrative areas. Dar-es-Salaam: National Bureau of Statistics; 2013.

16. Kinondoni Municipal Council. Kinondoni Municipal Profile 2011. Dar es Salaam: Kinondoni Municipality. 2012. p. 38-40.

17. World Health Organization. Pregnancy, childbirth, postpartum and newborn care: a guide for essential practice. 3rd ed. Geneva: B, QUICK CHECK, RAPID ASSESSMENT AND MANAGEMENT OF WOMEN OF CHILDBEARING AGE; 2015. https://www.ncbi.nlm.nih.gov/books/NBK326676/. Accessed 15 Aug 2017

18. World Health Organization. Adolescent Pregnancy Fact Sheet N°364, (Updated September 2014). http://www.who.int/mediacentre/factsheets/fs364/en/. Accessed 15 Aug 2017.

19. Atuyambe L, Mirembe F, Johansson A, Kirumira EK, Faxelid E. Experiences of pregnant adolescents-voices from Wakiso district, Uganda. Afr Health Sci. 2007;5(4):304–9.

20. Atuyambe L, Mirembe F, Mbona TN, Anika J, Kirumira KE, Faxelid E. Adolescent and adult first time mothers' health seeking practices during pregnancy and early motherhood in Wakiso District, Central Uganda. Repro Health. 2008; https://doi.org/10.1186/1742-4755-5-13. BMC Open Access.

21. Pembe AB, Carlstedt A, Urassa DP, Lindmark G, Nystrom L, Darj E. Quality of antenatal care in rural Tanzania: counselling on pregnancy danger signs. BMC Pregnancy Childbirth. 2010; https://doi.org/10.1186/1471-2393-10-35.

22. Magoma M, Requejo J, Merialdi M, Campbell OM, Cousens S, Filippi V. How much time is available for antenatal care consultations? Assessment of the quality of care in rural Tanzania. BMC Pregnancy Childbirth. 2011; https://doi.org/10.1186/1471-2393-11-64.

23. Aborigo RA, Moyer CA, Gupta M, Adongo PB, Williams J, Hodgson Allote P, Engmann CM. Obstetric danger signs and factors affecting health seeking behaviour among the Kassena-Nankani of northern Ghana: a qualitative study. Afr J Reprod Health. 2014;18(3):78–86.

24. Killewo J, Anwar I, Bashir I, Yunus M, Chakraborty J. Perceived delay in healthcare-seeking for episodes of serious illness and its implications for safe motherhood interventions in rural Bangladesh. J Health Popul Nutr. 2006;24(4):403–12.

9

Determination of medical abortion success by women and community health volunteers in Nepal using a symptom checklist

Kathryn L. Andersen[1*], Mary Fjerstad[2], Indira Basnett[3], Shailes Neupane[4], Valerie Acre[1], Sharad Sharma[3] and Emily Jackson[5]

Abstract

Background: We sought to determine if female community health volunteers (FCHVs) and literate women in Nepal can accurately determine success of medical abortion (MA) using a symptom checklist, compared to experienced abortion providers.

Methods: Women undergoing MA, and FCHVs, independently assessed the success of each woman's abortion using an 8-question symptom checklist. Any answers in a red-shaded box indicated that the abortion may not have been successful. Women's/FCHVs' assessments were compared to experienced abortion providers using standard of care.

Results: Women's (n = 1153) self-assessment of MA success agreed with abortion providers' determinations 85% of the time (positive predictive value = 90, 95% CI 88, 92); agreement between FCHVs and providers was 82% (positive predictive value = 90, 95% CI 88, 92). Of the 92 women (8%) requiring uterine evacuation with manual vacuum aspiration (n = 84, 7%) or medications (n = 8, 0.7%), 64% self-identified as needing additional care; FCHVs identified 61%. However, both women and FCHVs had difficulty recognizing that an answer in a red-shaded box indicated that the abortion may not have been successful. Of the 453 women with a red-shaded box marked, only 35% of women and 41% of FCHVs identified the need for additional care.

Conclusion: Use of a checklist to determine MA success is a promising strategy, however further refinement of such a tool, particularly for low-literacy settings, is needed before widespread use.

Keywords: Medical abortion, Abortion, Nepal, Self-assessment, Community health volunteers

Background

Medical abortion (MA) using a combined regimen of mifepristone followed by misoprostol is highly effective with few complications when used to terminate pregnancies up to, and after, 70 days gestation [1–5]. In low-resource settings where access to health care and trained abortion providers is limited, MA can increase the availability of safe abortion, and decrease morbidity and mortality related to unsafe abortion [6]. In Nepal, which continues to face high abortion-related morbidity and

mortality despite a liberal abortion law and government supported abortion services [7–10], provision of MA up to 63 days gestation has already been extended to include nurses and auxiliary nurse midwives trained as birth attendants, in addition to doctors [11, 12]. We evaluated the ability of a cadre of minimally-trained female community health volunteers (FCHVs) in Nepal and literate Nepali women to determine the success of MA with mifepristone and misoprostol using a checklist. Their assessments were compared to those made by comprehensive abortion care (CAC) trained providers using Nepal's current standard of care.

* Correspondence: andersenk@ipas.org
[1]Ipas, 300 Market Street, Suite 200, Chapel Hill, NC 27516, USA

Methods

This study was conducted in two phases. In the previously published first phase, women and FCHVs used a toolkit consisting of a modified gestational dating wheel and a nine-point checklist of MA contraindications or cautions to assess women's eligibility for MA, compared to experienced CAC-providers using standard of care in Nepal [13]. In the second phase, women and FCHVs used an eight-point checklist to determine if MA had been successful. For purposes of our study, success is defined as MA requiring no additional intervention, such as uterine aspiration or a repeat dose of misoprostol. Women and FCHV responses were compared to experienced CAC-providers. We report the second, success phase of the study in this paper.

Study facilities

Seven study facilities, public and NGO, in six Nepali districts were purposively selected based on adequate abortion caseload to meet sample size requirements. All study facilities were located in urban centers, drawing patients from the surrounding rural areas.

Study participants

Three thousand one hundred thirty-one literate women ≥16 years old (the age of consent in Nepal), with a positive pregnancy test, seeking safe abortion at a study facility were enrolled in the phase one, eligibility portion of this study. After completing the phase one study procedures, women received abortion by the method of her choice (uterine aspiration or MA with mifepristone and misoprostol) according to Nepali standard of care. All 1517 women who chose MA were invited to participate in the second, success phase of the study. These women were invited to return for a follow-up visit and evaluation in 2 weeks. Women received 400 Nepali rupees (approximately $5.20) and a month-supply of iron tablets for their participation in the success study. Those who agreed to participate in the success study but did not return for their 2-week follow-up visit were contacted by phone up to three times to encourage a return visit.

Nepal's FCHVs receive a total of 18 days of training in maternal and child health, including training in early pregnancy identification with urine pregnancy tests; they are a key referral link in their communities to antenatal care, safe abortion, or family planning as appropriate [14]. Literate FCHVs were selected randomly from the six study districts and were posted at each study facility for one to 2 weeks during data collection. Participating FCHVs received a stipend of 3000 Nepali rupees (approximately $39) per week.

CAC-providers included doctors and staff nurses trained and registered with the Nepal Ministry of Health to provide CAC with manual vacuum aspiration and MA. All providers at the included facilities were eligible to participate.

All participants provided written, informed consent to participate.

Sample size

Previous research indicates that > 90% of women receiving MA services will have a successful MA, and that the success checklist will have a 90% specificity to identify an unsuccessful MA [15]. We assumed a precision of 0.1 for both sensitivity (true positive rate) and specificity (true negative rate) of MA success determination, and a two-sided level of significance (α) of 0.5. Our calculated minimum sample size was 351 women. We continued to recruit beyond our minimum sample size until we had a minimum of 100 women for each public and 50 women for each private facility, and until we had a minimum of 50 women in each gestational age category, by weeks.

Success checklist

The success checklist (Fig. 1), adapted from Perriera et al. [16], is a series of eight questions assessing bleeding, cramping, and other symptoms following use of MA drugs, designed to determine if women have a continuing pregnancy or ongoing bleeding that would suggest the need for further care from a trained provider. In the real-world setting, if a woman or FCHV marks an answer in a red box on the checklist, the woman would be advised her abortion may not have been successful, and would be prompted to see a health care provider. If no red boxes are marked, the checklist indicates that the woman's abortion was successful.

We tested the checklist for construct validity, and pretested it with Nepali women, FCHVs and CAC-providers. We edited the checklist following each round of pretesting; pretesting was considered complete when no further substantive comments were elicited.

Study procedures

We collected data from September 2013 to March 2014. Each woman received a brief verbal orientation to the checklist, after which she used the checklist to self-determine whether or not her abortion had been successful. Demographic information and the woman's assessment of the ease of use of the checklist were also collected. Women's determinations of abortion success were sealed, and women were asked to not share their responses with the FCHV or CAC-provider they would subsequently meet. Next, an FCHV assessed the woman's MA success using the checklist; her assessment was also sealed. Finally, a CAC-provider used local standard of care (typically a history and physical examination, with ultrasound available only when indicated) to assess abortion

Use this checklist about two weeks after you've taken the first medical abortion tablet to assess whether or not you need additional medical care.

Success Checklist
Answer each question below by putting a tick in the appropriate box.

		Yes	No
1	Did you have cramping after you took all the medical abortion tablets?		
2	Did you have bleeding at least as heavy as your usual period after you took all the medical abortion tablets?		
3	Did you pass blood clots or tissue after you took all the medical abortion tablets?		
4	Have your pregnancy symptoms gone away?		
5	Do you think you are still pregnant?		
6	Are you having heavy bleeding today?		
7	Do you have a fever today?		
8	Are you having bad cramping or pain today?		

Success Assessment
If you have at least one tick in the red area, see a health care provider. You may still be pregnant or need additional medical care.
If you do not have any ticks in the red area, your medical abortion was successful. Use contraception to prevent an unwanted pregnancy.

Fig. 1 MA success checklist. The user answers each question. If any answer is in a red area, the woman may require additional care and should be seen by a provider

success. CAC-providers completed a brief questionnaire documenting their findings.

The Nepal Health Research Council and the Allendale Institutional Review Board in the United States reviewed this study for ethical considerations.

Data analysis

To assess how well participants understood the success checklist, information entered into the checklist by women and FCHVs was compared to how they ultimately interpreted that information. The assessments of MA success made by women and by FCHVs were compared to those made by CAC-providers using 2×2 tables. Diagnostic test statistics (positive predictive value [PPV], negative predictive value [NPV], sensitivity [Sn] and specificity [Sp]) where women/FCHVs correctly identifying success was considered a positive test were generated.

Results

Over three-quarters (76%) of the 1517 women enrolled in the phase one, eligibility portion of the study and who chose MA continued into the phase two, success portion of the study ($n = 1153$, Table 1). Women who continued into the success portion of the study were more likely to be married than women who did not participate in the second phase (97% vs 94%, $p = 0.008$); no other significant demographic differences were found (data not shown).

Comprehension and ease of use of success checklist

Overall, 74% of women accurately interpreted their responses on the success checklist. All but two women with no red items marked ($n = 698$ of 700, 99.7%) correctly interpreted their checklist result as 'successful'. However, of the 453 women who marked a red item, 295 (65%) did not identify that they may require additional care.

FCHVs interpreted the checklist correctly 100% of the time when no red boxes were marked as indicating a successful abortion, and misidentified women with a red box marked 59% of the time.

All women and FCHVs (100%) reported that the success checklist was easy to use. All women (100%) reported the checklist instructions were clear (yes/no), and

Table 1 Participant sociodemographic data

	Participants $n = 1153$
Age in years, mean (SD)	27.6 (5.4)
Pregnancies, mean (SD)	2.8 (1.3)
Some secondary school or higher, n (%)	1035 (90)
Married, n (%)	1113 (97)
Caste/Ethnicity, n (%)	
Disadvantaged Groups	351 (30)
Relatively Advantaged	190 (16)
Upper Caste Groups	612 (53)
Literacy, n (%)	1153 (100)

SD standard deviation
Disadvantaged groups includes dalit, disadvantaged janajaties, disadvantaged non-dalit Terai caste groups, and religious minorities

100% of FCHVs reported that the checklist instructions were either 'very clear' (54%) or 'somewhat clear' (46%).

MA success assessment among women, FCHVs, and CAC-providers

When assessing MA success, women and providers agreed 85% of the time (Table 2); PPV was 90% (95% CI 88, 92). Providers identified 176 women (15%) as potentially requiring additional care. Of these, 84 (7%) received observation only; the remaining 92 (8%) received either uterine aspiration ($n = 84$, 7%) or readministration of medications (n = 8, 0.7%). Of the 92 women who required additional intervention, 64% ($n = 59$, Table 3) of women themselves perceived that additional care was needed using the success checklist. Of the 33 women who believed that their abortion was successful, six had marked a red item on the checklist. These women misinterpreted their response to the success checklist and should have identified that they needed additional care. The remaining 27 women (2% overall) had no red items marked, and their need for additional care would have been missed if using the checklist alone to determine abortion success.

Agreement for MA success between FCHVs and CAC-providers was 82%; PPV was 90% (95% CI 88, 92). Of the 92 women requiring additional intervention, FCHVs identified 61% ($n = 56$). FCHVs incorrectly identified four women who had a red item marked on the Success Checklist as having had a successful abortion; 32 women (3% overall) had no red items marked and their need for additional care would have been missed if the checklist alone was used.

Discussion

We found that, when compared to CAC-trained providers using standard of care in Nepal to assess MA success, women using the success checklist agreed with CAC-providers 85% of the time, with a PPV of 90%. However these results must be interpreted with caution, given the significant difficulty that women had using the checklist. Although women reliably interpreted the checklist when no red items were marked (99.7%), more than half of the women who marked a red item (65%) did not realize they might need additional care, and should seek follow-up from a CAC-provider; FCHV results were similar. This is in contrast to earlier evidence indicating that women can accurately determine when their MA is successful using symptom-related questions. Indeed, in studies comparing women's assessments of expulsion to those made by clinicians [16–19] and ultrasound [18], particularly when standardized questions are used [15, 16, 19], women have repeatedly proven themselves to be nearly as accurate as both. Despite their demonstrated ability to read, it is likely that women and FCHVs in our study did not understand either the checklist instructions, or the checklist items themselves. Indeed, 'literacy' in Nepal, where 43% of the population is illiterate [20], often indicates the ability to read and write at a basic level; overall reading comprehension in such a population is likely to be more limited and may have affected our findings. This may be different from 'literacy' in the highly literate industrialized nations (United States [14, 15], Scotland [18]) where earlier studies have been conducted. It is also possible that women and FCHVs, regardless of literacy level, required additional orientation to our success checklist to use it effectively. A recent study [21] evaluating the ability of community health workers in Ethiopia, India and South Africa to assess women's eligibility for MA using a similar style of checklist oriented the workers to the checklist in a multi-day workshop. In contrast, the women and FCHVs in our study received a brief introduction,

Table 2 Women's ($n = 1153$) and FCHVs' ($n = 159$) assessments of MA success using the checklist are compared to CAC providers' ($n = 47$) determinations based on standard of care

	Provider assessment MA successful		Provider assessment additional care needed		Total		PPV	NPV	Sn	Sp
	n	%[a]	n	%[a]	n	%[a]	% (95%, CI)	% (95% CI)	% (95% CI)	% (95% CI)
Women's Assessment							90 (88, 92)	49 (41, 57)	92 (90, 93)	44 (36, 51)
MA successful	894	78	99	9	993	86				
Additional care needed	81	7	77	7	158	14				
Total	975	85	176	15	1151[b]	100				
FCHVs' Assessment							90 (88, 92)	41 (34, 49)	89 (87, 91)	44 (36, 51)
MA successful	868	75	99	9	967	84				
Additional care neded	109	9	77	7	186	16				
Total	977	85	176	15	1153	100				

PPV positive predictive value, *NPV* negative predictive value, *Sn* sensitivity, *Sp* specificity
[a]Numbers may not add up to 100% due to rounding
[b]2 women missing self-assessment of success

Table 3 Women's and FCHVs' assessments of MA success using the success checklist for the 92 women that CAC-providers determined required additional intervention to complete their abortion (either uterine aspiration or readministration of medications)

	Women receiving additional intervention	
	n	Overall %
Women's Assessment		
MA Successful	33	3
Additional care needed	59	5
Total	92	8
FCHVs' Assessment		
MA Successful	36	3
Additional care needed	56	5
Total	92	8

lasting only several minutes, to the checklist. Increasing comprehension of instructions and questions, reformatting of the checklist, moving away from the red = stop/green = go coloring scheme, which may not be suggestive enough in this setting, and use of newer technologies, such as a tablet computer, may make the checklist easier to use.

A small proportion of women who believed they had successful abortions based on the success checklist (2% of women's assessments and 3% of FCHV's assessments) were determined by CAC-providers to require additional intervention to complete their abortions. These women had marked no red items on their checklists. While it is possible that the checklist did not appropriately capture these as failures, it is also possible that the CAC-providers in our study were more conservative than expected in determining abortion success. The CAC-providers in our study did not utilize the success checklist when evaluating a patient, and instead relied on their own clinical practice and local standard of care. We found that CAC-providers in our study were more likely to provide additional treatment to women (8% of women received uterine evacuation with MVA or readministration of medications) than observed in other large MA efficacy trials up to 63 days gestation, where intervention rates are typically between 2 and 3% [22–24]. Given that an MA follow-up visit is optional in Nepal, it is possible that those women who returned for follow-up in our study were more likely to be experiencing complications, or were more anxious about experiencing complications. It is also possible, given that MA follow-up is not routine in Nepal, that CAC-providers may have been more inclined to intervene in women returning for interim care, a phenomenon that has been suggested in other studies [25]. We did not retrain the CAC-providers included in this study prior to study inception, which may

have led them to be more conservative when determining MA success than currently recommended practice. As we considered CAC-providers to be the 'gold standard' for determining success, this is a limitation of our study.

More difficult than determining MA success, both for women and clinicians, has been the identification of those few MA cases where pregnancy is ongoing. As continuing pregnancy after MA is rare, few studies are adequately powered to assess this outcome [26], however a case-control study by Jackson et al. (2012) comparing 53 women with ongoing pregnancies following medical abortion to 53 controls with successful abortions, determined that up to a third of ongoing pregnancies are missed when women's symptoms alone are used to assess completion [27]. While this would affect only a small absolute number of women, given potential teratogenicity of MA drugs and the need for timely uterine evacuation in these cases, the authors suggest that an objective measure of success, such as a urine pregnancy test, is still needed, in addition to report of women's symptoms after MA drug use. Studies in both high [15] and low-resource settings [25] have explored combining a low sensitivity pregnancy test with women's assessment of symptoms to determine MA success and identify rare, unrecognized continuing pregnancies. We did not include such a measure in this study, but this could be a consideration for future work.

Importantly, because of the high success rate of MA with mifepristone and misoprostol, WHO does not recommend routine follow-up after MA using the combined regimen. As provision of MA continues to be expanded to cadres of health care providers with less training [6], and perhaps even to women themselves, a reliable method of determining pregnancy expulsion and rare ongoing pregnancies, will be valuable.

Conclusions
Although a promising strategy, both literate women and a cadre of minimally trained community health volunteers in Nepal had difficulty correctly using a symptom checklist to determine the success of MA. Refinement of such a tool, particularly for low literacy settings, is needed before widespread use.

Abbreviations
CAC: Comprehensive abortion care; CI: Confidence interval; FCHV: Female community health volunteer; MA: Medical abortion; NGO: Non-governmental organization; NPV: Negative predictive value; PPV: Positive predictive value; Sn: Sensitivity; Sp: Specificity

Acknolwedgements
The authors wish to thank Alyson Hyman and Alexandra Teixiera for their early contributions to the conceptualization of this study.

Funding
This study was funded through the operating budget of IPAS; no donors were involved in the analysis or interpretation of findings.

Authors' contributions
KA led study design, analysis, interpretation and writing; MF contributed to design, analysis and interpretation; IB contributed to design, analysis and writing; SN contributed to design, implementation, and interpretation; VA contributed to analysis; SS contributed to design, implementation and interpretation; EJ contributed to analysis, interpretation and writing; all co-authors reviewed and approved the final manuscript.

Authors information
At the time of this study, Mary Fjerstad, Indira Basnett, and Sharad Sharma were all on staff with Ipas.

Competing interests
The authors declare that they have no competing interests.

Author details
[1]Ipas, 300 Market Street, Suite 200, Chapel Hill, NC 27516, USA. [2]San Diego, CA, USA. [3]Kathmandu, Nepal. [4]Valley Research Group (VaRG), Lalitpur, Nepal. [5]Los Angeles, CA, USA.

References
1. World Health Organisation Task Force on Post-ovulatory Methods of Fertility Regulation. Termination of pregnancy with reduced doses of mifepristone. BMJ. 1993;307(6903):532–7.
2. UK Multicentre Trial. The efficacy and tolerance of mifepristone and prostaglandin in first trimester termination of pregnancy. Br J Obstet Gynaecol 1990, 97(6):480–6.
3. Tang OS, Chan CCW, Ng EHY, Lee SWH, Ho PC. A prospective, randomized, placebo-controlled trial on the use of mifepristone with sublingual or vaginal misoprostol for medical abortions of less than 9 weeks gestation. Hum Reprod. 2003;18(11):2315–8.
4. Ashok PW, Penney GC, Flett GM, Templeton A. An effective regimen for early medical abortion: a report of 2000 consecutive cases. Hum Reprod. 1998;13(1O):2962–5.
5. Winikoff B, Dzuba IG, Chong E, Goldberg AB, Lichtenberg ES, Ball C, Dean G, Sacks D, Crowden WA, Swica Y. Extending outpatient medical abortion services through 70 days of gestational age. Obstet Gynecol. 2012;120(5):1070–6.
6. World Health Organization. Health worker roles in providing safe abortion care and post abortion contraception. Geneva: World Health Organization; 2015.
7. World Health Organization. Trends in maternal mortality: 1990 to 2010. In: WHO, UNICEF, UNFPA and the World Bank estimates. Geneva: WHO Press; 2012.
8. Samandari G, Wolf M, Basnett I, Hyman A, Andersen K. Implementation of legal abortion in Nepal: a model for rapid scale-up of high-quality care. Reprod Health. 2012;9(7):1742–4755.
9. Suvedi BK, Pradhan A, Barnett S, Puri M, Chitrakar SR, Poudel P, Sharma S, Hulton L. Nepal maternal mortality and morbidity study 2008/2009: summary of preliminary findings. Ministry of Health: Kathmandu; 2009.
10. Bhandari A, Gordon M, Shakya G. Reducing maternal mortality in Nepal. BJOG. 2011;2:26–30.
11. KC NP, Basnett I, Sharma SK, Bhusal CL, Parajuli RR, Andersen KL. Increasing access to safe abortion services through auxiliary nurse midwives trained as skilled birth attendants. Kathmandu Univ Med J. 2011;9(36):260–6.
12. Puri M, Tamang A, Shrestha P, Joshi D. The role of auxiliary nurse-midwives and community health volunteers in expanding access to medical abortion in rural Nepal. Reproductive Health Matters. 2014;22(Supplement 44):94–103.
13. Andersen K, Fjerstad M, Basnett I, Neupane S, Acre V, Sharma SK, Jackson E. Determination of medical abortion eligibility by women and community health volunteers in Nepal: a toolkit evaluation. PLoS One. 2017;12(9):e0178248.
14. Andersen K, Singh A, Shrestha MK, Shah M, Pearson E, Hessini L. Early pregnancy detection by female community health volunteers in Nepal facilitated referral for appropriate reproductive health services. Glob Health Sci Pract. 2013;1(3):372–81.
15. Clark W, Bracken H, Tanehaus J, Schweikert S, Lichtenberg S, Winikoff B. Alternative to a routine follow-up visit for early medical abortion. Obstet Gynecol. 2010;115(2):264–72.
16. Perriera LK, Reeves MF, Chen BA, Hohmann HL, Hayes J, Creinin MD. Feasibility of telephone follow-up after medical abortion. Contraception. 2010;81(2):143–9.
17. Bracken H, Clark W, Lichtenberg ES, Schweikert SM, Tanenhaus J, Barajas A, Alpert L, Winikoff B. Alternatives to routine ultrasound for eligibility assessment prior to early termination of pregnancy with mifepristone-misoprostol. BJOG. 2011;118(1):17–23.
18. Rossi B, Creinin MD, Meyn LA. Ability of the clinician and patient to predict the outcome of mifepristone and misoprostol medical abortion. Contraception. 2004;70(4):313–7.
19. Cameron ST, Glasier A, Dewart H, Johnstone A, Burnside A. Telephone follow-up and self-performed urine pregnancy testing after early medical abortion: a service evaluation. Contraception. 2012;86(1):67–73.
20. State of the World's Children 2015 Country Statistical Information [http://www.unicef.org/infobycountry/nepal_nepal_statistics.html]
21. Johnston HB, Ganatra B, Nguyen MH, Habib N, Afework MF, Harries J, Iyengar K, Moodley J, Lema HY, Constant D, et al. Accuracy of assessment of eligibility for early medical abortion by community health Workers in Ethiopia, India and South Africa. PloS one. 2016;11(1):e0146305.
22. Goldstone P, Michelson J, Williamson E. Early medical abortion using low-dose mifepristone followed by buccal misoprostol: a large Australian observational study. Med J Aust. 2012;197(5):282–6.
23. Gatter M, Cleland K, Nucatola DL. Efficacy and safety of medical abortion using mifepristone and buccal misoprostol through 63 days. Contraception. 2015;91(4):269–73.
24. Chen MJ, Creinin MD. Mifepristone with buccal misoprostol for medical abortion: a systematic review. Obstet Gynecol. 2015;126(1):12–21.
25. Iyengar K, Paul M, Iyengar SD, Klingberg-Allvin M, Essen B, Bring J, Germzell-Danielsson K. Self-assessment of the outcome of early medical abortion versus clinic follow-up in India: a randomised, controlled, non-inferiority trial. Lancet Glob Health. 2015;3(9):e537–3545.
26. Grossman D, Grindlay K. Alternatives to ultrasound for follow-up after medication abortion: a systematic review. Contraception. 2011;83(6):504–10.
27. Jackson AV, Dayananda I, Fortin JM, Fitzmaurice G, Goldberg AB. Can women accurately assess the outcome of medical abortion based on symptoms alone? Contraception. 2012;85(2):192–7.

10

Measurement error of mean sac diameter and crown-rump length among pregnant women at Mulago hospital, Uganda

Sam Ali[1,2]* ID, Rosemary Kusaba Byanyima[3], Sam Ononge[4], Jerry Ictho[1], Jean Nyamwiza[1],
Emmanuel Lako Ernesto Loro[1], John Mukisa[1], Angella Musewa[1], Annet Nalutaaya[1], Ronald Ssenyonga[1],
Ismael Kawooya[1], Benjamin Temper[1], Achilles Katamba[1,5], Joan Kalyango[1,6] and Charles Karamagi[1,7]

Abstract

Background: Ultrasonography is essential in the prenatal diagnosis and care for the pregnant mothers. However, the measurements obtained often contain a small percentage of unavoidable error that may have serious clinical implications if substantial. We therefore evaluated the level of intra and inter-observer error in measuring mean sac diameter (MSD) and crown-rump length (CRL) in women between 6 and 10 weeks' gestation at Mulago hospital.

Methods: This was a cross-sectional study conducted from January to March 2016. We enrolled 56 women with an intrauterine single viable embryo. The women were scanned using a transvaginal (TVS) technique by two observers who were blinded of each other's measurements. Each observer measured the CRL twice and the MSD once for each woman. Intra-class correlation coefficients (ICCs), 95% limits of agreement (LOA) and technical error of measurement (TEM) were used for analysis.

Results: Intra-observer ICCs for CRL measurements were 0.995 and 0.993 while inter-observer ICCs were 0.988 for CRL and 0.955 for MSD measurements. Intra-observer 95% LOA for CRL were ± 2.04 mm and ± 1.66 mm. Inter-observer LOA were ± 2.35 mm for CRL and ± 4.87 mm for MSD. The intra-observer relative TEM for CRL were 4.62% and 3.70% whereas inter-observer relative TEM were 5.88% and 5.93% for CRL and MSD respectively.

Conclusions: Intra- and inter-observer error of CRL and MSD measurements among pregnant women at Mulago hospital were acceptable. This implies that at Mulago hospital, the error in pregnancy dating is within acceptable margins of ±3 days in first trimester, and the CRL and MSD cut offs of ≥7 mm and ≥ 25 mm respectively are fit for diagnosis of miscarriage on TVS. These findings should be extrapolated to the whole country with caution. Sonographers can achieve acceptable and comparable diagnostic accuracy levels of MSD and CLR measurements with proper training and adherence to practice guidelines.

Keywords: Mean sac diameter, Crown-rump length, Measurement error

Background

The advent of ultrasonography and its swift advances has in the recent years significantly improved prenatal diagnosis and care globally [1, 2]. In the early stages of a pregnancy, ultrasound is essential in predicting the risk of adverse pregnancy outcomes such as aneuploidy, stillbirth, pre-eclampsia and the possibility of abnormal cord insertion visualization [3, 4]. It is also used for fetal anatomic surveys during a second-trimester scan to detect fetal malformations, monitoring fetal growth in utero and in pregnancy dating [5–7]. Therefore, given the essential role of ultrasonography in clinical decision making, it is imperative that sonographic parameters obtained are accurate and precise [8]. However, a small percentage of error in measurements or incompleteness of the information obtained is at times unavoidable. [9, 10]. In first trimester, measurement error of CRL and MSD has been reported

* Correspondence: alisambecker@gmail.com
[1]Clinical Epidemiology Unit, Makerere University College of Health Sciences, P.O. Box 7072, Kampala, Uganda
[2]Department of Radiology, UMC Victoria Hospital Bukoto, P.O. Box 72587, Kampala, Uganda

to be ±18.78% limits of agreement in United Kingdom (UK) [11]. If significant, this error has implications on the accuracy of estimates of the fetal gestation age obtained. And if not taken into account at MSD or CRL cut offs used for the diagnosis of miscarriage, some normal pregnancies may be erroneously deemed non-viable [11]. Consequently, this could lead to inadvertent termination of viable embryos and immense physical and emotional harm to the patient [11–13].

The unavoidable measurement error or incompleteness in information obtained during an ultrasound examination is related to various factors including but not limited to the skill of the sonographer and their level of training; technical factors related to the patient such as body habitus; the quality of the machine; fetal position; and the duration of the examination [14]. As in other low resourced settings, Uganda's healthcare system faces severe shortage of imaging experts [15–17]. This results in high workload which affects the performance and efficiency of health workers. In addition, majority of the low-income countries lack adequate resources to acquire high-end ultrasound machines with very good spatial resolution [16, 18]. With low spatial resolution machines, images appear blurred or enlarged, and due to this effect, calipers are placed beyond or may not cover the true dimensions leading to errors in measurements [19]. Errors arising from variation between machines have been found to be substantial [19]. The Ministry of Health Standards on Diagnostic Imaging and Therapeutic Radiology in Uganda recommends the use of CRL cut off of 5 mm to diagnose a miscarriage yet this has changed following recommendation by recent studies. The use of the outdated CRL cut off of 5 mm increases the risk of misdiagnosing normal pregnancies. This practice guidelines does not also provide clear guidance for measurement of MSD [20]. This may lead to significant variations in MSD measurements.

The reliability of CRL and MSD measurements in first trimester using modern ultrasound equipment has not been adequately explored in the low developed countries like in the developed nations [11, 19, 21]. This study sought to understand the level of intra- and inter-observer variability in measuring MSD and CRL in women between 6 and 10 weeks' gestation at Mulago National Referral Hospital.

Methods

This was a cross-sectional study conducted on pregnant women at the Department of Obstetrics and Gynecology, Mulago National Referral Hospital, Uganda from January to March 2016. We consecutively enrolled women with a single viable intrauterine embryo from 6 to 10 weeks of gestation and not bleeding. The first observer examined a woman who had consented, to assess if they were eligible for inclusion in this study. The second observer then further examined the eligible participant. The two observers examined each woman at the same point in time. Both observers used a Phillips Envisor (PHILIPS, USA, 2009) with a 7.5 MHz transvaginal probe for B-imaging to do all examinations.

For each examined participant, the observers took CRL measurements twice and MSD measurements once, and in between the two CRL measurements, the observers examined the ovaries and uterus. These measurements were obtained as described in the WHO Manual of diagnostic ultrasound, Volume 2 [5] (Fig. 1). To archive blinding, the measurements of the first observer were removed from the machine before the second observer was allowed to enter the examination room. The same two sonographers that examined all the women had good training in obstetric sonography and at least five years of experience in fetal ultrasound. A female nurse or professional was always brought into the examination room for all the transvaginal ultrasound scans done by the male sonographer to make the women feel comfortable and safe.

Statistical issues
Sample size
The sample size calculations were based on the formula below by considering 95% Limits of agreement (LOA) of ±18.78% as the cut off for clinical significance [11, 22, 23]. In the formula, n = desired sample size and s = standard deviation of the differences in CRL or MSD measurements [24].

$$1.96 \sqrt{\left[\frac{3s^2}{n}\right]} = \text{Desired confidence interval of limits of agreement [24]}.$$

Statistical analysis
Data was double entered and validated in Epidata version 3.1 to identify inconsistent entries before being exported to SPSS Version 19.0 for analysis. Scatterplots of paired sets of measurements created with the line of equality were visually assessed for potential systematic errors in the intra and inter-observer measurements. A paired t-test at 0.05 set level of significance was used to check if the paired sets of measurements were significantly different, to rule out any systematic errors in the measurements.

To assess the strength of the absolute agreement within and between observers, the intraclass correlation coefficient (ICC) was computed based on a two-way random effects model [24–26]. Normality, constant mean and variance assumptions for LOA were fulfilled. Therefore, the difference between paired sets of measurements were plotted against their mean in Bland–Altman plots

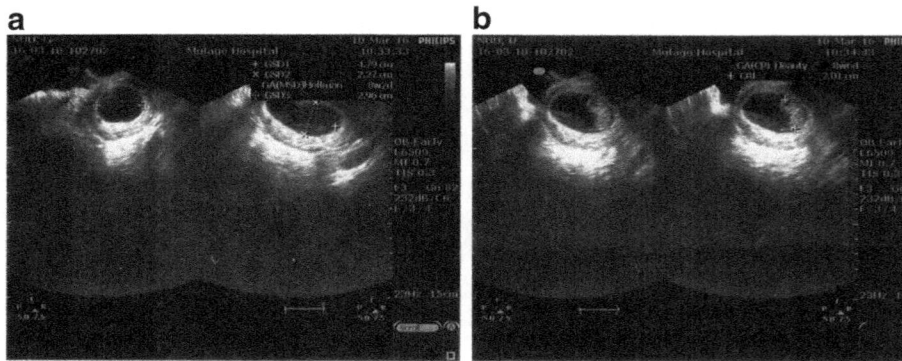

Fig. 1 a Measurement of mean sac diameter at 8 weeks' gestational age using transvaginal ultrasound scan. Gestational sac diameter was obtained by placing the calipers inner-to-inner on the sac wall, excluding the surrounding echogenic rim of tissue. MSD was calculated by first adding the longitudinal, anteroposterior and transverse dimensions of the chorionic cavity. Thereafter, the sum of the three measurements was divided by three. **b** Measurement of crown–rump length with transvaginal ultrasound at 8 weeks' gestational age. CRL was measured as the maximal straight-line length of the embryo, obtained along its longitudinal axis, with the embryo neither too flexed nor too extended

to assess the level of clinical agreement within and between the observers. The lack of agreement between measurements or observers becomes relevant only when the LOAs are wider than what is clinically acceptable [27, 28]. Technical error of measurements (TEM) within and between observers were calculated by taking the square root of the sum of the squares of the differences of the paired sets of measurements divided by twice the total number of participants measured.

Results

We screened 71 pregnant women suspected to be in first trimester and enrolled 56 in this study. Of the 15 women excluded from the study, one had a ruptured ectopic pregnancy; three had empty gestation sacs; six were more than 10 weeks of gestation pregnant; three were not pregnant and two declined to be examined after consenting. The mean (SD) maternal age was 25.8 (4.33) and mean (SD) gestation age was 7.5 (1.14) (Table 1).

Intra-observer ICCs were 0.993 and 0.995 for CRL measurements while inter-observer ICCs were 0.988 for CRL and 0.955 for MSD measurements (Table 2). Intra-observer 95% LOAs for CRL were ± 2.04 mm (Fig. 2) and ± 1.66 mm (Fig. 3). Inter-observer 95% LOAs were ± 2.35 mm (Fig. 4) for CRL and ± 4.87 mm for MSD (Fig. 5). Intra-observer relative TEM for CRL were 4.62% and 3.70%, while inter-observer relative TEM were 5.88% for CRL and 5.93% for MSD measurements respectively (Table 3).

Discussion

This study found a strong observer agreement with intra- and inter-observer ICCs ≥0.955 and this is similar to findings from other studies [29, 30]. Inter-observer 95% limits of agreement for MSD and CRL measurements were also

in tandem with findings from other studies [11]. However, intra-observer 95% limits of agreements for CRL measurements were about 2% higher than findings reported in a study by Pexters and colleagues [11]. They reported intra-observer limits of agreement of CRL of ±8.91 and ± 11.37% [11]. The minor differences observed could be attributed to the differences in settings such as observers, patient overload and the finite consistency and read-out

Table 1 Demographic characteristics of women between 6 and 10 weeks of gestation in Mulago Hospital, Kampala, 2016

Variable	Frequency (N = 56)	Percentage (%)
Age		
Mean(SD*)	25.8 (4.33)	
Gravidity		
Median (IQR*)	3 (1.5,4)	
Parity		
Median (IQR*)	1 (0,2)	
Number of previous abortions		
Median (IQR*)	0 (0,1)	
Weight		
Median (IQR*)	54 (50.5,61.0)	
Height		
Median (IQR*)	156.3 (154.0,160.1)	
Gestation age		
Mean (SD*)	7.5 (1.14)	
Body Mass Index		
Underweight (< 18.5)	5	8.9
Normal (18.5–24.9)	39	69.7
Overweight (25.0–29.9)	7	12.5
Obesity (≥ 30.0)	5	8.9

*SD standard deviation, *IQR interquartile range

Table 2 The intraclass correlation coefficients of CRL and MSD measurements of women between 6 and 10 weeks of gestation in Mulago Hospital, Kampala, 2016

Paired set of measurements	ICC*	95% CI*
Intra-observer variation (CRL*)		
Observer 1	0.993	(0.988, 0.996)
Observer 2	0.995	(0.992, 0.997)
Inter-observer variation		
CRL*	0.988	(0.980, 0.993)
MSD*	0.955	(0.924, 0.973)

*CI confidence interval, *ICC Intraclass correlation coefficient, *CRL Crown-rump length, *MSD Mean sac diameter

precision of the instrument used to measure the structures [9]. The study by Pexters et al. used an ultrasound machine with a 6–12-MHz transvaginal transducer for B-mode imaging while our machine was equipped with a 7.5-MHz probe [11]. Intra-observer inconsistencies highlight a lack of clear or uniform criteria of measurement and interpretation of embryonic landmarks [31]. Detailed instructions in locating landmarks are necessary to minimize intra- and inter-observer technique difference [31]. The majority of our study participants were between 6 to 7 weeks of gestation. At this stage, reproducibility of CRL measurements is better than it is later in the first trimester because of increased embryonic mobility at about 8 weeks' gestation and above [7]. This could also explain the optimal reliability observed in this study. The relative TEM observed were within clinically acceptable variability

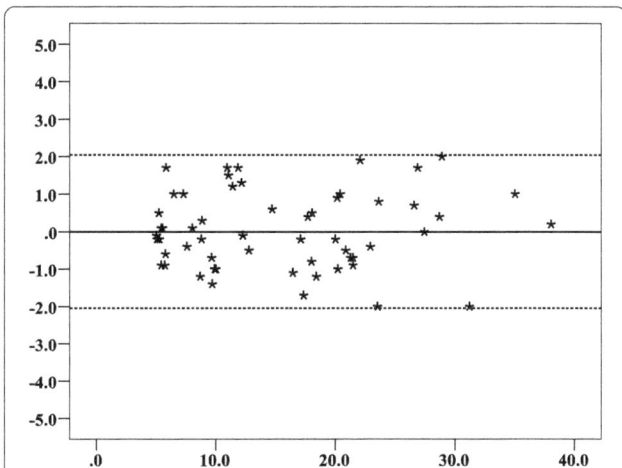

Fig. 3 Bland–Altman plots with 95% limits of agreement showing intra-observer agreement of crown–rump length measurements of observer 2. Y axis: Difference in CRL (mm). Y axis scale = 1. From − 5, − 4, − 3, − 2, − 1, 0, 1, 2, 3, 4, to 5. X axis: Mean of first and second CRL measurements of observer 2 (mm). X axis scale = 10. Start and end point: 0, 10, 20, 30, 40. ———— Reference point where the mean difference between repeated measures is equal to zero. — — — — — The upper and lower limit of the 95% confidence interval of limits of agreement

in the precision of anthropometric measurements of 5.0% and 7.5% for intra-observer and inter-observer variability respectively [10].

The strength in this study is that it utilized an ultrasound machine with a high spatial resolution. We used the best available ultrasound machine in our setting at

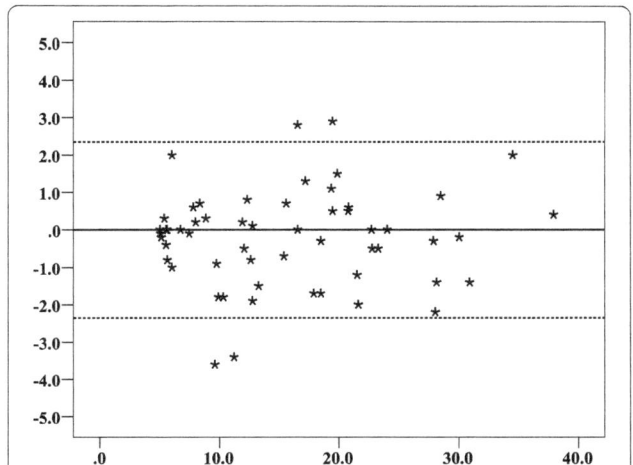

Fig. 2 Bland–Altman plots with 95% limits of agreement showing intra-observer agreement of crown–rump length measurements of observer 1. Y axis title: Difference in CRL (mm). Y axis scale = 1. From − 5, − 4, − 3, − 2, − 1, 0, 1, 2, 3, 4, to 5. X axis: Mean of first and second CRL measurements of observer 1 (mm). X axis scale = 10. Start and end point: 0, 10, 20, 30, 40. ———— Reference point where the mean difference between repeated measures is equal to zero. — — — — — The upper and lower limit of the 95% confidence interval of limits of agreement

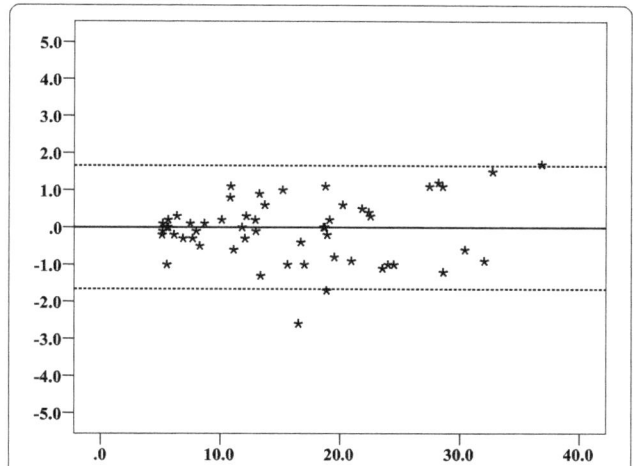

Fig. 4 Bland–Altman plots with 95% limits of agreement showing inter-observer agreement of crown–rump length measurements of observer 1 and observer 2. Y axis: Difference in CRL (mm). Y axis scale = 1. From − 5, − 4, − 3, − 2, − 1, 0, 1, 2, 3, 4, to 5. X axis: Mean of CRL measurements of observers 1 and 2 (mm). X axis scale = 10. Start and end point: 0, 10, 20, 30, 40. ———— Reference point where the mean difference between repeated measures is equal to zero. — — — — — The upper and lower limit of the 95% confidence interval of limits of agreement

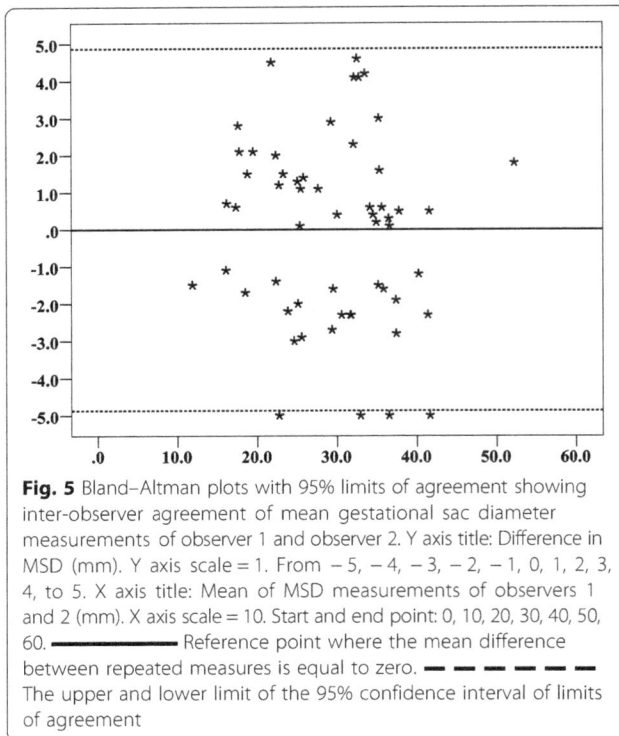

Fig. 5 Bland–Altman plots with 95% limits of agreement showing inter-observer agreement of mean gestational sac diameter measurements of observer 1 and observer 2. Y axis title: Difference in MSD (mm). Y axis scale = 1. From − 5, − 4, − 3, − 2, − 1, 0, 1, 2, 3, 4, to 5. X axis title: Mean of MSD measurements of observers 1 and 2 (mm). X axis scale = 10. Start and end point: 0, 10, 20, 30, 40, 50, 60. ————————— Reference point where the mean difference between repeated measures is equal to zero. ▬ ▬ ▬ ▬ ▬ ▬ The upper and lower limit of the 95% confidence interval of limits of agreement

the time this study was conducted. This allowed a clear delineation of the anatomical landmarks of the embryo and the gestational sac therefore minimizing measurement errors. In using the same machine, we also eliminated errors due to differences in the machines. The short time interval between intra-observer measurements was our major limitation.

The intra- and inter-observer differences in crown-rump length and mean sac diameter relates to the utility of these measurements in first trimester to accurately estimate gestation age and/or make a diagnosis of early pregnancy loss [5]. If the error is substantial, it may have serious clinical consequences. Our study has shown that intra and inter-observer error of CRL and MSD measurements among pregnant women in our

setting were within acceptable limits. Therefore, in relation to the accurate estimation of the gestation age, it is unlikely to result in large differences in days when dating a pregnancy. However, in relation to making a diagnosis of early miscarriage, even a difference of 1 mm can have an impact on the clinical decision [11]. Since our findings are within acceptable limits reported by Pexters et al. and other studies, an MSD cutoff of 25 mm and CRL cutoff of 7 mm for the diagnosis of early miscarriage should be suitable for use in our setting. These cut offs take into account measurement error and were amended as new guidelines [22, 23]. A large multicenter prospective study has demonstrated that these cutoffs are appropriate, with mean gestational sac diameter ≥ 25 mm with an empty sac (364/364 specificity: 100%, 95% confidence interval 99.0% to 100%), embryo with crown-rump length ≥ 7 mm without visible embryo heart activity (110/110 specificity: 100%, 96.7% to 100%) [32].

Conclusions

Intra- and inter-observer error of CRL and MSD measurements among pregnant women at Mulago hospital were within acceptable limits. This provides assurance that the error in the estimates of gestational age obtained are within acceptable margins of ±3 days in first trimester. The CRL and MSD cut offs of ≥7 mm and ≥ 25 mm are therefore reliable for diagnosis of miscarriage on TVS in our setting. However, these results should be generalized to the rest of the country with caution. Such diagnostic accuracy levels are achievable in Mulago hospital because it is a national referral hospital with sophisticated equipment and highly trained personnel. We recommend further studies in the lower health facilities to establish their diagnostic accuracy levels. Sonographers can achieve acceptable and comparable diagnostic accuracy levels of MSD and CLR measurements with proper training, regular audits and adherence to practice guidelines.

Table 3 The technical error of measurements of CRL and MSD of women between 6 and 10 weeks of gestation in Mulago Hospital, Kampala, 2016

Paired set of measurements	Absolute TEM*	VAV*	Relative TEM* (%)	Classification
Intra-observer variation (CRL*)				
Observer 1	0.72	15.54	4.62	Acceptable
Observer 2	0.58	15.81	3.70	Acceptable
Inter-observer variation				
CRL*	0.92	15.66	5.88	Acceptable
MSD*	1.74	29.36	5.93	Acceptable

*TEM Technical error of measurement, *VAV Variable average value, *CRL Crown-rump length, *MSD Mean sac diameter

Abbreviations
CRL: Crown-rump length; ICC: Intra-class correlation coefficient; LOA: Limits of agreement; MSD: Mean sac diameter; TEM: Technical error of measurements

Acknowledgments
The authors wish to thank the mothers and their spouses, Mulago hospital staff, and whoever contributed to the success of this study.

Authors' contributions
SA participated in the conception, design, study implementation, statistical analysis, interpretation of data and drafting of the manuscript. JI, JN, ELEL, JM, AM, AN, RS, IK and BT participated in polishing the study design, analysis and interpretation of data and reviewing the manuscript. RKB, SO, AK, JK and CK participated in study conception, design and critically reviewing the manuscript for important intellectual content. All authors read and approved the final manuscript.

Competing interests
The authors declare that they have no competing interests.

Author details
[1]Clinical Epidemiology Unit, Makerere University College of Health Sciences, P.O. Box 7072, Kampala, Uganda. [2]Department of Radiology, UMC Victoria Hospital Bukoto, P.O. Box 72587, Kampala, Uganda. [3]Department of Radiology, Mulago Hospital Complex, P.O. Box 7051, Kampala, Uganda. [4]Department of Obstetrics and Gynaecology, Makerere University College of Health Sciences, P.O. Box 7072, Kampala, Uganda. [5]Department of Medicine, Makerere University College of Health Sciences, P.O. Box 7072, Kampala, Uganda. [6]Department of Pharmacy, Makerere University College of Health Sciences, P.O. Box 7072, Kampala, Uganda. [7]Department of Pediatrics and Child Health, Makerere University College of Health Sciences, P.O. Box 7072, Kampala, Uganda.

References
1. McNay MB, Fleming JE: Forty years of obstetric ultrasound 1957–1997: from A-scope to three dimensions. Ultrasound Med Bio 1999, 25(1):3–56.
2. Alan B, Goya C, Tunc S, Teke M, Hattapoglu S. Assessment of placental stiffness using acoustic radiation force impulse Elastography in pregnant women with fetal anomalies. Korean J Radiol. 2016;17(2):218–23.
3. Padula F, Laganà A, Vitale S, Mangiafico L, D'Emidio L, Cignini P, Giorlandino M, Gulino F, Capriglione S, Giorlandino C. Ultrasonographic evaluation of placental cord insertion at different gestational ages in low-risk singleton pregnancies: a predictive algorithm. Facts Views Vis ObGyn. 2016;8(1):3.
4. Andrietti S, Carlucci S, Wright A, Wright D, Nicolaides KH. Repeat measurements of uterine artery pulsatility index, mean arterial pressure and serum placental growth factor at 12, 22 and 32 weeks in prediction of pre-eclampsia. Ultrasound Obstet Gynecol. 2017;50(2):221–7.
5. WHO. WHO manual of diagnostic ultrasound, vol. 2. 2nd ed. Geneva: Switzerland World Health Organization: World Health Organization & World Federation for Ultrasound in Medicine and Biology; 2013.
6. Rumack CM: Diagnostic ultrasound, vol. Vol. 1: Elsevier/Mosby; 2011.
7. Chudleigh Trish, Thilaganathan B: obstetric ultrasound: how, why and when, third edn: Churchill Livingstone; 2004.
8. Padula F, Capriglione S, Magliarditi M, De Sole R, Nuara R, Santonocito VC, Teodoro MC, Giorlandino C. Goal-directed junior ultrasound training in quantitative measurement of crown-rump length and fetal nuchal translucency: evaluation of a specific training program in a specialized center for prenatal diagnosis. Eur J Obstet Gynecol Reprod Biol. 2015;186:112–3.
9. Harris EF, Smith RN. Accounting for measurement error: a critical but often overlooked process. Arch Oral Biol. 2009;54(Suppl 1):S107–17.
10. Perini TA, Oliveira GL, Ornellas JD, Oliveira FP. Technical error of measurement in anthropometry. Rev Bras Med Esporte. 2005;11(1):81–5.
11. Pexsters A, Luts J, Van Schoubroeck D, Bottomley C, Van Calster B, Van Huffel S, Abdallah Y, D'Hooghe T, Lees C, Timmerman D, et al. Clinical implications of intra- and interobserver reproducibility of transvaginal sonographic measurement of gestational sac and crown-rump length at 6-9 weeks' gestation. Ultrasound Obstet Gynecol. 2011;38(5):510–5.
12. Bickhaus J, Perry E, Schust DJ. Re-examining sonographic cut-off values for diagnosing early pregnancy loss. Gynecol Obstet (Sunnyvale, Calif). 2013;3(1):141.
13. Lubinga SJ, Levine GA, Jenny AM, Ngonzi J, Mukasa-Kivunike P, Stergachis A, Babigumira JB. Health-related quality of life and social support among women treated for abortion complications in western Uganda. Health Qual Life Outcomes. 2013;11:118.
14. Padula F, Gulino FA, Capriglione S, Giorlandino M, Cignini P, Mastrandrea ML, D'Emidio L, Giorlandino C. What is the rate of incomplete fetal anatomic surveys during a second-trimester scan? J Ultrasound Med. 2015;34(12):2187–91.
15. MoH: Health sector development plan 2015-16_2019–20. In. Ministry of Health, Uganda; 2015.
16. WHO: Medical devices: managing the mismatch: an outcome of the priority medical devices project: World Health Organization; 2010.
17. Kawooya MG. Training for rural radiology and imaging in sub-saharan Africa: addressing the mismatch between services and population. J Clin Imaging Sci. 2012;2:37.
18. Maru DS-R, Schwarz R, Andrews J, Basu S, Sharma A, Moore C. Turning a blind eye: the mobilization of radiology services in resource-poor regions. Glob Health. 2010;6(1):1.
19. Sarris I, Ioannou C, Chamberlain P, Ohuma E, Roseman F, Hoch L, Altman DG, Papageorghiou AT. Intra- and interobserver variability in fetal ultrasound measurements. Ultrasound Obstet Gynecol. 2012;39(3):266–73.
20. MoH: Standards on Diagnostic Imaging and Therapeutic Radiology in Uganda In.: Ministry of Health 2012: 146.
21. Souka AP, Pilalis A, Papastefanou I, Salamalekis G, Kassanos D. Reproducibility study of crown-rump length and biparietal diameter measurements in the first trimester. Prenat Diagn. 2012;32(12):1158–65.
22. Lane BF, Wong-You-Cheong JJ, Javitt MC, Glanc P, Brown DL, Dubinsky T, Harisinghani MG, Harris RD, Khati NJ, Mitchell DG, et al. ACR appropriateness criteria® first trimester bleeding. Ultrasound Quarterly. 2013;29(2):91–6.
23. RCOG: Clinical practice guideline; management of early pregnancy miscarriage. In: Royal College of Obstetricians and Gynaecologists. Edited by Farah Nadine, Nadine Andrea Nugent, Anglim M; 2014.
24. McAlinden C, Khadka J, Pesudovs K. Statistical methods for conducting agreement (comparison of clinical tests) and precision (repeatability or reproducibility) studies in optometry and ophthalmology. Ophthalmic Physiol Opt. 2011;31(4):330–8.
25. Weir JP: Quantifying test-retest reliability using the intraclass correlation coefficient and the SEM. J Strength Cond Res 2005, 19(1):231–240.
26. Shrout PE, Fleiss JL. Intraclass correlations: uses in assessing rater reliability. Psychol Bull. 1979;86(2):420.
27. Bland JM, Altman DG. Applying the right statistics: analyses of measurement studies. Ultrasound Obstet Gynecol. 2003;22(1):85–93.
28. Bland JM, Altman D. Statistical methods for assessing agreement between two methods of clinical measurement. Lancet. 1986;327(8476):307–10.
29. Verburg BO, Mulder PG, Hofman A, Jaddoe VW, Witteman JC, Steegers EA. Intra- and interobserver reproducibility study of early fetal growth parameters. Prenat Diagn. 2008;28(4):323–31.
30. Verwoerd-Dikkeboom CM, Koning AH, Hop WC, Rousian M, Van Der Spek PJ, Exalto N, Steegers EA. Reliability of three-dimensional sonographic measurements in early pregnancy using virtual reality. Ultrasound Obstet Gynecol. 2008;32(7):910–6.
31. Kouchi M, Mochimaru M, Tsuzuki K, Yokoi T. Interobserver errors in anthropometry. J Hum Ergol. 1999;28(1/2):15–24.
32. Preisler J, Kopeika J, Ismail L, Vathanan V, Farren J, Abdallah Y, Battacharjee P, Van Holsbeke C, Bottomley C, Gould D. Defining safe criteria to diagnose miscarriage: prospective observational multicentre study. BMJ. 2015;351:h4579.

11

Prevalence of and risk factors associated with sexual health issues in primiparous women at 6 and 12 months postpartum; a longitudinal prospective cohort study (the MAMMI study)

Deirdre O'Malley[1], Agnes Higgins[2], Cecily Begley[2,3], Deirdre Daly[2] and Valerie Smith[2*] (ID)

Abstract

Background: Many women are not prepared for changes to their sexual health after childbirth. The aim of this paper is to report on the prevalence of and the potential risk factors (pre-pregnancy dyspareunia, mode of birth, perineal trauma and breastfeeding) for sexual health issues (dyspareunia, lack of vaginal lubrication and a loss of interest in sexual activity) at 6 and 12 months postpartum.

Methods: A longitudinal cohort study of 832 first-time mothers who were recruited in early pregnancy and returned postnatal surveys at 3, 6, 9 and 12 months postpartum were assessed for sexual health issues and associated risk factors.

Results: Nearly half of the women (46.3%) reported a lack of interest in sexual activity, 43% experienced a lack of vaginal lubrication and 37.5% of included women had dyspareunia 6 months after birth. On univariate analysis, vacuum-assisted birth, 2nd degree perineal tears, 3rd degree perineal tears and episiotomy were all associated with dyspareunia 6 months postpartum, but, of these only 3rd degree tears, in association with breastfeeding and pre-existing dyspareunia, remained significant on multivariable analysis. Breastfeeding, in combination, with other significant factors, was associated with dyspareunia, a lack of vaginal lubrication and a loss of interest in sexual activity 6 months postpartum, and, dissatisfaction with body image emerged as a significant factor associated with lack of interest in sexual activity at 12 months postpartum. Pre-pregnancy dyspareunia and breastfeeding emerged as common factors associated with all three outcomes of dyspareunia, a lack of vaginal lubrication and a loss of interest in sexual activity at 6 months postpartum.

Conclusion: Breastfeeding and pre-existing dyspareunia are associated with sexual health issues at 6 months postpartum. Pre-existing dyspareunia is associated with a lack of vaginal lubrication at 12 months postpartum and breastfeeding is associated with dissatisfaction with body image. Preparing women and their partners during the antenatal period and advising on simple measures, such as use of lubrication to avoid or minimise sexual health issues, could potentially remove stress, anxiety and fears regarding intimacy after birth. Introducing the topic of pre-existing sexual health issues antenatally may facilitate appropriate support, treatment or counselling for women.

Keywords: Sexual health postpartum, Prevalence, Dyspareunia, Sexual activity, Perineal trauma, Breastfeeding, Regression analysis

* Correspondence: smithv1@tcd.ie
[2]School of Nursing and Midwifery, Trinity College Dublin, Dublin, Ireland
Full list of author information is available at the end of the article

Background

Discourse on women's sexual health after birth is gaining momentum across diverse disciplines, for example, midwifery, obstetric, sexology and psychology disciplines [1–5]. This increased interest and body of research in perinatal sexual health, however, is not evidenced in sexual health policy [6, 7] or maternity care policy [8, 9], although data demonstrating that women are not prepared for changes to their sexual health after birth [10], are available. Lack of knowledge and preparation for sexual health issues postpartum can be distressing for women, and their partner, while also negatively impacting on their ability to adapt to their new role as mothers [10–12]. Postpartum sexual health is challenging to theoretically define but cannot be separated from sexuality and sexual function, and is thought to be influenced by labour and birth events [13]. Attributes of good postpartum sexual health include; sexual desire, resumption of sexual intercourse after birth, pain free sex and orgasm. Several studies to date have focused on factors such as timing of resumption of sexual intercourse [4, 14] and frequency of sexual intercourse [15, 16] and are often limited to the first 3 to 6 months postpartum [17–20]. Others, in measuring women's postpartum sexual health tend to do so with instruments not validated for use in a postpartum population; for example, the Female Sexual Function Index [21–23], the Arizona Sexual Experience Scale [24] and the Golombok Rust Inventory of Sexual Satisfaction [25]. Furthermore, health professionals themselves have identified a lack of expertise on advising women about potential changes to sexual health after birth [26]. Studying women's sexual health for a lengthy period of time postpartum, for example, up to 1 year postpartum, from the perspectives of women themselves (i.e. self-report) is paramount so as to gain a deeper understanding of potential sexual health issues affecting women, insight into any issues that may persist or worsen over time and an understanding of factors that are associated with emergent issues. Gaining an understanding of issues can assist healthcare professionals plan healthcare practices or interventions to address these, and, in doing so, positively impact the sexual health of women who give birth.

The Maternal health And Maternal Morbidity in Ireland (MAMMI) study, launched in February 2012 (www.mammi.ie) is a longitudinal cohort study investigating the existence, extent and prevalence of an array of morbidities (mental health issues, sexual health issues, urinary incontinence, faecal incontinence, pelvic girdle pain, etc.) in nulliparous women antenatally and up to 1 year postpartum across three maternity units in Ireland. The survey was launched in the three maternity units on a rolling basis; February 2012 (site 1), September 2013 (site 2) and August 2015 (site 3). Data were collected via self-reported questionnaires in early pregnancy and at 3, 6, 9 and 12 months postpartum, and from hospital records, so that changes over time might be evaluated. Women received the study information, consent form and Survey 1 on their first visit (the booking visit) to the hospital. Those who completed and returned Survey 1 and the consent form were sent Surveys 2 to 5 by post with a stamped addressed envelope provided for return, at 3, 6, 9 and 12 months postpartum, respectively, unless they indicated, during this time, that they wished to withdraw from the study. At time of analysis, a total of 2764 women joined the study, representing 38% of all those who were invited to take part ($n = 7348$) and future plans involve following this cohort of women up to 5 years postpartum.

In this paper we report on the prevalence of sexual health issues (i.e., dyspareunia, lack of vaginal lubrication, a loss of interest in sexual activity) and the potential factors (pre-pregnancy dyspareunia, mode of birth, perineal trauma, and breastfeeding) that might be associated with these at 6 and 12 months postpartum in a cohort of 832 women from one study site (site 1) who completed all 5 MAMMI study surveys between February 2012 and July 2015. Limiting to this site was necessary as data collection and entry in sites 2 and 3 was ongoing at the time of the analysis and complete data were only available from site 1.

Methods

Study design

A longitudinal prospective cohort study was conducted, evaluating sexual health issues self-reported by women, at 6 and 12 months postpartum, recruited to the MAMMI study from one large urban maternity hospital in Ireland. Surveys, providing the study data, were returned between February 2012 and July 2015 (see http://mammi.ie/surveys.php for downloadable copies of the MAMMI surveys).

Sample

Women were eligible to take part if they were nulliparous (no previous live birth or pregnancy ending in stillbirth), aged 18 years or over and had sufficient English to complete the surveys. No additional exclusion criteria were applied. Midwives and midwifery students offered eligible women the study invitation pack at women's first antenatal appointment, which takes place usually between 12 and 16 weeks gestation, and all women who accepted the study information were telephoned within 1–2 weeks of their booking visit. The purpose of this call was to offer women additional information on the study, answer questions, and determine their interest in taking part. Women were regarded as recruited to the study when they returned the completed consent form and Survey 1.

Ethical approval

Ethical approval for the study was granted by the Faculty of Health Sciences Research Ethics Committee, Trinity College Dublin and the Research Ethics Committee of the participating hospital study site.

Data collection and outcomes measures

The MAMMI study surveys are A4 booklets of approximately 60 pages in length, taking 40–50 min to complete. All surveys sought information on sexual health issues, within a discrete survey section, and women's demographics (e.g. age, relationship status, employment status, highest level of education) were additionally collected in Survey 1. The surveys were developed from surveys used in a similar cohort study, the Maternal Health Study, in Melbourne, Australia [27], and were subsequently assessed for face validity (with 15 women), content validity (with 18 experts), tested for reliability using the test-retest method (with 11 women) (Cohen's Kappa co-efficient 0.87 to 1.0), piloted (with a sample of 33 women) and modified accordingly for use in an Irish maternity population with permission from The Maternal Health study team. Specific information that related to sexual health morbidity centred on issues such as the occurrence of a lack of vaginal lubrication, dyspareunia (pain during sexual intercourse), difficulty in reaching orgasm, inability to reach orgasm, vaginal tightness, vaginal looseness and a loss of interest in sexual activity. In Survey 1 women were asked to report on these symptoms, if any, in the previous 12 months and since becoming pregnant. In the four postpartum surveys women were again asked to self-report on any of these issues for the 3 months preceding their 3, 6, 9 and 12 months postpartum time-frames.

Data on mode of birth, perineal trauma and birth events were collected from the hospital records using a detailed pre-designed data extraction form and in the first postpartum (3 month) survey. Mode of birth was classified into 5 categories; spontaneous vaginal birth, vacuum birth, forceps birth (including failed vacuum birth), emergency caesarean section (CS) (included failed forceps birth) and elective CS (includes elective CS in labour). Grades of perineal trauma were classified into 6 categories; intact perineum (includes women who had a CS), 1st degree tear (includes women who had both sutured and unsutured 1st degree tears), 2nd degree tears, episiotomy (includes women who had an extended episiotomy), 3rd degree tears and labial and vaginal wall lacerations. Breastfeeding at each time point was ascertained through one question *'Are you still breastfeeding your baby or giving expressed breastmilk'?* Women were also asked to rate their satisfaction with their body image at each time point, indicating if they were *'always satisfied', 'sometimes satisfied'* or *'never satisfied'* with their body image.

Statistical analysis

Data were analysed using IBM SPSS (version 23). Frequencies and descriptive statistics were used to present prevalence rates of sexual health issues in the year before this pregnancy, in early pregnancy and at 6 and 12 months postpartum. To determine if there was any statistically significant change over time in sexual health issues, McNemar's Chi-squared test for differences in correlated proportions was calculated [28].

Univariate and multivariable logistic regression analyses, using Odds Ratio (OR) and 95% Confidence Intervals (CI) were used to assess associations between pre-pregnancy dyspareunia, mode of birth, perineal trauma and breastfeeding, and, dyspareunia, a lack of vaginal lubrication and a loss of interest in sexual activity at 6 and 12 months. These three sexual health issues were chosen for the analyses as they are the more commonly reported of all sexual health issues. The multivariable logistic regression analysis model included the variables; age, pre pregnancy body mass index (BMI) and level of education. The Omnibus Test of Model Coefficients and the Hosmer and Lemeshow Test supported the models used.

Results

Characteristics of the study participants

Women included in this study report (n = 1477) all gave birth between August 2012 and end of July 2014. Of these 1477 women who were recruited in early pregnancy, 1408 were eligible for follow-up. For those 69 women not available for follow-up, reasons included, gave birth elsewhere, withdrew at Survey 1, experienced a late miscarriage or stillbirth, and no consent provided. Subsequent 2, 3, 4 and 5 survey return rates were 1180 (84%) 1094 (80%), 1027 (77%) and 971 (74%), respectively. To determine, accurately, any changes over time only data from women who returned all five surveys (n = 866, 59%) and consented to having their hospital records accessed (n = 832, 56%) were included in these analyses (Fig. 1).

Where it was possible to do so, study data were compared to data in the Irish National Perinatal Statistics Report for 2013 [29]. This allowed for an assessment of the national representativeness of the study participants. The National Perinatal Statistics Report is produced annually and collates data (hereafter referred to as national data) on the obstetric and social characteristics of every woman who gave birth in Ireland in the year preceding the report. Comparative assessments demonstrated that the study sample had proportionately fewer women under 24 years of age and more 30–34 and 35–39 year old women when compared to national statistics (30–39 years: 70.1% in the MAMMI study versus 52.5% in the national data). Greater than two-thirds (n = 566, 68.1%) of women in the MAMMI study are Irish with just over a quarter

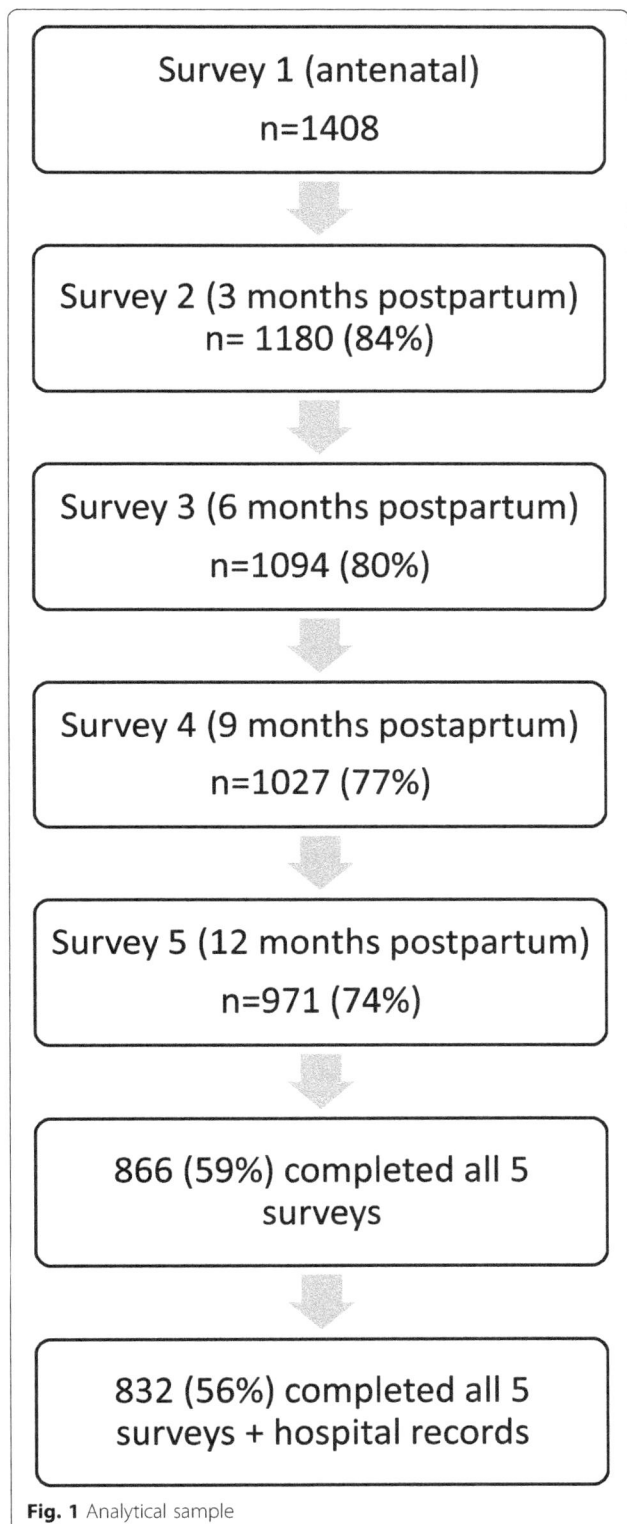

Fig. 1 Analytical sample

Survey 1 (antenatal)
n=1408

Survey 2 (3 months postpartum)
n= 1180 (84%)

Survey 3 (6 months postpartum)
n=1094 (80%)

Survey 4 (9 months postaprtum)
n=1027 (77%)

Survey 5 (12 months postpartum)
n=971 (74%)

866 (59%) completed all 5 surveys

832 (56%) completed all 5 surveys + hospital records

(n = 216, 25.9%) born in another European country. The five most common countries of birth after Ireland were; Poland (n = 58, 7%), United Kingdom (n = 45, 5.4%), France

(n = 13, 1.6%), Germany (n = 12, 1.5%) and Romania (n = 12, 1.5%). Seventy-one percent of participants had a university degree or higher (n = 588, 70.6%). No data were available for this item from the National Perinatal Statistics Report; however, the Central Statistics Office reports a national rate of women aged 25–34 with a third level qualification in Ireland of 55.3% in 2014 [30].

Women in the MAMMI study were under represented in terms of spontaneous vaginal birth (35.6% versus 45.5% nationally), over represented for forceps births (12% versus 5.6% nationally) and representative for caesarean section rates (31.6% versus 27.2% nationally). One third (n = 301, 36.1%) of study participants had an episiotomy compared to nearly half (n = 1187, 46.3%) of nulliparous women at the hospital site in 2013. The study sample were representative in all other categories of perineal trauma compared to the research site. Table 1 presents the characteristics of the MAMMI study sample.

Prevalence of self-reported sexual health issues over time
Table 2 presents the number and proportion of women who experienced sexual health issues pre-pregnancy, in early pregnancy and at 6 and 12 months postpartum. The prevalence of loss of interest in sexual activity was considerably elevated 6 months postpartum (46.3%) and remained significantly so at 12 months postpartum compared to pre-pregnancy levels (39.8% versus 33% $p < 0.001$). The proportion of women reporting dyspareunia at 6 months was significantly higher than those who experienced it pre-pregnancy (37.5% versus 29.3%, $p < 0.001$). Contrastingly, this was significantly lower than pre-pregnancy levels at 12 months postpartum (20.5% versus 29.3% $p < 0.001$). Six months postpartum 43% of women reported a lack of vaginal lubrication compared to 36.6% pre-pregnancy ($p = 0.002$). This decreased to 35.4% 12 months after birth ($p = 0.761$). Pregnancy and birth appeared to resolve difficulties women experienced with orgasm, as, pre-pregnancy, 34.1% of women experienced difficulty achieving orgasm and 19.7% were unable to achieve orgasm. The prevalence of these sexual health issues were significantly less, however at 12 months after birth (23.5% ($p < 0.001$) and 13.8% ($p = 0.001$), respectively). Figure 2 illustrates the prevalence of sexual health issues experienced by women at the different time points.

Univariate logistic regression analysis
Mode of birth as a risk factor for postpartum sexual health issues
Six months postpartum, vacuum-assisted birth was significantly associated with dyspareunia (OR 1.6, 95% CI 1.1–2.4), elective CS was associated with a reduced odds of experiencing dyspareunia (OR 0.5, 95% CI 0.3–0.9), and an emergency CS was protective of experiencing a loss of interest in sexual activity 6 months postpartum;

Table 1 Characteristics of study participants

Characteristics of study participants		Study participants	
		n	%
Age	Up to 24	41	4.9
	25 to 29	179	21.5
	30 to 34	376	45.2
	35 to 39	207	24.9
	40 and over	29	3.5
Place of birth	Irish	566	68.1
	Europe (excluding Ireland and UK)	171	20.5
	UK	45	5.4
	America	17	2
	Asia	10	1.2
	Africa	8	0.9
	Australia	3	0.4
	Missing	12	1.4
Highest level of education	School - second level	89	10.7
	Apprenticeship	75	9.1
	Certificate or Diploma	77	9.3
	Undergraduate degree	254	30.5
	Postgraduate degree	334	40.1
	Missing	3	0.3
Mode of birth	Spontaneous vaginal birth	296	35.6
	Vacuum birth	172	20.7
	Forceps birth	101	12
	Elective Caesarean Section	74	8.9
	Emergency Caesarean Section	189	22.7
Perineal trauma	Intact	268	32.2[a]
	1st degree tear	43	5.2
	2nd degree tear	168	20.2
	3rd degree tear	26	3.1
	Episiotomy	301	36.1
	Labial/vaginal wall tears	26	3.1

[a]includes participants who had a CS

these associations did not persist to 12 months postpartum. There was no significant association between vacuum-assisted birth and an increased lack of vaginal lubrication at 6 (OR 1.3, 95% CI 0.9–2.0) and 12 months postpartum (OR 1.3, 95% CI 0.9–1.9) (Table 3).

Perineal trauma as a risk factor for postpartum sexual health issues

Compared to women with an intact perineum, women who had 2nd degree perineal tears (OR 1.6, 95% CI 1.0–2.3), episiotomy (OR 1.7, 95% CI 1.2–2.5) or 3rd degree perineal tears (OR 3.7, 95% CI 1.5–9.3), were significantly more likely to experience dyspareunia at 6 months postpartum. This association persisted to 12 months for both episiotomies and 3rd degree perineal tears (Table 4). At 6 months postpartum a loss of interest in sexual activity was associated with both 2nd and 3rd degree perineal tears (Table 4).

Breastfeeding as a risk factor for postpartum sexual health issues

When data on women who were breastfeeding and not breastfeeding were compared, the results showed that women who were breastfeeding were significantly more likely to experience dyspareunia (OR 1.9, 95% CI 1.3–2.6), a lack of vaginal lubrication (OR 1.7, 95% CI 1.2–2.3) and a loss of interest in sexual activity (OR 1.7, 95% CI 1.3–2.3) 6 months postpartum. This association was not significant at 12 months postpartum, likely due, perhaps, to the low numbers still breastfeeding 12 months after birth. It is noteworthy that for those breastfeeding, the ORs for dyspareunia, a lack of vaginal lubrication and a loss of interest in sexual activity were all greater than 1.0 at 12 months postpartum, although none reached a level of significance (Table 5).

Pre-pregnancy dyspareunia as a risk factor for postpartum sexual health issues

Women who reported pre-pregnancy dyspareunia were significantly more likely to report several postpartum sexual health issues including dyspareunia at 6 and 12 months postpartum, a lack of vaginal lubrication at 6 and 12 months and

Table 2 Prevalence of self-reported sexual health issues pre pregnancy, in early pregnancy and at 6 and 12 months postpartum

	Pre pregnancy n (%)	Early pregnancy n (%)	6 months pp. n (%)	12 months pp. n (%)
Lack of vaginal lubrication m = 174	241/658 (36.6)	167/658 (25.4)	283/658 (43)	233/658 (35.4)
Pain during sexual intercourse m = 203	184/629 (29.3)	155/629 (24.6)	236/629 (37.5)	129/629 (20.5)
Difficulty reaching orgasm m = 236	203/596 (34.1)	156/596 (26.2)	183/596 (30.7)	140/596 (23.5)
Unable to reach orgasm m = 254	114/578 (19.7)	98/578 (17)	90/578 (15.6)	80/578 (13.8)
Vaginal tightness m = 216	138/616 (22.4)	130/616 (21.1)	200/616 (32.5)	107/616 (17.4)
Vaginal looseness / lack of muscle tone m = 243	10/589 (1.7)	10/589 (1.7)	79/589 (13.4)	53/589 (9)
Loss of interest in sexual activity compared with before pregnancy m = 187	216/654 (33)	349/654 (53.4)	303/654 (46.3)	260/654 (39.8)

m missing responses; pp. postpartum

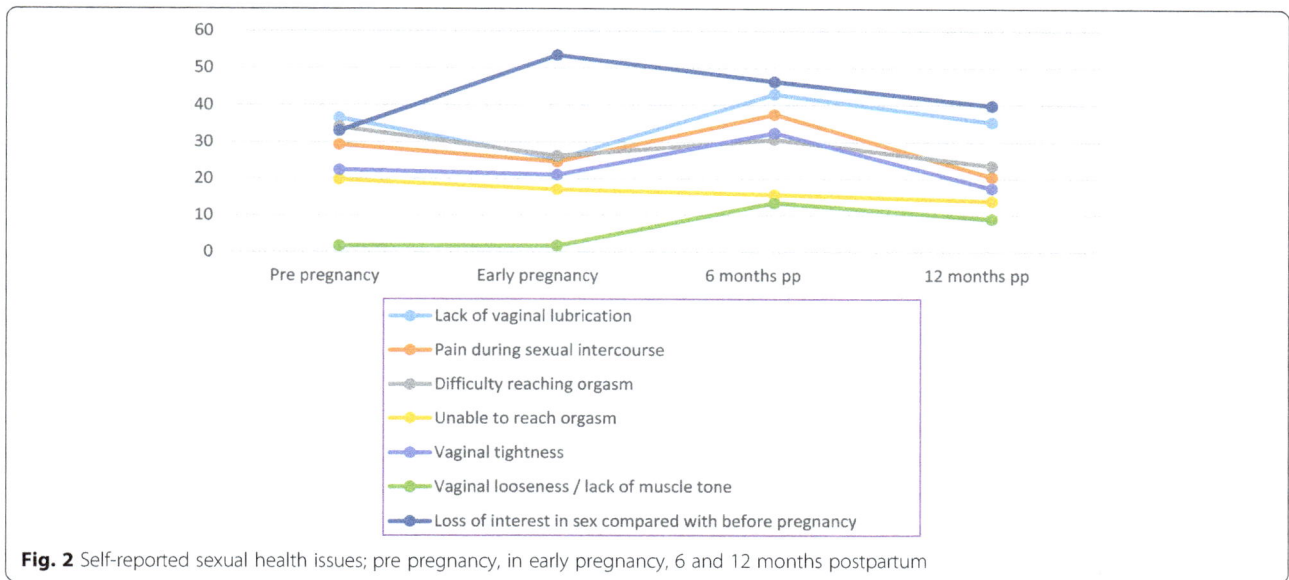

Fig. 2 Self-reported sexual health issues; pre pregnancy, in early pregnancy, 6 and 12 months postpartum

a loss of interest in sexual activity at 6 and 12 months postpartum compared to those who did not report it (Table 6).

Multivariable logistic regression analysis
Dyspareunia at 6 and 12 months postpartum
Pre-existing dyspareunia was strongly associated with dyspareunia (over two and half times more likely) at 6 months postpartum (Adjusted OR (AOR) 2.6, 95% CI

1.8–3.6), and this association was even more pronounced at 12 months (AOR 3.8, 95% CI 2.5–5.8). Breastfeeding and a 3rd degree perineal tear were both associated with experiencing dyspareunia 6 months after birth. Having a vacuum-assisted birth was not a significantly associated risk factor for dyspareunia 6 months postpartum (AOR 1.7, 95% CI 0.9–2.7). Compared to women aged 18–29 years, women aged ≥30 years were

Table 3 Mode of birth as a risk factor for sexual health issues at 6 and 12 months postpartum

	6 months postpartum					12 months postpartum				
	n/total	%	Unadjusted OR	95% CI	p value	n/total	%	Unadjusted OR	95% CI	p value
Dyspareunia										
Spontaneous vaginal birth	108/279	38.7	1.0 (ref.)			60/280	21.4	1.0 (ref.)		
Vacuum birth	83/163	50.9	1.6	1.1–2.4	0.013*	47/164	28.7	1.5	0.9–2.3	0.086
Forceps birth	30/89	33.7	0.8	0.5–1.3	0.397	18/96	18.8	0.8	0.4–1.5	0.577
Elective CS	16/66	24.2	0.5	0.3–0.9	0.03*	10/64	15.6	0.7	0.3–1.4	0.3
Emergency CS	61/181	33.7	0.8	0.5–1.2	0.277	31/181	17.1	0.8	0.5–1.2	0.258
Lack of vaginal lubrication										
Spontaneous vaginal birth	122/285	42.8	1.0 (ref.)			93/286	32.5	1.0 (ref.)		
Vacuum birth	83/166	50	1.3	0.9–2.0	0.139	63/164	33	1.3	0.9–1.9	0.206
Forceps birth	36/92	39.1	0.9	0.5–1.4	0.535	33/96	34.4	1.1	0.7–1.8	0.738
Elective CS	22/65	33.8	0.7	0.4–1.2	0.187	20/64	31.3	0.9	0.5–1.7	0.845
Emergency CS	77/181	42.5	1.0	0.7–1.4	0.955	69/185	37.3	1.2	0.8–1.8	0.287
Loss of interest in sexual activity										
Spontaneous vaginal birth	145/285	50.9	1.0 (ref.)			112/286	39.2	1.0 (ref.)		
Vacuum birth	88/165	53.3	1.1	0.7–1.6	0.615	69/165	41.8	1.1	0.8–1.6	0.579
Forceps birth	40/95	42.1	0.7	0.4–1.2	0.139	40/96	41.7	1.1	0.7–1.8	0.664
Elective CS	25/67	37.3	0.6	0.3–1.0	0.047	29/65	44.6	1.2	0.7–2.1	0.419
Emergency CS	73/181	40.3	0.6	0.4–0.9	0.027*	63/179	35.2	0.8	0.6–1.2	0.391

*indicates statistical signficance at p < 0.05

Table 4 Perineal trauma as a risk factor for sexual health issues at 6 and 12 months postpartum

	6 months postpartum					12 months postpartum				
	n/total	%	Unadjusted OR	95% CI	p value	n/total	%	Unadjusted OR	95% CI	p value
Dyspareunia										
Intact	77/252	30.6	1.0 (ref.)			40/250	16	1.0 (ref.)		
1st degree tear	11/39	28.2	0.9	0.4–1.9	0.766	7/40	17.5	1.1	0.5–2.7	0.811
2nd degree tear	66/161	41	1.6	1.0–2.3	0.03*	35/158	22.2	1.5	0.9–2.5	0.119
3rd degree tear	13/21	61.9	3.7	1.5–9.3	0.005*	8/25	32	2.5	1.0–6.1	0.05*
Episiotomy	121/281	43.1	1.7	1.2–2.5	0.003*	69/288	24	1.6	1.1–2.6	0.023*
Labial or vaginal wall tear	10/24	41.7	1.6	0.7–3.8	0.267	7/24	29.2	2.1	0.8–5.6	0.109
Lack of vaginal lubrication										
Intact	101/251	40.2	1.0 (ref.)			91/254	35.8	1.0 (ref.)		
1st degree tear	16/39	41	1.0	0.5–2.1	0.926	14/42	33.3	0.89	0.5–1.8	0.754
2nd degree tear	72/163	44.2	1.2	0.8–1.8	0.428	57/162	35.2	1.0	0.6–1.5	0.894
3rd degree tear	12/23	52.2	1.6	0.7–3.8	0.269	9/24	37.5	1.0	0.4–2.6	0.87
Episiotomy	128/288	44.4	1.2	0.8–1.7	0.325	97/289	33.6	0.9	0.6–1.3	0.58
Labial or vaginal wall tear	11/25	44	1.2	0.5–2.7	0.715	10/24	41.7	1.3	0.5–3.0	0.57
Loss of interest in sexual activity										
Intact	103/253	40.7	1.0 (ref.)			94/249	37.8	1.0 (ref.)		
1st degree tear	17/41	41.5	1.0	0.5–2.0	0.928	19/42	45.2	1.4	0.7–2.6	0.358
2nd degree tear	88/163	54	1.7	1.1–2.5	0.008*	69/162	42.6	1.2	0.8–1.8	0.327
3rd degree tear	15/24	62.5	2.4	1.0–5.8	0.044*	9/25	36	0.9	0.4–2.2	0.863
Episiotomy	138/288	47.9	1.3	0.9–1.9	0.093	114/289	39.4	1.1	0.8–1.5	0.687
Labial or vaginal wall tear	10/24	41.7	1.0	0.4–2.4	0.927	8/24	33.3	0.8	0.3–2.0	0.67

*indicates statistical signficance at $p < 0.05$

less likely to experience dyspareunia at 6 and 12 months. This was most pronounced at 12 months for women ≥35 years of age (Table 7).

Lack of vaginal lubrication at 6 and 12 months postpartum

Pre-existing dyspareunia was strongly associated with a lack of vaginal lubrication at 6 months (AOR 1.6, 95% CI 1.1–2.2) and the association persisted to 12 months postpartum (AOR 1.7, 95% CI 1.2–2.5). Breastfeeding, being sometimes satisfied with one's body image and never satisfied with one's body image were all associated with a lack of vaginal lubrication 6 months postpartum. Compared to ideal weight women, being overweight or obese was protective of experiencing a lack of vaginal lubrication 6 months after birth. A non-significant

association between a vacuum-assisted birth and an increased lack of vaginal lubrication at 12 months was also found (Table 8).

Loss of interest in sexual activity at 6 and 12 months postpartum

Breastfeeding at 6 months and 12 months postpartum were associated with experiencing a loss of interest in sexual activity at these time-points (AOR 2.2, 95% CI 1.6–3.0 and AOR 1.6, 95% CI 1.0–2.1, respectively). Being sometimes satisfied and never satisfied with one's body image was a risk factor for a loss of interest in sexual activity 6 months after birth. This association persisted for women who were never satisfied with their body image to 12 months postpartum (AOR 3.6, 95% CI

Table 5 Breastfeeding as a risk factor for sexual health issues at 6 and 12 months postpartum

	6 months postpartum					12 months postpartum				
	n/total	%	Unadjusted OR	95% CI	p value	n/total	%	Unadjusted OR	95% CI	p value
Dyspareunia	139/292	47.6	1.9	1.3–2.6	< 0.001*	33/133	24.8	1.2	0.7–1.8	0.477
Lack of vaginal lubrication	159/295	52.9	1.7	1.2–2.3	0.001*	55/135	40.7	1.3	0.9–1.9	0.221
Loss of interest in sexual activity	168/298	56.4	1.7	1.3–2.3	0.001*	62/135	45.9	1.4	1.0–2.1	0.064

*indicates statistical signficance at $p < 0.05$

Table 6 Pre-existing dyspareunia as a risk factor for sexual health issues 6 and 12 months postpartum

	6 months postpartum					12 months postpartum				
	n/total	%	Unadjusted OR	95% CI	p value	n/total	%	Unadjusted OR	95% CI	p value
Dyspareunia	126/234	53.8	2.5	1.8–3.5	< 0.001*	85/235	36.2	3.2	2.3–4.6	< 0.001*
Lack of vaginal lubrication	123/242	50.8	1.6	1.1–2.1	0.004*	106/237	44.7	1.8	1.3–2.5	< 0.001*
Loss of interest in sexual activity	127/242	52.5	1.4	1.0–1.9	0.025*	110/237	46.4	1.5	1.1–2.0	0.01*

*indicates statistical signficance at p < 0.05

1.9–6.7). Compared with women without degree-level educational qualifications, women who had a postgraduate qualifiction were more likely to experience a loss of interest in sexual activity 6 months after birth (AOR 1.5, 95% CI 1.0–2.3) (Table 9).

Discussion

Discourse on women's sexual health after birth is gaining momentum across diverse disciplines, for example, midwifery, obstetric, sexology and psychology disciplines [1–5]. This increased interest and body of research in perinatal sexual health, however, is not evidenced in sexual health policy [6, 7] or maternity care policy [8, 9], although data demonstrating that women are not prepared for changes to their sexual health after birth [10], are available. Lack of knowledge and preparation for sexual health issues postpartum can be distressing for women, and their partner, while also negatively impacting on their ability to adapt

Table 7 Multivariable logistic regression of dyspareunia at 6 and 12 months postpartum

Associated factors		6/12 postpartum Total n = 748			12/12 postpartum Total n = 585		
		OR	95% CI	p value	OR	95% CI	p value
Age Groups	18–29 years	1.0 (ref.)			1.0 (ref.)		
	30–34 years	0.7	0.4–1.0	0.059	0.7	0.4–1.2	0.222
	35+ years	0.7	0.4–1.0	0.096	0.4	0.2–0.8	0.009*
BMI Groups	Ideal	1.0 (ref.)			1.0 (ref.)		
	Overweight	1.0	0.6–1.6	0.947	0.9	0.5–1.7	0.773
	Obese	1.1	0.6–1.8	0.841	0.8	0.4–1.7	0.545
	Underweight	1.4	0.7–2.7	0.325	1.4	0.6–3.4	0.387
	Unknown BMI	0.7	0.3–1.4	0.366	0.9	0.4–2.5	0.926
Highest level of education	No degree	1.0 (ref.)			1.0 (ref.)		
	Primary degree	1.4	0.9–2.1	0.11	1.3	0.7–2.3	0.35
	Postgrad qualification	1.1	0.7–1.6	0.698	1.3	0.8–2.3	0.283
Pre-existing dyspareunia	Yes	2.6	1.8–3.6	< 0.001*	3.8	2.5–5.8	< 0.001*
Mode of birth	SVB	1.0 (ref.)			1.0 (ref.)		
	Vacuum birth	1.7	0.9–2.7	0.053	1.5	0.7–2.8	0.225
	Forceps birth	0.7	0.3–1.4	0.384	0.8	0.3–1.8	0.611
	Elective CS	0.7	0.3–1.7	0.491	1.9	0.6–5.7	0.255
	Emergency CS	1.1	0.6–2.2	0.605	1.537	0.6–3.7	0.344
Perineal trauma	Intact[a]	1.0 (ref.)			1.0 (ref.)		
	2nd degree	1.6	0.8–3.1	0.133	1.4	0.5–3.4	0.466
	3rd degree	4.1	1.3–12.3	0.013*	2.7	0.7–10.1	0.143
	Episiotomy	1.4	0.7–2.7	0.336	1.5	0.6–3.6	0.374
Still breastfeeding	Yes	1.9	1.3–2.7	< 0.001*	1.1	0.7–1.9	0.56
Perception of body image	Always satisfied	1.0 (ref.)			1.0 (ref.)		0.993
	Sometimes satisfied	0.9	0.6–1.5	0.96	1.0	0.6–1.7	0.941
	Never satisfied	1.4	0.8–2.4	0.211	1.0	0.5–2.2	0.905

[a]includes 1st degree tears and vaginal wall and labial tears
*indicates statistical signficance at p < 0.05

Table 8 Multivariable logistic regression of lack of vaginal lubrication at 6 and 12 months postpartum

Associated factors		6/12 postpartum Total $n = 758$			12/12 postpartum Total $n = 591$		
		OR	95% CI	p value	OR	95% CI	p value
Age Groups	18–29 years	1.0 (ref.)			1.0 (ref.)		
	30–34 years	0.9	0.7–1.4	0.994	0.8	0.5–1.3	0.383
	35+ years	0.9	0.6–1.4	0.799	0.7	0.4–1.1	0.149
BMI Groups	Ideal	1.0 (ref.)			1.0 (ref.)		
	Overweight	0.5	0.3–0.8	0.003*	0.7	0.3–1.1	0.129
	Obese	0.5	0.3–1.0	0.038*	0.6	0.3–1.2	0.148
	Underweight	1.5	0.8–2.9	0.226	1.8	0.9–3.7	0.117
	Unknown BMI	0.6	0.3–1.2	0.182	0.9	0.4–2.0	0.896
Highest level of education	No degree	1.0 (ref.)			1.0 (ref.)		
	Primary degree	1.0	0.6–1.5	0.985	1.0	0.6–1.7	0.862
	Postgrad qualification	1.1	0.8–1.7	0.496	1.2	0.8–2.0	0.332
Pre-existing dyspareunia	Yes	1.6	1.1–2.2	0.005*	1.7	1.2–2.5	0.004*
Mode of birth	SVB	1.0 (ref.)			1.0 (ref.)		
	Vacuum birth	1.4	0.9–2.4	0.145	1.7	1.0–3.0	0.062
	Forceps birth	1.0	0.6–1.9	0.932	1.4	0.7–2.9	0.308
	Elective CS	0.7	0.3–1.5	0.339	1.2	0.5–2.9	0.677
	Emergency CS	0.9	0.5–1.7	0.874	1.3	0.6–2.7	0.405
Perineal trauma	Intact[a]	1.0 (ref.)			1.0 (ref.)		
	2nd degree	1.0	0.5–1.8	0.963	1.0	0.5–2.0	0.945
	3rd degree	1.4	0.5–3.7	0.55	1.2	0.4–3.8	0.787
	Episiotomy	0.8	0.4–1.5	0.449	0.7	0.3–1.4	0.325
Still breastfeeding	Yes	2.1	1.5–2.9	< 0.001*	1.3	0.8–1.9	0.27
Perception of body image	Always satisfied	1.0 (ref.)			1.0 (ref.)		
	Sometimes satisfied	1.8	1.2–2.8	0.005*	1.2	0.7–1.9	0.444
	Never satisfied	2.4	1.4–4.0	0.001*	1.5	0.8–2.8	0.233

[a]includes 1st degree tears and vaginal wall and labial tears
*indicates statistical signficance at $p < 0.05$

to their new role as mothers [10–12]. Postpartum sexual health is challenging to theoretically define but cannot be separated from sexuality and sexual function, and is thought to be influenced by labour and birth events [13]. Attributes of good postpartum sexual health include; sexual desire, resumption of sexual intercourse after birth, pain free sex and orgasm.

Key findings

This study provides a further body of evidence demonstrating that women experience considerable sexual health issues after pregnancy and childbirth, and adds to the discourse on women's sexual health after birth from a maternity (midwifery and obstetric) perspective. Almost half of the women included in this study reported sexual health issues 6 months postpartum with more than 40% doing so 12 months after birth. A loss of interest in sexual activity was the most commonly reported

issue (46.3% at 6 months and 39.8% at 12 months). This is somewhat less than that reported in the Australian Maternal Health Study (60.3% at 6 and 51.3% at 12 months) [1] and more than that reported by Barrett and colleagues at 6 months postpartum (37%) [17]. Information relating to sexual health issues that was sought in these 3 studies were almost identical; however, there is a 15-year interval from data collection in our study and that of Barrett and colleagues. It is, therefore, possible that over the past 15 years women have become more comfortable and confident in recognising sexual health issues, possibly as a result of the increased interest in the social media, weekender magazines and in other media which discuss women's sexual lives after birth [31, 32]. Experiencing a loss of interest in sexual activity during the first year after birth is relatively common, which suggests that altered desire for sex is a normal part of adapting to motherhood and new roles of

Table 9 Multivariable logistic regression of loss of interest in sexual activity at 6 and 12 months postpartum

Associated factors		6/12 postpartum Total n = 762			12/12 postpartum Total n = 588		
		OR	95% CI	p value	OR	95% CI	p value
Age Groups	18–29 years	1.0(ref.)			1.0(ref.)		
	30–34 years	0.8	0.6–1.2	0.396	1.0	0.7–1.6	0.836
	35+ years	0.8	0.5–1.3	0.436	1.2	0.7–2.0	0.441
BMI Groups	Ideal	1.0(ref.)			1.0(ref.)		
	Overweight	0.9	0.6–1.4	0.562	0.7	0.4–1.3	0.276
	Obese	1.6	1.0–2.8	0.07	0.8	0.4–1.5	0.42
	Underweight	0.9	0.5–1.9	0.982	0.9	0.4–2.0	0.882
	Unknown BMI	0.7	0.4–1.4	0.337	0.9	0.4–2.1	0.931
Highest level of education	No degree	1.0(ref.)			1.0(ref.)		
	Primary degree	1.0	0.7–1.5	0.916	1.3	0.8–2.0	0.326
	Postgrad qualification	1.5	1.0–2.3	0.021*	1.3	0.8–2.0	0.249
Pre-existing dyspareunia	Yes	1.4	1.0–1.9	0.05*	1.3	0.9–1.9	0.127
Mode of birth	SVB	1.0(ref.)			1.0(ref.)		
	Vacuum birth	1.1	0.7–1.8	0.686	1.4	0.8–2.4	0.235
	Forceps birth	0.7	0.4–1.3	0.244	1.3	0.6–2.5	0.489
	Elective CS	0.7	0.4–1.6	0.446	1.0	0.4–2.2	0.933
	Emergency CS	0.8	0.4–1.5	0.464	0.7	0.3–1.3	0.266
Perineal trauma	Intact[a]	1.0(ref.)			1.0(ref.)		
	2nd degree	1.6	0.9–2.9	0.125	1.0	0.5–2.0	0.941
	3rd degree	2.6	0.9–7.2	0.065	0.9	0.3–2.8	0.853
	Episiotomy	1.2	0.6–2.3	0.595	0.7	0.3–1.4	0.272
Still breastfeeding	Yes	2.2	1.6–3.0	< 0.001*	1.6	1.0–2.4	0.029*
Perception of body image	Always satisfied	1.0(ref.)			1.0(ref.)		
	Sometimes satisfied	1.6	1.0–2.4	0.035*	1.5	0.9–2.3	0.082
	Never satisfied	2.8	1.6–4.6	< 0.001*	3.6	1.9–6.7	< 0.001*

[a]includes 1st degree tears and vaginal wall and labial tears
*indicates statistical signficance at p < 0.05

both parents in the household. If viewed through the adaptation lens, one is left with questions around the appropriateness of including lack of sexual activity as an indicator of 'sexual dysfunction' in the DSM-5 definition of sexual dysfunctions [33], especially for this cohort of postpartum women. The high rate of reported loss of interest in sexual activity also points to the need for women and their partners to be forewarned of this potential change, as a routine part of perinatal care. By so doing much of the stress and anxiety identified by women interviewed by Olsson [10] and guilt reported by women in Woolhouse and colleague's study [11] around intimacy would be reduced.

In our study 37.5% of women experienced dyspareunia 6 months after birth, compared to 43.4% reported in the Maternal Health Study [1] and 31% in Barrett et al.'s (2000) study [17]. Our findings demonstrate that events that occur during labour and birth influence the extent

with which women report dyspareunia 6 months after birth. The likelihood of women experiencing dyspareunia at 6 months was substantially higher in women whose birth was vacuum-assisted, had 2nd degree tears, 3rd degree tears and episiotomies compared to those who had a spontaneous vaginal birth and an intact perineum; although, when all other factors were considered, 3rd degree tears, only, along with pre-existing dyspareunia and breastfeeding emerged as significant factors for dyspareunia at 6 months postpartum. Our univariate results reflect the findings from previous studies which also report an association with episiotomy and poor sexual health outcomes [15], instrumental birth and dyspareunia [19, 34]. In addition, it raises questions about the rates of obstetric intervention experienced by women in Ireland. In our study 20.7% of women experienced a vacuum-assisted birth, similar to a national rate of 21.2% [29], double the rate of 10.4% in the Maternal Health

Study in Australia [34] and much higher than the 5% in the nulliparous sample used by Connolly and colleagues [35]. Our high rate of vacuum-assisted birth could be related to the equally high uptake of epidural anaesthesia in Irish maternity settings, as 78% of women in this study used epidural analgesia (similar to the 72% of nulliparous women at the research site), and a 2011 Cochrane review identified that epidural analgesia increased the risk of an instrumental birth [36]. The association between episiotomy and persistent dyspareunia up to 12 months was found in our study, although it did not emerge as a risk factor for dyspareunia in multivariable analysis. In our study 36.1% of women had an episiotomy, while this may appear elevated it is worth noting that 33% of women had an instrumental birth which is commonly associated with an episiotomy. Our high rate of episiotomy (36.1%) compares poorly, internationally, where 16% of women in the Maternal Health Study had an episiotomy [34] and 14% in Connolly's research [35]. This finding does not necessarily suggest there is routine use of episiotomy but rather poses concern over the high rate of epidural uptake, consequent instrumental births, perineal trauma and associated long term dyspareunia.

Little has been published on the influence of breastfeeding on postpartum sexual health, with many studies choosing to focus on breastfeeding as a means of contraception [37] or the influence of breastfeeding on resumption of sexual activity and frequency of sexual activity [38–40]. In our study, breastfeeding, in association with other related factors, remained significantly present for all three of the outcomes of dyspareunia, a lack of vaginal lubrication and a loss of interest in sexual activity 6 months postpartum. This finding highlights the potential for cognitive dissonance to occur. Cognitive dissonance occurs when people experience inconsistency between cognitions or between cognitions and behaviour [41]. In a professional or practice context that emphasises women-centred care and disclosure, and a policy context that promotes breastfeeding, there is potential for internal conflict to arise. Practitioners may struggle with the professional imperative to inform women of the impact of breastfeeding on sexual activity, dyspareunia and vaginal lubrication at the same time as fearing a decrease in women's willingness to breastfeed if impact is known. However, information regarding breastfeeding needs to take account of these findings, if care is to be 'woman-centred' as opposed to 'breast-feeding centred' [42]. Without this information women may blame themselves for their loss of sexual interest, or struggle alone without information on the array of vaginal lubricants available to alleviate vaginal dryness.

Little attention has been given to pre-existing dyspareunia and its influence on sexual health after birth to date, however two studies found a similar association

between pre-existing dyspareunia and experiencing sexual health issues after birth [17, 34]. In our study 29.3% of women experienced dyspareunia in the 12 months before becoming pregnant, and this, with other significantly related factors (e.g. 3rd degree tears and breastfeeding at 6 months and age > 35 years at 12 months) contributed to dyspareunia 6 and 12 months after birth. The majority of women do not seek professional support for postpartum sexual health issues, 15% in Barrett et al.'s study spoke to a health professional [17] and 24% in the Australian study were asked directly by a health professional about their sexual health postpartum [1]. This corresponds to conclusions from qualitative studies that demonstrated that women find it difficult to bring up sexual health issues with health professionals [10, 11, 43] and this occurs at a time when women have direct contact with a variety of health professionals during the postpartum period. Therefore it is very likely that women do not seek help for dyspareunia experienced before pregnancy as there may be limited contact with health services. The antenatal period, a time when women have frequent consultations with health professionals appears to be an ideal opportunity to ask them about their sexual health and discuss any problems, such as pain during sexual intercourse, they may be experiencing. It is potentially an ideal time to refer women to the most appropriate professional for help, be it the women's health physiotherapist attached to the maternity services, sexual health therapist or couples therapy. However, previous studies of healthcare professionals have shown that many lack competence and confidence in their abilities to help with sexual problems [44], which may be why so many women had not been asked. Managing dyspareunia during pregnancy will go some way to reducing the identified association between pre-pregnancy dyspareunia and a lack of vaginal lubrication and a loss of interest in sexual activity seen in this study. Similarly, it is probable that persistent postpartum dyspareunia at 6 and 12 months would be reduced if managed antenatally or at the very least women should be asked about sexual health issues, and would then know where to seek appropriate help.

This study is unique in its investigation of an association between perception of body image and sexual health issues after birth. In this study women with a poor perception of their body images 6 and 12 months postpartum were more likely to experience a lack of vaginal lubrication (in the context of being overweight, obese, breastfeeding and pre-existing dyspareunia) and a loss of interest in sexual activity (in the context of breastfeeding and pre-existing dyspareunia). The complex nature of the concept of postpartum body image and its influence on postpartum sexual health is poorly researched, and this led the first author of this paper to carry out qualitative one-to-one semi-structured interviews with some of the women who completed the survey and identified themselves as experiencing sexual health problems. Analysis of these data is in progress and will be reported at a later date.

Strengths and limitations

The strengths of this study include the recruitment of a large sample of nulliparous women in early pregnancy, regular follow-up and a high retention rate to 12 months postpartum. The frequency of follow-up reduces the likelihood of recall bias and provides reliable data on changes to women's sexual health over time following birth. Some findings in our study are similar to other comparable studies. This strengthens the argument for introducing sexual health to antenatal and postnatal care pathways well beyond the traditional 6 week postnatal assessment.

A number of potential limitations have been identified that may influence the data. The study sample is from one maternity unit in Ireland, which is not entirely representative of a national sample. The survey did not include definitions of concepts such as lack of vaginal lubrication, hence they are open to individual interpretation on meaning. The association of breastfeeding and sexual health issues may be questionable as Ireland has a low breastfeeding continuation rate; for example, in a national study of infant feeding in Ireland, only 19% ($n = 347$) of women were exclusively breastfeeding at 3–4 months postpartum [45]. Data on other factors such as medications (e.g., psychotropic drugs) that may affect interest in sexual activity [46] were not collected. A further limitation is the lack of data on the sexual orientation of women in our study, thus it was not possible to identify if there was any difference between women in same sex relationships and those in opposite sex relationships.

Conclusion

The findings from this large prospective cohort study of nulliparous demonstrates that women experience considerable sexual health issues after pregnancy and childbirth. Dyspareunia, lack of vaginal lubrication and loss of interest in sexual activity at 6 months postpartum were all significantly associated with pre-existing dyspareunia and breastfeeding. Additionally dyspareunia was associated with 3rd degree tears, lack of vaginal lubrication was associated with being overweight, obese and dissatisfaction with body image was a risk factor for a lack of vaginal lubrication and a loss of interest in sexual activity. Preparing women and their partners for this during the antenatal period and advising on simple measures, such as use of lubrication to avoid issues, could potentially remove stress, anxiety and fears regarding intimacy after birth. Pregnancy and the frequent interactions it brings with health professionals provide an ideal opportunity to discuss pre-existing sexual health issues

with women and their partners and suitable care pathways can be put in place with appropriate referrals made.

Abbreviations
AOR: Adjusted Odds Ratio; BMI: Body Mass Index; CI: Confidence Interval; CS: Caesarean Section; MAMMI: Maternal health And Maternal Morbidity in Ireland; OR: Odds ratio; PP: Postpartum; SPSS: Statistical Package for the Social Sciences

Acknowledgements
We are grateful to all of the women who participated in the MAMMI study, the midwives and midwifery students who recruited women to the study and to other members of the MAMMI research team who have contributed to data collection and data management.

Funding
This research was funded by a Health Research Board Healthcare Professional Fellowship grant awarded to Deirdre O'Malley (HRB HPF/2013/477-Begley). The funders had no role in the design of the study and collection, analysis, and interpretation of data and in writing the manuscript.

Authors' contributions
DOM planned and conducted the analyses, interpreted data and contributed to writing the paper. VS and AH supervised the analysis, contributed to interpretation of data and reviewed and commented on all drafts of the paper. DD wrote the study protocol and took primary responsibility for the design and conduct of the MAMMI study, in conjunction with CB was original supervisor to DOM and is the grant holder for this research. All authors have approved the final draft of the paper prior to submission.

Competing interests
Valerie Smith is a member of the BMC Pregnancy and Childbirth Editorial Board. All remaining authors declare that they have no competing interests.

Author details
[1]Health Research Board, Research Fellow, School of Nursing and Midwifery, Trinity College Dublin, Dublin, Ireland. [2]School of Nursing and Midwifery, Trinity College Dublin, Dublin, Ireland. [3]Institute of Health and Care Sciences, The Sahlgrenska Academy, University of Gothenburg, Gothenburg, Sweden.

References
1. McDonald E, Woolhouse H, Brown SJ. Consultation about sexual health issues in the year after childbirth: a cohort study. Birth. 2015;42(4):354–61.
2. Schlagintweit HE, Bailey K, Rosen NO. A new baby in the bedroom: frequency and severity of postpartum sexual concerns and their associations with relationship satisfaction in new parent couples. Journal of Sexual Medicine. 2016;13(10):1455–65.
3. Fehniger JEMD, Brown JSMD, Creasman JMM, Van Den Eeden SKP, Thom DHMDP, Subak LLMD, et al. Childbirth and female sexual function later in life. Obstet Gynecol. 2013;122(5):988–97.
4. Fodstad K, Staff AC, Laine K. Sexual activity and dyspareunia the first year postpartum in relation to degree of perineal trauma. Int Urogynecol J Pelvic Floor Dysfunct. 2016;27(10):1513–23.
5. DeJudicibus MA, McCabe MP. Psychological factors and the sexuality of pregnant and postpartum women. Journal of Sex Research. 2002;39(2):94–103.
6. Department of Health. A Framework for Sex Health Improvement in England London: Department of Health, 2013.
7. Department of Health. National Sexual Health Strategy 2015–2020. Dublin: Department of Health; 2015.
8. Department of Health. Creating a better future together. National Maternity Strategy 2016–2026. Dublin: Department of Health; 2016.

9. National Health Service England. The National Maternity Review. Better births. Improving outcomes of maternity services in England. England: National Health Service; 2016.

10. Olsson A, Lundqvist M, Faxelid E, Nissen E. Women's thoughts about sexual life after childbirth: focus group discussions with women after childbirth. Scand J Caring Sci. 2005;19(4):381–7.

11. Woolhouse H, McDonald E, Brown S. Women's experiences of sex and intimacy after childbirth: making the adjustment to motherhood. J Psychosom Obstet Gynecol. 2012;33(4):185–90.

12. Pastore L, Owens A, Raymond C. Postpartum sexuality concerns among first-time parents from one U.S. academic hospital. J Sex Med. 2007;4(1):115–23.

13. O'Malley D, Higgins A, Smith V. Postpartum sexual health: a principle-based concept analysis. J Adv Nurs. 2015;71(10):2247–57.

14. McDonald EA, Brown SJ. Does method of birth make a difference to when women resume sex after childbirth. BJOG: An International Journal of Obstetrics and Gynaecology. 2013;120(7):823–30.

15. Baksu B, Davas I, Agar E, Akyol A, Varolan A. The effect of mode of delivery on postpartum sexual functioning in primiparous women. Int Urogynecol J Pelvic Floor Dysfunct. 2007;18(4):401–6.

16. Safarinejad MR, Kolahi AA, Hosseini L. The effect of the mode of delivery on the quality of life, sexual function, and sexual satisfaction in primiparous women and their husbands. Journal of Sexual Medicine. 2009;6(6):1645–67.

17. Barrett G, Pendry E, Peacock J, Victor CR, Thakar R. Women's sexual health after childbirth. Br J Obstet Gynaecol. 2000;107(2):186–95.

18. Rathfisch G, Dikencik BK, Kizilkaya Beji N, Comert N, Tekirdag AI, Kadioglu A. Effects of perineal trauma on postpartum sexual function. J Adv Nurs. 2010;66(12):2640–9.

19. Signorello LB, Harlow BL, Chekos AK, Repke JT. Postpartum sexual functioning and its relationship to perineal trauma: a retrospective cohort study of primiparous women. Am J Obstet Gynecol. 2001;184(5):881–8. discussion 8-90

20. Chang SR, Chen KH, Lin HH, Chao YM, Lai YH. Comparison of the effects of episiotomy and no episiotomy on pain, urinary incontinence, and sexual function 3 months postpartum: a prospective follow-up study. Int J Nurs Stud. 2011;48(4):409–18.

21. Hosseini L, Iran-Pour E, Safarinejad MR. Sexual function of primiparous women after elective cesarean section and normal vaginal delivery. Urol J. 2012;9(2):498–504.

22. Baud D, Meyer S, Vial Y, Hohlfeld P, Achtari C. Pelvic floor dysfunction 6 years post-anal sphincter tear at the time of vaginal delivery. Int Urogynecol J Pelvic Floor Dysfunct. 2011;22(9):1127–34.

23. Chivers ML, Pittini R, Grigoriadis S, Villegas L, Ross LE. The relationship between sexual functioning and depressive symptomatology in postpartum women: a pilot study. Journal of Sexual Medicine. 2011;8(3):792–9.

24. Acele EO, Karacam Z. Sexual problems in women during the first postpartum year and related conditions. J Clin Nurs. 2011;21(7–8):929–37.

25. Dean N, Wilson D, Herbison P, Glazener C, Aung T, Macarthur C. Sexual function, delivery mode history, pelvic floor muscle exercises and incontinence: a cross-sectional study six years post-partum. Aust N Z J Obstet Gynaecol. 2008;48(3):302–11.

26. Olsson A, Robertson E, Falk K, Nissen E. Assessing women's sexual life after childbirth: the role of the postnatal check. Midwifery. 2011;27(2):195–202.

27. Brown SJL, M J, McDonald EA, Krastev AH, Bessell C, Brennecke S, Burrows R, Gunn J, Mitchell C, Watson L, Wein P, MacArthur C, Klein M, Luoto R, Hegarty K. Maternal health study: a prospective cohort study of nulliparous women recruited in early pregnancy. BMC Pregnancy and Childbirth. 2006;6

28. Field A. Discovering Statistics using SPSS. 2nd ed. London: Sage Publications; 2005.

29. Health Service Executive. Perinatal Statistics Report 2013. Dublin: Health Service Executive; 2014.

30. Central Statistics Office Men and women in Ireland. Dublin: Stationary Office, 2014.

31. Shanahan C. Sex after baby: groundbreaking research on what happens in the bedroom after birth. Irish examiner. In: 2016 10th; 2016.

32. Dillner L. How long after giving birth should I wait before having sex again. The Guardian. 2013;

33. American Psychiatric Association. Diagnostic and statistical manual of mental disorders. 5th ed. Arlington, VA: American Psychiatric Publishing; 2013.

34. McDonald EA, Gartland D, Small R, Brown SJ. Dyspareunia and childbirth: a prospective cohort study. BJOG Int J Obstet Gynaecol. 2015;122(5):672–9.

35. Connolly A, Thorp J, Pahel L. Effects of pregnancy and childbirth on postpartum sexual function: a longitudinal prospective study. Int Urogynecol J Pelvic Floor Dysfunct. 2005;16(4):263–7.

36. Anim-Somuah M, Smyth RMD, Jones L. Epidural versus non-epidural or no analgesia in labour. Cochrane Database Syst Rev. 2011;12

37. Van der Wijden CKJ, Van den Berk T. Lactational amenorrhea for family planning. Cochrane database of systematic reviews. 2003;4 CD001329

38. Yee LM, Kaimal AJ, Nakagawa S, Houston K, Kuppermann M. Predictors of postpartum sexual activity and function in a diverse population of women. Journal of Midwifery & Women's Health. 2013;58(6):654–61.

39. Visness CMK K I. The frequency of coitus during breastfeeding. Birth-issues in. Perinatal Care. 1997;24(4):253–7.

40. Rowland M, Foxcroft L, Hopman WM, Breastfeeding PR. Sexuality immediately post partum. Can Fam Physician. 2005;51:1366–7.

41. Festinger L. A theory of cognitive dissonance. In: Stanford CA: Stanford university press; 1957.

42. Carroll M, Gallagher L, Clarke M, Millar S, Begley C. Artificial milk-feeding women's views of their feeding choice in Ireland. Midwifery. 2015;31(6):640–6.

43. Buurman MBR, Lagro-Janssen ALM. Women's perception of postpartum pelvic floor dysfunction and their help-seeking behaviour: a qualitative interview study. Scand J Caring Sci. 2013;27(2):406–13.

44. Higgins A, Barker P, Begley CM. Sexuality: the challenge to espoused holistic care. Int J Nurs Pract. 2006;12(6):345–51.

45. Begley C, Gallagher L, Clarke M, Carroll M, Millar S. The National Infant Feeding Survey 2008. School of Nursing and Midwifery, Trinity College Dublin: 2010.

46. Higgins A. Impact of psychotropic medication on sexuality: literature review. Br J Nurs. 2007;16(9):545–50.

12

Prevalence of behavioral risk factors of cardiovascular diseases and associated socio-economic factors among pregnant women in a rural area in Southern Nepal

Rajan Paudel[1], Kwan Lee[2], Jitendra Kumar Singh[3], Seok-Ju Yoo[2], Dilaram Acharya[2,8]* (iD), Rajendra Kadel[4], Samaj Adhikari[5], Mohan Paudel[6] and Narayan Mahotra[7]

Abstract

Background: Cardiovascular diseases (CVDs) have dramatically infiltrated populations living in abject poverty in Low- and Middle-income Countries (LMICs), and poor maternal and child health outcomes have been frequently reported for those with CVD risk factors. However, few studies have explored the behavioral risk factors of CVDs among pregnant women in rural settings. This study aimed at determining the prevalence and identifying the socio-economic predictors of behavioral risk factors of CVDs among pregnant women in rural area in Southern Nepal.

Methods: A Community-based cross-sectional study was conducted in 52 clusters of Dhanusha District of Nepal in a total of 426 pregnant women in their second trimester using multistage cluster sampling method. Multivariable logistic regression model was used to assess independent associations between behavioral risk factors during pregnancy and maternal socio-economic characteristics.

Results: Of the 426 study participants, 86.9, 53.9, 21.3 and 13.3%, respectively, reported insufficient fruits and vegetables consumption, insufficient physical activity, tobacco use, and harmful alcohol drinking. Socio-economic factors significantly associated with more than one behavioral risk factors in expectant mothers with a primary level education (adjusted odds ratio (AOR) 2.78; 95% Confidence Interval (CI) (1.35–5.72)), 20–34 years age group (Adjusted Odds Ratio (AOR) 0.27; 95% CI (0.13–0.56)), and those with the highest wealth index (AOR 0.36; 95% CI (0.16–0.84)).

Conclusion: Higher prevalence of behavioral risk factors for CVDs and their socio-economic factors prevailing among pregnant women living in rural Nepal call for immediate health promotion interventions such as community awareness and appropriate antenatal counseling.

Keywords: Behavioral risk factors, Cardiovascular disease, Pregnant women, Socio-economic predictors, Nepal

Introduction

Cardiovascular diseases (CVDs) include disorders of heart and blood vessels, and are usually associated with atherosclerosis, heart attacks, strokes, valvular diseases, congenital heart diseases and arrhythmia [1]. Mortality resulting from CVDs reached 17.7 million globally in 2015, which represented 31% of all global deaths. Of the

CVD deaths, more than three quarters took place in low- and middle-income countries (LMICs) [2]. Cardiovascular diseases, which are typically viewed as diseases of the wealthy, have dramatically infiltrated those living in abject poverty in LMICs [3], and accounted for a substantial burden of non-communicable diseases in Nepal. Studies [4, 5] revealed a prevalence of about 5% for coronary heart diseases among adult population in Nepal. A study by Dhungana et al. found high prevalence of risk factors of CVDs such as smoking, alcohol consumption, insufficient fruit and vegetable intake, daily salt intake, overweight

* Correspondence: dilaramacharya123@gmail.com
[2]Department of Preventive Medicine, College of Medicine, Dongguk University, 123 Dongdae-ro, Gyeongju-si 38066, Republic of Korea
[8]Department of Community Medicine, Kathmandu University, Devdaha Medical College and Research Institute, Rupandehi, Nepal

and obesity, and hypertension among rural Nepalese residents [6].

Smoking, alcohol consumption, inadequate physical activity and inadequate fruit and vegetable intake are well-established modifiable behavioral risk factors of CVDs [7]. Globally smoking accounts for 10% of deaths attributed to CVDs, and this figure is gradually increasing in LMICs, alcohol is responsible for 6 and 1% of deaths among men and women, respectively, whereas inadequate physical activity and insufficient fruit and vegetable intake contribute nearly 33 and 10%, respectively, to the burden of ischemic heart disease [7].

The spectrum of CVDs in pregnancy encompasses congenital heart disease, valvular heart disease, ischemic heart disease, peripartum cardiomyopathy, hypertensive disorders, and venous thromboembolism. Furthermore, the global burden of CVDs in pregnancy has increased alarmingly in parallel with the rising prevalence of behavioral risk factors among women of reproductive age [8].

Addressing the risk factors of CVDs in pregnant mothers is crucial not just for reducing adverse pregnancy outcomes such as low birth weight, fetal and infant mortalities, and potential congenital defects, but for reduction of CVDs among mothers as well [8–11]. Cardiovascular diseases are exacerbated by physiological changes in pregnancy and contribute to maternal mortality and morbidity, and delay in health care response [12, 13], which has important impacts in resource constrained settings as rural Nepal. In Nepal, the 2013 non-communicable disease risk factor survey (STEPS) revealed national prevalence of tobacco use of 30.8%, alcohol consumption of 17.4%, inadequate fruit and vegetable consumption of 98.9%, and inadequate physical activity of 3.5% [14]. Studies on impact of the combined effects of behavioral health risk factors on longevity showed that these risk factors increased mortality rates in both genders [15, 16]. In addition, a higher percentage (9 to 15%) of pregnant women have been reported to drink alcohol during pregnancy in Nepal [17, 18]. However, these studies were limited in terms of describing the prevalence of behavioral risk factors and their predictors.

Identification of the behavioral risk factors of CVDs among pregnant women is an important global public health issue, but very limited studies have sought to identify behavioral risk factors of CVDs in pregnant women residing in rural settings. In this study, we aimed to determine the prevalence and to identify socio-economic predictors of behavioral risk factors of CVDs among pregnant women living in rural southern Terai of Nepal.

Methods
Study design, setting and sampling
We employed community-based cross-sectional study design. We used baseline data obtained from the

'MATRI-SUMAN', a randomized controlled trial of a capacity building and text messaging intervention designed to enhance maternal and child health service utilization among pregnant women residing in rural Nepal [19]. The baseline data included socio-demographic information and CVD risk factors - tobacco use, alcohol consumption, fruits and vegetables intake and physical activities.

The study was conducted in Dhanusha district of Nepal. Dhanusha, one of the 75 districts of Nepal, is situated in the southern part of the country (also known as 'Terai' in local language). Dhanusha is a district of considerable cultural and historic importance. It occupies an area of 1180 sq. km in southern Terai province and is located at an altitude of between 61 and 610 m. It borders three districts – Siraha, Mahottari and Sindhuli to the east, west, and north, respectively, and India to the south. The main residents of Terai are from the Maithili ethnic group and the adult literacy rate is 69% [20]. Administratively, this district comprises one municipality and 101 Village Development Committees (VDCs) and has an estimated population of 754,777 in 2011. VDC is the smallest administrative unit of a district [20, 21]. Data for this study were collected from eligible pregnant women from July to September 2015.

We used multi-stage cluster sampling technique to identify study participants. One primary health care center and one health post of Dhanusha district were selected purposively for the study. These health facilities were chosen because these were the only government-funded maternal and child health (MCH) services facilities available in these areas. No healthcare services were available from the private or not-for-profit sectors, which helped to evaluate the true impact of the government MCH services. These two health facilities consisted of 12 VDCs (54 wards), and populations in these VDCs ranged from 3500 to 19,000 [22, 23]. From each health facility, three VDCs were randomly selected so that study area constituted a total of six VDCs. In total, there were 54 clusters (nine in each VDC), but we excluded two clusters because they were situated in semi-urban areas. Complete enumeration of all households having pregnant women with gestational period between 13 to 28 weeks (2nd trimester) from the selected clusters of six VDCs was performed. Pregnant women were identified using antenatal care register maintained by Female Community Health Volunteers (FCHVs). Of the 453 eligible pregnant women, 426 gave consent to participate in the study. The details of study design can be found elsewhere [19].

Data collection
Structured interview questionnaire was used to collect information from a pregnant woman and the interview

was taken place at participant's home. Enumerators were trained in research tools, interview process and measurement of variables. Field coordinators experienced in CVD risk factors supervised enumerators to ensure the quality of information. Preliminary questionnaires were checked and pre-tested in an adjacent district and necessary modifications were made. The questionnaire consisted of two parts: i) baseline characteristics of respondents; and ii) behavioral risk factors of cardiovascular diseases (tobacco use, alcohol consumption, fruit and vegetable consumption and physical activity).

The major outcome variables were behavioral risk factors of CVDs among pregnant women. CVDs risk factors were operationalized based on the standard definitions to ensure their comparability and to minimize error. If the participants had been using tobacco of any form (smoke or smokeless) and alcohol for last 30 days, they were considered as current users. Women who were using tobacco daily were defined as current daily tobacco users. Likewise, women having five or more drinks a day in past 30 days were labeled as current episodic heavy drinker. Consuming 341 ml of beer or 43 ml of home-made alcohol was equivalent to one standard drink (13.6 g of pure alcohol) [24]. If a person took at least five portions (400 g) of fruits and vegetables per day, it was considered as sufficient. One cup (250 ml) of raw green leafy vegetables and a half cup (125 ml) of cooked or chopped raw vegetables was equivalent to one serving of vegetables. Similarly, one portion of fruits was defined as one whole medium sized fruits like apple, banana or orange and ½ cup of chopped, cooked, canned fruit or a half cup of fruit juice [25]. We used "show cards" associated with food frequency questionnaire to collect data regarding fruits and vegetables intake during pregnancy.

We adopted World Health Organization (WHO) global recommendations on physical activity for health (adult) guideline to measure physical activity level among pregnant women in our study. Physical activity includes activities during travel, recreation and work. It was evident from this guideline that more active people are less likely to have metabolic and cardiovascular risks. WHO recommended moderate-intensity physical activity (at least 150 minutes per week) can help to reduce such risks among adults [26]. In rural (Terai) Nepal, women are generally engaged in the household chores and farm activities, and these activities fairly meet the criteria of moderate-intensity physical activity level [14]. Participants were asked various questions regarding their physical activity levels and based on their response the enumerator recorded hours spent on daily household, travel, recreational and occupational activities. Based on recorded hours of time on various activities, the researchers then recoded these activities into two equalized categories (i) less than 150 minutes per week of moderate-intensity physical activity (Physical inactivity) and (ii) more than 150 minutes per week moderate-intensity physical activity (Active physical activity).

The independent variables comprised: age, caste/ethnicity, place of origin, religion, education, occupation, wealth index, and parity, which were adapted from the Nepal demographic and population health survey 2011 [27]. Caste/ethnicity was based on the caste base system in Nepal: disadvantaged-Dalit, disadvantaged-Adibasi/Janajati, and advantaged-Brahmin and Chhetri [28].

Data analysis

Data were compiled, checked, cleaned and verified carefully to ensure consistency and then entered into database systems using Epi-info data version 3.1. Data analysis was carried out using SPSS version 20 for Windows. Univariate analysis was performed to describe the distributions of the four risk factors of cardiovascular diseases (tobacco use, alcohol consumption, physical inactivity and insufficient fruit and vegetable consumption). Associations between various factors such as, ethnicity, women education and wealth index and CVDs risk factors were analyzed first by bivariate analyses using chi-square test. A multivariate regression model was used to assess independent associations between risk factors during pregnancy and maternal socio-economic characteristics. Factors which were significant ($p < 0.05$) in bivariate analysis were selected for multivariable analysis and adjusted odds ratios (OR) and 95% confidence intervals (95% CI) were obtained. A p-value of < 0.05 was considered statistically significant. Further, to determine the simultaneous presence of behavioral risk factors and possible predictors, a number of risk factors in each pregnant woman was recorded (range of 0–4 behavioral risk factors). A model was used for a number of simultaneous risk factors; each woman was dichotomized as having less than two or having two or more behavioral risk factors (< 2 vs. ≥ 2). This dichotomized variable was used as outcome variable [29].

Ethical considerations

Ethical approval for Matri-Suman trial was obtained from the Nepal Health Research Council, Nepal (Approval no: 101), the ethics committee of the Institute of Medical Sciences, Banaras Hindu University, India (approval no: ECR/526/Inst/UP/2014 Dt.31.1.14), and from the District Public Health Office, Dhanusha, Nepal (Ref. 2245). The objectives of the study were clearly explained to all participants and written informed consent was obtained before data collection. Personal identifiers were removed before data analysis.

Results

Table 1 shows the prevalence of behavioral risk factors for cardiovascular diseases. Of the 426 study subjects, majority (86.9%) of them reported insufficient fruits and vegetables consumption, more than half (53.9%) mentioned insufficient physical activity, 21.3% reported tobacco use of any form (smoke or smokeless), and 13.3% as having harmful alcohol consumption.

Table 2 presents the socio-demographic details and the prevalence of behavioral risk factors for cardiovascular diseases among expectant mothers. The highest percentage of the study subjects (68.1%) were from 20 to 34 years of age. Most study subjects were from upper caste (62.0%), of Terai origin (71.8%), and Hindus (91.8%). Slightly more than a quarter of the study subjects had never been to school (25.4%), 68.5% were engaged in occupation other than agriculture, 29.1% belonging to lower socioeconomic strata, and 39.2% were primipara (pregnant for the first time).

Chi-square test demonstrated that participants' baseline characteristics-(age, caste/ethnicity, women education, and wealth index), (age, caste/ethnicity, birth origin, women education, women occupation, wealth index and parity), (caste/ethnicity, women education and wealth index), and (age, caste/ethnicity, women education, and wealth index) were respectively, strongly associated with tobacco use, alcohol use, insufficient fruit and vegetable intake, and insufficient physical activity ($p < 0.05$) (Table 2).

The results of multiple regression analyses for risk factors of CVD are presented in Table 3. Expectant mothers aged 20–34 (AOR 2.11; 95% CI (0.97–4.57)), 35–45 (AOR 2.31; 95% CI (0.83–6.41)), of Terai origin (AOR 1.18; 95% CI (0.67–2.08)), Muslim/Buddhist (AOR 1.33; 95% CI (0.55–3.20)), engaged in agriculture (AOR 2.89; 95% CI (1.3–6.15)), belonging to the second wealth index (AOR 2.73; 95% CI (1.12–6.64)) were more likely to consume tobacco than their counterparts. Pregnant women in upper caste group (AOR 0.50; 95% CI (0.25–0.99)), and with a primary (AOR 0.20; 95% CI (0.8–0.50)) or higher education (AOR 0.32; 95% CI (0.12–0.81)) were less likely to consume tobacco compared with Dalit caste group and no education, respectively. Women with parity > 3(AOR 4.80;

95% CI (1.15–19.95)) were more likely to consume alcohol than those with ≤ 3 parity. However, women from Terai origin (AOR 0.43; 95% CI (0.21–0.90) and having primary education (AOR 0.15; 95% CI (0.52–0.48)) were associated with less alcohol consumption.

Women from Terai origin (AOR 2.06; 95% CI (1.07–3.9)), primigravida (AOR 2.88; 95% CI (1.16–7.13)), primary education (AOR 0.15; 95% CI (0.52–0.48)), second wealth index (AOR 0.16; 95% CI (0.04–0.68)) and fourth wealth index (AOR 0.13; 95% CI (0.03–0.54)) were less likely to consume fruit and vegetable.

Regarding physical inactivity, respondents aged 20–34 years (AOR 4.84; 95% CI (2.22–10.57)), Adibashi/Janajati women (AOR 5.14; 95% CI (2.29–11.53)), upper caste (AOR 3.19; 95% CI (1.72–5.92)), Muslim/Buddhist (AOR 2.94; 95% CI (1.14–7.57)), primary education (AOR 3.59; 95% CI (1.58–8.14)), secondary education (AOR 0.45; 95% CI (0.21–0.94)), wealth indices middle (AOR 0.40; 95% CI (0.16–0.95)) and fourth (AOR 0.29; 95% CI (0.14–0.74)) were less likely to be physically inactive.

The results of multiple regression analyses for behavioral risk factors of CVDs among pregnant women with associated risk factors are presented in Table 4. Expectant mothers with primary level education (AOR 2.78; 95% CI (1.35–5.72)) were more likely to have ≥ 2 behavioral risk factors than illiterate women or women with a higher educational level.

Women aged 20–34 years (AOR 0.27; 95% CI (0.13–0.56)) had a lower chance for more than one behavioral risk factors than those of either lower or higher age group. Similarly, women belonging to the highest wealth index (AOR 0.36; 95% CI (0.16–0.84)) were less likely to have more than one behavioral risk factors compared to lower wealth quintile.

Discussion

This study provides the prevalence and socio-economic predictors of the four major behavioral risk factors of CVDs: insufficient fruit and vegetable consumption, insufficient physical activity, use of tobacco and harmful alcohol consumption by pregnant women. We noted this as the first ever study from rural Nepal that focused on predicting behavioral risk factors of CVDs among pregnant women.

The most common behavioral risk factor of CVD in pregnant women is the insufficient intake of fruits and vegetables, which concurs with the findings from a nationwide survey on risk factors of non-communicable diseases and with other studies conducted in different parts of Nepal [6, 14, 30]. These studies reported that insufficient fruits and vegetables consumption among pregnant women could be attributed to poverty that might have caused rural women not to afford adequate amount of fruits and vegetables. The other studies also

Table 1 Behavioral Risk factors of the study subjects

Behavioral risk factors	Yes	No	Total
	n (%)	n (%)	N (%)
Use of Tobacco (any form)	91 (21.4)	335 (78.6)	426 (100)
Use of alcohol	57 (13.4)	369 (86.6)	426 (100)
Insufficient fruit & vegetable intake	370 (86.9)	56 (13.1)	426 (100)
Insufficient physical activities	230 (53.9)	196 (46.1)	426 (100)

Table 2 Behavioral Risk factors associated with baseline characteristics among the study subjects

Variable	Total	Behavioral risk Factors for cardiovascular diseases (Yes, %)			
		Use of tobacco	Use of alcohol	Insufficient fruit & Veg.	physical inactivity
	N (%)	Yes, n (%)	Yes, n (%)	Yes, n (%)	Yes, n (%)
	426 (100)	91(21.36)	57 (13.38)	370 (86.9)	230 (53.99)
Age (years)		$p = 0.006$	$p < 0.0001$	$p = 0.686$	$p = 0.004$
< 20	102 (23.9)	33 (32.4)	22 (21.6)	86 (84.3)	65 (63.7)
20–34	290 (68.1)	45 (17.2)	21 (8.0)	254 (87.5)	143 (46.2)
35–45	34 (8.0)	13 (21.0)	14 (22.6)	30 (88.2)	22 (64.7)
Caste/ethnicity		$p < 0.0001$	$p < 0.0001$	$p = 0.044$	$p < 0.0001$
Dalit	71 (16.7)	31 (43.7)	30 (42.3)	68 (95.8)	17 (23.9)
Adibasi/ Janajati	91 (21.4)	27 (29.7)	7 (7.7)	79 (86.8)	37 (40.7)
Upper caste group	264 (62.0)	33 (12.5)	20 (7.6)	223 (84.5)	176 (66.7)
Origin		$p = 0.542$	$p = 0.01$	$p = 0.235$	$p = 0.466$
Hill	120 (28.2)	34 (19.9)	31 (18.1)	100 (83.3)	96 (56.1)
Terai	306 (71.8)	57 (22.4)	26 (10.2)	270 (88.2)	134 (52.5)
Religion		$p = 0.05$	$p = 0.086$	$p = 0.835$	$p = 0.146$
Hindu	391 (91.8)	79 (20.2)	49 (12.5)	340 (87.0)	207 (52.9)
Muslim/Buddhist	35 (8.2)	12 (34.3)	8 (22.9)	30 (85.7)	23 (65.7)
Women education		$p < 0.0001$	$p < 0.0001$	$p = 0.005$	$p < 0.0001$
No education	108 (25.4)	49 (35.3)	42 (30.2)	99 (91.6)	50 (36.0)
Primary	149 (35.0)	23 (19.5)	3 (2.5)	136 (91.2)	76 (64.4)
Secondary	79 (18.5)	7 (8.9)	5 (6.3)	65 (82.2)	52 (65.8)
Higher	90 (21.1)	12 (13.3)	7 (7.8)	70 (77.7)	52 (57.8)
Women occupation		$p = 0.545$	$p = 0.002$	$p = 0.971$	$p = 0.623$
Non-agriculture	292 (68.5)	60 (20.5)	29 (9.9)	254 (87.0)	132 (45.2)
Agriculture	134 (31.5)	31 (23.1)	28 (20.9)	116 (86.6)	64 (47.8)
Wealth Index		$p < 0.0001$	$p < 0.0001$	$P < 0.0001$	$p < 0.0001$
Lower	124 (29.1)	48 (38.7)	38 (30.6)	119 (93.5)	43 (34.7)
Second	100 (23.5)	13 (13.0)	5 (5.0)	80 (83.0)	53 (53.0)
Middle	84 (19.7)	12 (14.3)	4 (4.8)	80 (95.2)	53 (63.1)
Fourth	61 (14.3)	6 (9.8)	4 6.6)	52 (85.2)	47 (77.0)
Highest	57 (13.4)	12 (21.1)	6 (10.5)	39 (63.1)	34 (59.6)
Parity		$p = 0.540$	$p = 0.021$	$p = 0.334$	$p = 0.329$
Primi	167 (39.20)	32 (19.2)	17 (10.2)	149 (89.2)	91 (54.5)
1	112 (26.29)	29 (25.9)	19 (17.0)	98 (87.5)	63 (56.2)
2	58 (13.62)	13 (22.4)	3 (5.2)	61 (87.9)	35 (60.3)
3+	89 (20.89)	17 (19.1)	18 (20.2)	82 (92.1)	41 (46.1)

Note: $p < 0.05$ for statistical significance

supported that low income level prevents from consuming adequate fruits and vegetables [31, 32]. Another possible reason for less intake of fruits and vegetables during pregnancy could be associated with seasonal and geographical availability of such foods. In Nepalese culture, fruits consumption is not considered a priority compared to main cereals in their daily meals, most importantly rice and wheat. Cultural practices to avoid more hot foods during pregnancy is prevalent due to the belief that pregnancy is considered as hot state [33]. A study conducted by Christian et al. [34] described that foods such as peppers, lime and tamarind, sweet foods and green leafy vegetables that are fibrous and hard to digest, have been avoided during pregnancy in Terai, Nepal. Likewise, it is believed that eating sufficient mangoes is considered as a cause of abortion. Some of the cultural beliefs for not eating sufficient

Table 3 Adjusted Odds Ratios (aOR) for behavioral risk factors of CVD among rural women

Variable	Behavioral risk Factors for cardiovascular diseases (aOR, 95% CI)			
	Use of tobacco	Use of Alcohol	Insufficient Fruits and Vegetables	Physical inactivity
Age (Years)				
< 20	1.00	1.00	1.00	1.00
20–34	2.11 (0.97–4.57)	1.15 (0.33–3.96)	1.19 (0.32–4.43)	4.84 (2.22–10.57)**
35–45	2.31 (0.83–6.41)	1.99 (0.73–5.41)	1.41 (0.43–4.64)	0.6 (0.2–1.8)
Caste/ethnicity				
Dalit	1.00	1.00	1.00	1.00
Adibasi/ Janajati	0.31 (0.14–0.67)	0.26 (0.10–0.64)	0.51 (0.12–2.18)	5.14 (2.29–11.53)**
Upper caste group	0.50 (0.25–0.99)**	1.67 (0.58–4.82)	0.42 (0.14–1.24)	3.19 (1.72–5.92)**
Origin				
Hill	1.00	1.00	1.00	1.00
Terai	1.18 (0.67–2.08)	0.43 (0.21–0.90)**	2.06 (1.07–3.9)**	0.84 (0.51–1.3)
Religion				
Hindu	1.00	1.00	1.00	1.00
Muslim/others	1.33 (0.55–3.20)	1.01 (0.36–2.80)	2.1 (0.44–10.33)	2.94 (1.14–7.57)**
Women Education				
No education	1.00	1.00	1.00	1.00
Primary	0.20 (0.8–0.50)**	0.15 (0.52–0.48)**	0.36 (0.18–0.74)**	3.59 (1.58–8.14)**
Secondary	1.17 (0.40–3.38)	1.82 (0.39–8.52)	0.28 (0.18–3.65)	0.45 (0.21–0.94)**
Higher	0.32 (0.12–0.81)**	0.59 (0.16–2.24)	0.14 (0.07–2.33)	0.72 (0.33–1.55)
Women Occupation				
Non-agriculture	1.00	1.00	1.00	1.00
Agriculture	2.89 (1.3–6.15)**	2.02 (0.82–4.95)	0.70 (0.24–2.05)	1.4 (0.7–3.0)
Wealth Index				
Lower	1.00	1.00	1.00	1.00
Second	2.73 (1.12–6.64)**	0.77 (0.23–2.55)	0.16 (0.04–0.68)**	0.90 (0.40–2.03)
Middle	1.61 (0.64–4.08)	2.22 (0.51–9.68)	0.43 (0.12–1.43)	0.40 (0.16–0.95)**
Fourth	2.13 (0.71–6.39)	1.68 (0.37–7.63)	0.13 (0.03–0.54)**	0.29 (0.14–0.74)**
Highest	0.75 (0.29–1.94)	1.41 (0.33–6.01)	0.54 (0.18–1.61)	1.19 (0.48–2.91)
Parity (years)				
Primi	1.00	1.00	1.00	1.00
One	1.05 (0.53–2.08)	1.82 (0.65–5.07)	2.88 (1.16–7.13)**	0.85 (0.46–1.55)
Two	0.75 (0.31–1.82)	1.46 (0.48–4.39)	1.86 (0.60–5.73)	0.66 (0.30–1.45)
Three and above	1.13 (0.49–2.59)	4.80 (1.15–9.95)**	1.40 (0.46–4.28)	1.26 (0.63–2.55)

**p value < 0.05 (Significant)

foods include 'causing harm to mother and/or baby' and 'not enough space for baby in stomach' [34].

Lack of physical activity during pregnancy was the second most common behavioral risk factor of CVDs among our study subjects with a prevalence of 53.9%, which is similar to that found in other Nepalese studies [6, 35], but significantly greater than those found in nationwide non-communicable disease survey [36]. This could result from the general belief among Nepalese and promoted by some grassroot level health care providers that physical activity leads to miscarriage, poor fetal growth or premature delivery. A systematic review on physical activity during pregnancy suggests that some light-to-moderate physical activity is protective for maternal and child health outcomes such as pre-eclampsia, gestational hypertension and premature birth [37]. Physical activity guidelines around the world has recommended moderate intensity exercise such as brisk walking and other leisure time activities for pregnant women [38], therefore, appropriate counseling regarding optimal

Table 4 Prevalence and Adjusted Odds Ratios (aORs) of ≥ 2 behavioral risk factors for CVD among pregnant rural women

Variable	≥ 2 Behavioral risk Factors for cardiovascular diseases (aORs, 95% CI)		
	N (%)	aORs	95%CI
Age (Years)			
< 20	77 (75.5)	1.00	–
20–34	160 (61.1)	0.27	0.13–0.56**
35–49	46 (74.2)	0.91	0.37–2.24
Caste/ethnicity			
Dalit	49 (69.0)	1.00	–
Adibasi/Janajati	60 (65.9)	0.84	0.40–1.77
Upper caste group	174 (65.9)	0.94	0.45–1.97
Place of Origin			
Hill	115 (67.3)	1.00	–
Terai	168 (65.9)	0.89	0.55–1.44
Religion			
Hindu	256 (65.5)	1.00	–
Muslim/others	27 (77.1)	1.87	0.76–4.58
Women Education			
No education	88 (63.3)	1.00	–
Primary	89 (75.4)	2.78	1.35–5.72**
Secondary	50 (63.3)	1.28	0.63–2.61
Higher	56 (62.2)	1.15	0.56–2.35
Women Occupation			
Non-agriculture	197 (67.5)	1.00	–
Agriculture	86 (64.2)	0.59	0.31–1.11
Wealth Index			
Lower	87 (70.2)	1.00	–
Second	64 (64.0)	0.59	0.27–1.2
Middle	59 (70.2)	1.22	0.55–2.73
Fourth	42 (68.9)	0.98	0.41–2.30
Highest	31 (54.4)	0.36	0.16–0.84**
Parity (years)			
Primi	112 (67.1)	1.00	–
1	75 (67.0)	0.74	0.42–1.32
2	41 (70.7)	1.20	0.58–2.49
3+	55 (61.8)	0.77	0.40–1.47
Total	283 (100)	–	–

**p value < 0.05 (Significant)

physical activity during pregnancy could reduce the risk of CVDs associated with inadequate physical activity.

High rates of tobacco use (21.3%) and alcohol consumption (13.3%) among pregnant women are other key findings from the present study. Previous studies from Nepal also identified a higher prevalence of tobacco and alcohol use during pregnancy [17, 39]. The reason behind increasing tobacco use could be the widespread availability of a range of tobacco products, which made it easier to access for everyone even in rural areas. One of the most common form of tobacco used in rural parts of south Asian countries, including Nepal is Bidi (a dried and crushed tobacco flakes rolled by hand in *tendu* (*Diospyrus*) leaf) that contains higher amount of nicotine and tar than cigarette [40].

Similarly, brewing different types of traditional alcoholic beverages at home in rural Nepal [41], most commonly by women, could be one of the common reasons of a high rate of alcohol consumption by pregnant women. In Nepal, a nationwide study reported that cereals (rice, barley and millet) and sugar are commonly used ingredients to prepare home-brewed alcohol. Ethanol concentration on home-brewed alcohol were 14.0% (3 to 40%) for distilled and 5.2% (1 to 18.9%) for non-distilled forms [41]. Locally brewed alcoholic beverages are considered culturally acceptable to drink even by pregnant women in some ethnic groups. This could be due to lack of awareness about the harmful effects of these products to mother and fetus during pregnancy. Health promotion strategies should, therefore, include general awareness programme to reduce these maternal behavior risk factors of CVDs.

Interestingly, our study demonstrated the association between educational level, age and wealth index of respondents with more than one behavioral risk factors of CVDs. Adjusting for potential confounders yielded more direct evidence of the contribution of these parameters to the prevalence of risk factors for CVDs among pregnant women in rural Nepal. Poor level of awareness on negative effects of behavioral risk factors of CVDs during pregnancy could be associated with low level of literacy. Similarly, poor access to adequate fruits and vegetables could be associated with poverty in rural areas. Several studies [39, 42, 43] are in line with our study findings. For example, level of education and age factors were associated with physical inactivity [42, 43]. Targeted educational campaigns and poverty reduction strategies should be recommended to reduce behavioral risk factors of CVDs among women in rural settings.

Despite our efforts to explore this important topic in the Nepalese context, this study should be evaluated in the light of some limitations. First, the information we collected was obtained by self-reporting, and thus, is subject to informant bias. Second, our study did not consider information about nutritional status of pregnant women (e.g. under or over nutrition status by body mass index) which is considered to be one of the major factors of understanding these risk factors [44]. Third, because the study was performed in southern plain area, its findings may not be generalizable for hilly or mountainous regions. Thus, it would be imperative to conduct similar types of studies in hilly and mountainous regions of Nepal, taking into consideration of the limitations of this study. Further, intervention studies to reduce prevalence of behavioral risk factors of CVDs during pregnancy and to improve birth outcome is recommended for Nepal.

Conclusion

This study identifies a high prevalence of fruits and vegetables insufficiency, insufficient physical activity, tobacco use and alcohol consumption as behavioral risk factors of CVDs among pregnant women residing in rural Nepal and highlights the predictors of these behavioral risk factors. Health promotion strategies such as community-based awareness activities on how to reduce behavioral risk factors of CVDs and appropriate counseling regarding cardiovascular risk reduction ought to be routinely performed in antenatal clinics in rural Nepal. Furthermore, interventional studies should be considered to reduce risky behaviors in pregnancy associated with CVDs to improve maternal and child health outcomes.

Abbreviations
AOR: Adjusted Odds Ratio; CI: Confidence Interval; CVDs: Cardiovascular Diseases; FCHVs: Female Community Health Volunteers; LMICs: Low- and Middle-income Countries; MCH: Maternal and Child Health; VDCs: Village Development Committees; WHO: World Health Organization

Acknowledgements
We acknowledge all study participants and academics at the Institute of Medical Sciences, Banarus Hindu University, India for their, guidance and support.

Funding
We declare that we have no funding help to perform and publish this research including writing of the manuscript.

Authors' contributions
RP, JKS and DA conceptualized the study, performed statistical analysis and drafted the initial manuscript. KL, SY, RK, SA, MP, and NM, contributed to the critical inputs for data analysis and interpretation of results, and substantial revision of the manuscript contents. All authors read and approved the final manuscript.

Competing interests
The authors declare that they have no competing interests.

Author details
[1]Department of Community Medicine and Public Health, Maharajgunj Medical Campus, Institute of Medicine, Tribhuvan University, Kathmandu, Nepal. [2]Department of Preventive Medicine, College of Medicine, Dongguk University, 123 Dongdae-ro, Gyeongju-si 38066, Republic of Korea. [3]Department of Community Medicine and Public Health, Janaki Medical College, Tribhuvan University, Janakpur, Nepal. [4]Personal Social Services Research Unit, London School of Economics and Political Science, London, UK. [5]Maharajgunj Medical Campus, Institute of Medicine, Tribhuvan University, Kathmandu, Nepal. [6]Southgate Institute for Health, Society and Equity, Flinders University, Adelaide, Australia. [7]Department of Physiology, Maharajgunj Medical Campus, Institute of Medicine, Tribhuvan University, Kathmandu, Nepal. [8]Department of Community Medicine, Kathmandu University, Devdaha Medical College and Research Institute, Rupandehi, Nepal.

References
1.   American Heart Association. What is cardiovascular disease? Available from: http://www.heart.org/en/health-topics/consumer-healthcare/what-is-cardiovascular-disease. Accessed 18 Dec 2017.
2.   World Health Organization. Cardiovascular diseases (CVD) fact sheet. Available from: http://www.who.int/en/news-room/fact-sheets/detail/cardiovascular-diseases-(cvds). Accessed 18 Dec 2017.
3.   Mendis S, Puska P, Norrving B. Global atlas on cardiovascular disease prevention and control. Geneva: World Health Organization; 2011.
4.   Vaidya A, Pokharel PK, Nagesh S, Karki P, Kumar S, Majhi S. Prevalence of coronary heart disease in the urban adult males of eastern Nepal: a population-based analytical cross-sectional study. Indian Heart J. 2009;61(4):341–7.
5.   Maskey A, Sayami A, Pandey M. Coronary artery disease: an emerging epidemic in Nepal. J Nepal Med Assoc. 2003;42(146):122–4.
6.   Dhungana RR, Devkota S, Khanal MK, Gurung Y, Giri RK, Parajuli RK, Adhikari A, Joshi S, Hada B, Shayami A. Prevalence of cardiovascular health risk behaviors in a remote rural community of Sindhuli district, Nepal. BMC Cardiovasc Disord. 2014;14(1):1.
7.   World Health Organization. Global health risks: mortality and burden of disease attributable to selected major risks. Geneva: World Health Organization; 2009.
8.   Faden VB, Graubard BI, Dufour M. The relationship of drinking and birth outcome in a US national sample of expectant mothers. Paediatr Perinat Epidemiol. 1997;11(2):167–80.
9.   Bailey BA, Sokol RJ. Prenatal alcohol exposure and miscarriage, stillbirth, preterm delivery, and sudden infant death syndrome. Alcohol Res Health. 2011;34(1):86–91.
10. Grewal J, Carmichael SL, Ma C, Lammer EJ, Shaw GM. Maternal periconceptional smoking and alcohol consumption and risk for select congenital anomalies. Birth Defects Res A Clin Mol Teratol. 2008;82(7):519–26.
11. Hackshaw A, Rodeck C, Boniface S. Maternal smoking in pregnancy and birth defects: a systematic review based on 173 687 malformed cases and 11.7 million controls. Hum Reprod Update. 2011. https://doi.org/10.1093/humupd/dmr022.
12. Gelson E, Gatzoulis MA, Steer P, Johnson MR. Heart disease—why is maternal mortality increasing? BJOG. 2009;116(5):609–11.
13. Hall ME, George EM, Granger JP. The heart during pregnancy. Rev Esp Cardiol. 2011;64(11):1045–50.
14. Aryal K, Neupane S, Mehata S, Vaidya A, Singh S, Paulin F, Madanlal R, Riley L, Cowan M, Guthold R, et al. Non communicable diseases risk factors: STEPS Survey Nepal 2013. Kathmandu: Nepal Health Research Council; 2014.
15. Khaw KT, Wareham N, Bingham S, Welch A, Luben R, Day N. Combined impact of health behaviours and mortality in men and women: the EPIC-Norfolk prospective population study. PLoS Med. 2008;5(1):e12.
16. Martin-Diener E, Meyer J, Braun J, Tarnutzer S, Faeh D, Rohrmann S, Martin BW. The combined effect on survival of four main behavioural risk factors for non-communicable diseases. Prev Med. 2014;65:148–52.
17. Niraul S, Jha N, Shyangwa P. Alcohol consumption among women in a district of Eastern Nepal. Health Renaiss. 2014;11(3):205–12.
18. Niraula SR, Shyangwa P, Jha N, Paudel R, Pokharel P. Alcohol use among women in a town of eastern Nepal. J Nepal Med Assoc. 2004;43(155):244–49.
19. Singh JK, Kadel R, Acharya D, Lombard D, Khanal S, Singh SP. 'MATRI-SUMAN' a capacity building and text messaging intervention to enhance maternal and child health service utilization among pregnant women from rural Nepal: study protocol for a cluster randomised controlled trial. BMC Health Serv Res. 2018;18(1):018–3223.
20. District Development Committee Dhanusha. District Profile of Dhanusha, District Development Committee. Janakpur: Ministry of Local Development, & District Development Committee, Dhanusha; 2012. p. 1–4.
21. Central Bureau Statistics. General and Social Characteristics Tables: Household and Population, Age-Sex Distribution, Relationship, Marital Status and Religion,

National Population and Housing Census 2011, vol. 5. Kathmandu: Government of Nepal, National Planning Commission Secretariat, Central Bureau of Statistics; 2014.
22. District Health Office Dhanusha. District health profile of Dhanusha, Nepal. Edited by Office MoHaPDH, Dhanusha; 2013.
23. District Development Committee Dhanusha, Ministry of Local Development. A profile of Dhanusha District of Nepal. Edited by Ministry of Local Development, Janakpur and District Development Committee, Dhanusha; 2012.
24. Karki K, Dahal B, Regmi A, Poudel A, Gurung Y. WHO STEPS Surveillance: Non Communicable Diseases Risk Factors Survey. 2008. Kathmandu: Ministry of Health and Population, GoN, Society for Local Integrated Development Nepal (SOLID Nepal) and WHO; 2008.
25. Agudo A, Joint F. Measuring intake of fruit and vegetables [electronic resource]; 2005.
26. Organization WH. Obesity: preventing and managing the global epidemic. Geneva: World Health Organization; 2000.
27. Ministry of Health and Population NE, ICF International. Nepal Demographic and Health Survey 2011. Kathmandu: Nepal Ministry of Health and Population, New ERA and Maryland: ICF International Calverton; 2012.
28. Acharya D, Khanal V, Singh JK, Adhikari M, Gautam S. Impact of mass media on the utilization of antenatal care services among women of rural community in Nepal. BMC Res Notes. 2015;8(1):345.
29. Barbosa Filho VC, de Campos W, Bozza R, da Silva LA. The prevalence and correlates of behavioral risk factors for cardiovascular health among Southern Brazil adolescents: a cross-sectional study. BMC Pediatr. 2012;12(1):130.
30. Oli N, Vaidya A, Thapa G. Behavioural risk factors of noncommunicable diseases among Nepalese urban poor: a descriptive study from a slum area of Kathmandu. Epidemiol Res Int. 2013;2013:13.
31. Hall JN, Moore S, Harper SB, Lynch JW. Global variability in fruit and vegetable consumption. Am J Prev Med. 2009;36(5):402–409.e5.
32. Valmórbida JL, Vitolo MR. Factors associated with low consumption of fruits and vegetables by preschoolers of low socio-economic level. J Pediatr. 2014;90(5):464–71.
33. Christian P, West K, Katz J, Kimbrough-Pradhan E, LeClerq S, Khatry S, Shrestha S. Cigarette smoking during pregnancy in rural Nepal. Risk factors and effects of β-carotene and vitamin A supplementation. Eur J Clin Nutr. 2004;58(2):204–11.
34. Christian P, Bunjun Srihari S, Thorne-Lyman A, Khatry SK, LeClerq SC, Shrestha SR. Eating down in pregnancy: exploring food-related beliefs and practices of pregnancy in rural Nepal. Ecol Food Nutr. 2006;45(4):253–78.
35. Bhandari B, Bhattarai M, Bhandari M, Ghimire A, Pokharel PK. Prevalence of other associated risk factors of Cardiovascular Disease among Hypertensive patients in Eastern Nepal. Nepal Heart J. 2014;11(1):27–31.
36. Aryal K, Thapa P, Mehata S, Vaidya A, Pandey A, Bista B, Pandit A, Dhakal P, Karki K, Dhimal M. Alcohol Use by Nepalese Women: Evidence from Non Communicable Disease Risk Factors STEPS Survey Nepal 2013. J Nepal Health Res Counc. 2015;13(29):1–6.
37. Schlüssel MM, Souza EB, Reichenheim ME, Kac G. Physical activity during pregnancy and maternal-child health outcomes: a systematic literature review. Cad Saude Publica. 2008;24:s531–44.
38. Evenson KR, Barakat R, Brown WJ, Dargent-Molina P, Haruna M, Mikkelsen EM, Mottola MF, Owe KM, Rousham EK, Yeo S. Guidelines for physical activity during pregnancy: comparisons from around the world. Am J Lifestyle Med. 2014;8(2):102–21.
39. Chasan-Taber L, Schmidt MD, Pekow P, Sternfeld B, Manson J, Markenson G. Correlates of physical activity in pregnancy among Latina women. Matern Child Health J. 2007;11(4):353–63.
40. Rahman M, Fukui T. Bidi smoking and health. Public Health. 2000;114(2):123–7.
41. Thapa N, Aryal KK, Paudel M, Puri R, Thapa P, Shrestha S, Shrestha S, Stray-Pedersen B. Nepalese homebrewed alcoholic beverages: types, ingredients, and ethanol concentration from a nation wide survey. J Nepal Health Res Counc. 2015;13(29):59–65.
42. Dumith SC, Domingues MR, Mendoza-Sassi RA, Cesar JA. Physical activity during pregnancy and its association with maternal and child health indicators. Rev Saude Publica. 2012;46(2):327–33.
43. Nascimento SL, Surita FG, Godoy AC, Kasawara KT, Morais SS. Physical activity patterns and factors related to exercise during pregnancy: a cross sectional study. PLoS One. 2015;10(6):e0128953.
44. Hashmi AH, Paw MK, Nosten S, Darakamon MC, Gilder ME, Charunwatthana P, Carrara VI, Wickramasinghe K, Angkurawaranon C, Plugge E, et al. 'Because the baby asks for it': a mixed-methods study on local perceptions toward nutrition during pregnancy among marginalised migrant women along the Myanmar-Thailand border. Glob Health Action. 2018;11(1):1473104.

13

High pregnancy incidence and low contraceptive use among a prospective cohort of female entertainment and sex workers in Phnom Penh, Cambodia

Putu Duff[1,2,5], Jennifer L. Evans[3], Ellen S. Stein[3], Kimberly Page[3,4], Lisa Maher[5]* on behalf of the Young Women's Health Study Collaborative

Abstract

Background: While HIV and unintended pregnancies are both occupational risks faced by female sex workers, the epidemiology of pregnancy and its drivers in this population remains understudied. This includes Cambodia, where the drivers of pregnancy among female entertainment and sex workers (FESW) remain unknown. The current study aimed to examine factors associated with incident pregnancy, as well as describe contraceptive use among FESW in Phnom Penh, Cambodia.

Methods: This analysis drew from the Young Women's Health Study (YWHS)-2, a 12-month observational cohort of 220 FESW aged 15–29 years, conducted between August 2009 and August 2010. Interviewer-administered questionnaires were conducted at baseline and quarterly thereafter, alongside HIV and pregnancy testing. Bivariate and multivariable extended Cox regression analysis was used to examine correlates of incident pregnancy.

Results: At baseline, 6.8% of participants were pregnant, and only 10.8% reported using hormonal contraceptives, with 11.3% reporting an abortion in the past 3 months. Pregnancy incidence was high, at 22/100 person-years (95% CI: 16.3–30.1). In multivariable analysis, younger age (19–24 years versus 25–29 years) (Adjusted Hazards Ratio (AHR): 2.28; 95% Confidence Interval (CI) 1.22–4.27), lower income (400,000–600,000 Riel (≤150$USD) versus > 600,000 Riel (> 150$USD)) (AHR 2.63; 95% CI 1.02–6.77) positively predicted pregnancy, while higher self-reported condom self-efficacy were associated with reduced pregnancy incidence (AHR 0.89; 95% CI 0.81–0.98).

Conclusions: Results document high incidence of pregnancy and unmet reproductive health needs among FESWs in Cambodia. Findings point to an urgent need for multi-level interventions, including venue-based HIV/STI and violence prevention interventions, in the context of legal and policy reform. High pregnancy incidence in this population may also undermine recruitment and retention into HIV prevention intervention trials. The exploration of innovative and comprehensive sex worker-tailored sexual and reproductive health service models, also as part of HIV prevention intervention trials, is warranted.

Keywords: Pregnancy, Reproductive health, Sex work, Cambodia, Cohort study, prevention trials

* Correspondence: lmaher@kirby.unsw.edu.au; http://www.kirby.unsw.edu.au
[5]Kirby Institute for Infection and Immunity (formerly the National Centre in HIV Epidemiology and Clinical Research), UNSW Australia I, Wallace Wurth Building, Sydney, NSW 2052, Australia
Full list of author information is available at the end of the article

Background

Pregnancy in women at high risk of HIV is an important issue, with unprotected sex as the primary exposure for both HIV and pregnancy. While previous epidemiological research among women engaged in transactional sex has largely focused on risk of HIV and other sexually transmitted infections (STIs), a growing number of studies have begun to examine the broader reproductive health need of women engaged in transactional sex, including pregnancy [1–4]. Recent studies among women in engaged in transactional sex have documented lifetime pregnancy prevalence ranging between 70% and 90% [1, 3, 5–7], many of which are unintended pregnancies [7, 8]. The prevalence of unintended pregnancies among women engaged in transactional sex is high - up to 86% in some studies [3] – yet recent research indicates that many women engaged in transactional sex have a strong desire to have children [9], with pregnancy intentions similar to those of women in other occupations [10].

The high prevalence of pregnancy among women engaged in transactional sex also has important implications for the success of HIV prevention trials, which often enroll high-risk sexually active women, some of which target women engaged in transactional sex. Understanding the incidence and correlates of pregnancy among women involved in transactional sex is therefore critical, as pregnancy intention is often an exclusion criterion and actual pregnancy typically results in study product discontinuation (if the study product is considered potentially harmful to a pregnant woman or her fetus), potentially impacting the success of the trial, as well as the efficacy of subsequent interventions. Increased understanding of the drivers of pregnancy among women engaged in transactional sex is critical in developing sexual and reproductive health (SRH) services tailored to the specific needs of women engaged in transactional sex [11]. However, there remains a research gap on the prevalence and correlates of pregnancy among women working in entertainment venues with high-risk sexual patterns as well as women engaged in commercial sex. The few studies that have examined correlates of pregnancy, have found that individual and interpersonal factors such as previous history of abortion, having a steady intimate partner [12], experiencing violence [13] and alcohol/illicit drug use [12, 14] were associated with unintended pregnancy in this population.

In Cambodia, women engaged in high-risk and transactional sex are a heterogeneous group working in variety of environments and venues, whom collectively can be referred to as female entertainment and sex workers (FESW) [15, 16]. Empirical data on pregnancy among FESW remain limited. Previous work by Delvaux [8] and colleagues highlighted low knowledge around SRH and limited access to reproductive health services among brothel-based women engaged in transactional sex in Phnom Penh, underscoring a need to examine the drivers of pregnancy in this population. Moreover, little is known about the pregnancy outcomes of FESW following the implementation of the 2008 'Law on Suppression of Human Trafficking and Sexual Exploitation' [17]. The 'Trafficking Law' effectively criminalized the selling and purchase of sex, by prohibiting almost all aspects of sex work including: public solicitation, procurement of prostitution, management of a sex work venue and the provision of premises for prostitution [18]. The passage of this law resulted in increased police crackdowns and brothel closures, and led to the displacement of FESW to entertainment venues, streets and guesthouses, where they lacked protections from peers and management [16]. In these new settings, FESW have reported increased vulnerability to client-perpetrated violence and a reduced ability to negotiate client condom use [16]. The displacement of FESW to diverse settings and the associated disruption of peer networks has been found to reduce the reach of HIV prevention and service delivery [16, 19], access to health services and condoms [16], and may also have had an impact on unintended pregnancy rates.

Given the dearth of research examining the correlates of pregnancy, particularly within the Cambodian context, this longitudinal study aimed to determine the factors associated with time to pregnancy among FESWs working in Phnom Penh, Cambodia over a twelve-month period. While our overall goal was to determine the set of factors that best describe incident pregnancy, we hypothesized that the following could potentially be associated with reduced time to pregnancy: marital status, young age and low parity, alcohol/illicit drug use, intimate partner violence and condom non-use by non-paying partners and clients.

Methods
Study design and setting

The data from this study were drawn from the Young Women's Health Study 2 (YWHS-2), a prospective cohort of young women engaged in sex work across a variety of venues and settings in Phnom Penh, Cambodia. [15] The YWHS was led by a multidisciplinary team including Cambodian Women's Development Association (CWDA), the National Center for HIV/AIDS, Dermatology and STD (NCHADS), the University of California, San Francisco (UCSF) in the United States, and the Kirby Institute at the University of New South Wales (UNSW) in Australia.

The study design and recruitment procedures are described in detail elsewhere [15]. Briefly, eligibility criteria included: being biologically female (aged 15–29), Khmer language comprehension, working in a sex work or entertainment venue and having two or more sexual partners in the last month *or* engaging in transactional sex (defined as having exchanged sex for money, drugs, or other goods or services) in the past three months, with plans of remaining in Phnom Penh throughout the course of the one-year study. Trained staff members recruited a convenience sample of women engaged in sex work from a variety of locations including: 1) YWHS information meetings held by CWDA; 2) neighbourhood-based outreach; and 3) referrals by previous participants or community groups. All study participants provided voluntary informed consent prior to enrolment in the study.

Data collection
Between 2009 and 2010, study participants visited the YWHS clinic at baseline and quarterly thereafter, where they completed a structured questionnaire, administered in Khmer by trained interviewers. The questionnaire elicited a wide range of information including socio-demographic characteristics (e.g., age, education, marital status), individual and interpersonal factors such as alcohol and drug use, interpersonal violence as well as sex work factors including occupational and sexual risk history, reproductive health and STI/HIV prevention (e.g., STI infection, contraceptive use and pregnancy). Staffed by a team of health care professionals, including a physician, nurses, counselors and a laboratory technician, all study participants attending the YWHS clinic for interviews were also tested for HPV and provided with STI treatment free of charge. Participants who tested positive for HPV or HIV were referred to local health providers for no-cost medical assessment and treatment.

All participants underwent voluntary client-centred risk-reduction counseling prior to testing. HIV serology testing, using two rapid tests: Uni-Gold Recombigen HIV rapid HIV test (Trinity Biotech USA, Jamestown, New York, USA) and the Clairview HIV ½ STAT-PAK (Inverness Medical Diagnostics, Waltham, Massachusetts, USA). HIV-1 immunoblot was used to confirm HIV serodiscordant samples. All participants who tested negative for HIV and were not pregnant were offered HPV vaccination. Study participants were provided free transport to interview sites and remunerated (US$5) for their time and expertise, regardless of whether they had or had not received the HPV vaccine. Ethical approval was obtained from the Institutional Review Board of the Committee on Human Research at the University of California, San Francisco, the Cambodian National Ethics Committee and the University of New South Wales Human Research Ethics Committee, aligned with both national and institutional ethical standards and the Helsinki Declaration of 1975 (revised in 2000). The Cambodian and U.S. IRB deemed the inclusion of minors ethical and waived requirement for parental consent based on the minimal risk posed by study procedures and potential for direct benefit to participants. Informed consent procedures following

international guidelines (Declaration of Helsinki, and Council for International Organizations of Medical Sciences (CIOMS) with WHO)) were conducted in Khmer, by trained research personnel and with ongoing consultative supervision and training from staff of Cambodia National Center for HIV AIDS, and STDs (NCHADS) STD Clinic in Phnom Penh, Cambodia.

Measures
Dependent variable
The primary dependent variable, incident pregnancy, was based on a 'Yes' response to the question, 'As far as you know, are you pregnant now?' which was asked at each three-monthly follow-up.

Independent variables
Independent variables were considered based on a priori knowledge of their associations with pregnancy, including among women engaged in transactional sex, in the literature. Age and education (number of years in school) were considered fixed variables, and all other variables were considered time-variant and updated at every quarterly follow-up. Other socio-demographic variables included marital status (defined as living together (married), living together (not married) and living alone (divorced, widowed and single)) and number of children (measured continuously). Individual sexual and substance use patterns were also considered, such as number of days participants drank alcohol in the last month (measured continuously), self reported amphetamine-type stimulant (ATS) use in the last 3 months, including crystal (ice) and *yama*. We also included a 6-item scale for measuring self-efficacy for negotiating condom use, modified for the sex work context [20]. The scale included questions such as: "I can ask a new private partner to use condoms" and "I can refuse sex when I don't have a condom available". Participants indicated their agreement with each of the five items measured on a five-point Likert scale ranging from strongly agree (for a score of 4) to strongly disagree (for a score of 0). A continuous score for condom self-efficacy was used, by summing the scores for all five items. Sex work variables included: number of sex clients in the past month and income in the last month. Women indicated if they currently worked as: a beer promoter, in a beer garden, as a waitress or hostess in a karaoke bar, nightclub, in a massage parlour, brothel, or as a freelance worker in the park, street or another location. FESWs were categorized as entertainment venue-based (i.e., working as beer promoter, in a beer garden, as a waitress or hostess in a karaoke bar, nightclub, in a massage parlour) versus non-entertainment venue-based (i.e., working on the street, brothel or public spaces). In light of the literature linking gender-based violence (from clients and

intimate partners) with reduced condom negotiation, use and pregnancy [21, 22], we also examined the relationship between physical and sexual violence by clients and intimate partners, in the last year.

Statistical analyses
Pregnancy incidence was calculated using the person-years method. Frequencies and proportions were calculated at baseline for categorical variables, and measures of central tendency (i.e., mean, median and IQR) were used to describe continuous variables. To examine the relationships between potential confounders on time to pregnancy, time-dependent Cox regression analyses were used. First, bivariate analyses using an extended Cox regression model were run to estimate the time to pregnancy using unadjusted hazard ratios. Using a conservative p-value cut-off of 0.10, a priori potential confounders that were also significant at $p < 0.10$ were included in a full multivariable model (model 1). A second model was constructed with variables significant at $p < 0.05$ in bivariate analysis (model 2). All statistical analyses were performed using SAS software version 9.3 (SAS Institute, Cary, NC, USA).

Results
A total of 204 FESWs were included in our sample, yielding 799 observations over the one-year/12-month follow-up period. More than two thirds of participants (60.3%) were between the ages of 25–29, with 119 (58.3%) reporting between one to six years of education. Most participants (63.2%) were single, divorced, widowed or separated and the median number of children was three (IQR: 2–4) (See Table 1). At baseline, 14 (6.8%) participants were pregnant, and only 22 (10.8%) reported using hormonal contraceptives (i.e., oral contraceptive pills or injectable hormones), and 23 (11.3%) reporting an abortion in the past 3 months (Table 2). Pregnancy incidence was high, at 22/100 person-years (py) (95% CI: 16.3–30.1). The number of new pregnancies at each quarterly time point were as follows: 13, 9, 6 and 13. In bivariate analysis, variables associated with increased pregnancy incidence (at $p < 0.10$) included: age (19–24 years versus 25–29 years); income in the last month (≤600,000 Riel versus > 600,000 Riel; the equivalent of ≤ \$USD 150 versus >&USD 150); numbers of years in school (1–6 years versus 7+ years), cohabiting with a partner (not legally married) compared to living alone (single, widowed, divorced or separated) and hormonal contraceptive use in the last 3 months (measured at baseline). Factors associated with lower pregnancy incidence were HIV-positive serostatus, condom self-efficacy and condom use at last sex.

In multivariable analysis (Model 1), younger age (Adjusted Hazards Ratio (AHR): 2.28; 95% CI 1.22–4.27), and lower income (AHR 2.63; 95% CI 1.02–6.77) were independently associated with decreased time to pregnancy.

Self-reported condom self-efficacy was associated with a longer time to incident pregnancy (AHR 0.89; 95% CI 0.81–0.98). As displayed in Table 3, similar associations were present in Model 2, a more parsimonious model restricted to factors significant at $p < 0.05$ in bivariate analysis.

Discussion
The one-year pregnancy incidence in this cohort of young FESW was high, even when compared to Cambodia's crude birth rate of 22 live births per 1000 women/year [23]. Moreover, despite the young age of our sample, the median number of children (three) in our cohort exceeded the estimated number of births for urban Cambodian women (2.1 children) over their entire reproductive lives [23]. The finding of high number of pregnancies corroborates a growing body of research, including unintended pregnancies (using abortion rates as a proxy), among women engaged in transactional sex in various settings [4, 8]. For example, 408/475 (86%) of women in transactional sex in Kenya and 264/514 (53%) of Colombian women engaged in sex work reported at least one induced abortion [2, 3]. In Uzbekistan, 109/448(24.3%) of women engaged in transactional sex reported three or more lifetime abortions [7]. While there is a need to examine pregnancy intentions among FESW in Cambodia, the high number of abortions in the past three months suggests that many pregnancies in this sample were unintended. Alongside previous research that documented 166/592 (28.2%) of brothel-based sex workers in Cambodia (in 2007) attending STI care in Phnom Penh had an induced abortion in the last year [24], these findings highlight large reproductive health needs among Cambodian women engaged in commercial sex.

The low use of hormonal contraceptives further underscores the reproductive health gap among FESW in this setting. The baseline prevalence of hormonal contraceptive use in our sample was roughly 23/204 (11%) compared to 642/2069 (31%) among Cambodian women living in urban areas [25]. This is especially low when compared to married women in Phnom Penh, (616/1099) 56% of whom were documented to use hormonal contraceptives in 2010 [25]. Previous research among brothel-based Cambodian women engaged in transactional sex revealed low SRH knowledge, with very few having attended family planning services [26]. Future research into the barriers to SRH services access, including hormonal contraceptives and safe abortion services is warranted. While hormonal contraceptive use in this sample was low, most participants reported using condoms to prevent pregnancy and HIV/STIs. This is not surprising given the dual function of condoms in preventing HIV/STIs and pregnancy, and their relative availability and low cost compared to hormonal contraceptives. The preference for condoms may also reflect Cambodia's 100% condom use

Table 1 Baseline characteristics of 204 Female and Entertainment Sex Workers (FESWs) in the YWHS-II study, Phnom Penh, Cambodia

Characteristic	Total (%) (n = 204)	Participants who were pregnant at least once over follow-up Yes (%) (n = 41)	p-value
Socio-demographics, biological and individual factors			
Age (years)			
16–18	14 (6.9)	2 (14.3)	0.997
19–24	67 (32.8)	20 (29.9)	0.010
25–29	123 (60.3)	19 (15.5)	–
Income, last month ($USD)			
≤ 150	128 (63.1)	26 (20.3)	0.061
> 150	75 (36.9)	15 (20.0)	–
Education			
No schooling	44 (21.6)	7 (15.9)	0.610
1–6 years	119 (58.3)	30 (25.2)	0.096
7+ years	41 (20.1)	4 (9.8)	–
Marital status			
Legally married	8 (3.9)	1 (12.5)	0.321
Living together, not legally married	67 (32.8)	17 (25.4)	0.026
Single, widowed, divorced or separated	129 (63.2)	23 (17.8)	–
Number of previous children (continuous) Median, IQR	3 (2–4)	3 (2–3)	0.079
HIV status			
HIV positive	33 (16.2)	3 (7.3)	0.086
HIV negative	171 (83.8)	38 (92.7)	–
Days drank alcohol, last month	15 (3.5–29.0)	24 (3–30)	0.226
ATS use, last 3 months (self-report)	55 (27.0)	12 (21.8)	0.569
Condom self-efficacy (median score; IQR)	21 (18–24)	20 (17–21)	0.035
Hormonal contraceptive use, last 3 months	22 (10.8)	1 (4.6)	0.088
Interpersonal factors			
Used condom at last sex (yes)	128 (62.8)	23 (18.0)	0.020
Condom use, last client (yes)	117 (90.0)	23 (19.7)	0.772
Condom use, last non-paying partner	11 (14.9)	0 (0.0)	0.393
Number of sexual partners, last month Median, IQR	4 (2–10)	3 (2–10)	0.790
Any client physical or sexual violence, last year	53 (26.0)	14 (26.4)	0.189
Any intimate partner physical or sexual violence, last year	41 (20.1)	9 (22.0)	0.957
Sex work factors			
Entertainment venue-based sex work, last month	131 (67.2)	24 (18.3)	0.241
Non-entertainment venue-based sex work, last month	64 (32.8)	16 (25.0)	–
Had a manager	145 (71.4)	29 (20.0)	0.172

policy for women engaged in transactional sex work, previously enforced widely in brothels; however there is evidence that nation's 2008 anti-trafficking legislation has impeded condom access and use [27]. Condoms as the sole method of contraception can be problematic, given their reduced effectiveness in preventing pregnancy compared to hormonal methods. Dual contraceptive methods

(hormonal contraceptives in addition to condom use) are indicated to prevent both HIV/STI and pregnancy in this population. There is an urgent need to explore innovative sex worker-specific service delivery models to improve Cambodian FESWs' access to non-judgmental SRH services that promote dual contraceptive use and safe abortion services.

Table 2 Pregnancy and HIV/STI prevention methods in the last 3 months, reported at baseline

	Total (100%) (n = 204)	Participants who were pregnant at least once over the study period	
Method for pregnancy prevention, last 3 months		Yes (20.1%) (n = 41)	No (79.9%) (n = 163)
Male condom	203 (99.5)	41 (20.2)	162 (79.8)
Withdrawal	71 (34.8)	11 (15.5)	60 (84.5)
Oral sex/sex without penetration	37 (18.1)	6 (16.2)	31 (83.8)
Birth control pills	16 (7.84)	1 (6.2)	15 (93.8)
Injectable contraceptives	6 (2.9)	0 (0.0)	6 (100.0)
Abortion	23 (11.3)	6 (26.1)	17 (73.9)
Other method	2 (0.98)	0 (0.0)	2 (100.0)
Method for HIV/STI prevention, last 3 months			
Male condom	204 (100.0)	41 (20.1)	163 (79.9)
Oral sex/sex without penetration	40 (19.6)	8 (20.0)	32 (80.0)
Masturbation	75 (36.8)	18 (24.0)	57 (76.0)

FESW who reported increased self-efficacy or control over condom use had significantly lower pregnancy incidence, likely due to more consistent condom use by sexual partners. While FESWs' ability to negotiate safe sex is critical, growing evidence suggests this needs to be coupled with venue-based interventions that provide access to condoms and support the safe negotiation of condom use by clients [27, 28]. It is well documented that condom negotiation and use is often beyond the control of women engaged in transactional sex, often due to gender-based violence (and fear of violence), and coerced unprotected sex [29–32]. In this analysis, client physical/sexual violence was associated with elevated pregnancy incidence, though this was not statistically significant. Multi-pronged combined interventions (e.g., safer indoor work spaces, supportive management, FESW mobilization and empowerment) [33] that offer protection against violence within environments that support condom negotiation and use are needed. Cambodia's anti-trafficking legislation and the subsequent displacement of women formerly working in brothels to diverse and sometimes clandestine venues continues to act as an impediment to condom access, venue-based HIV prevention interventions [34] and undermines condom negotiation and access to HIV prevention and SRH services [16, 35]. Indeed, qualitative research among Cambodian FESW has revealed increased vulnerability to sexual and physical violence among those operating out of guesthouses and hotels, in part due to the lack of protection mechanisms previously offered by peers and management in more formal settings [27]. Barriers to HIV care service delivery have also been reported by NGOs following the legislative shift, as FESW have become more difficult to identify and reach [27].

The association between lower income and pregnancy incidence accords with literature documenting greater inconsistent condom use among women engaged in transactional sex with lower socioeconomic status [36].

Possible explanations for this association include the prohibitive costs of hormonal contraceptives and/or barriers to accessing reproductive health services. Lower-income FESW may also be more willing to accept client requests for unprotected sex in an effort to make more money per transaction. Finally, while the association between younger age (19–24 versus 25–29 years) and increased pregnancy incidence in our study warrants further investigation, possible explanations for this association include reduced knowledge of SRH, limited access to SRH services and supplies (e.g., condoms) and lower fertility intentions among older, parous FESW. Given the link between income and pregnancy incidence, structural approaches, such as microfinance or income-generating opportunities warrant investigation [37, 38].

Our findings also have important implications for HIV prevention trials that target FESW. Specifically, high pregnancy incidence may impact recruitment, retention and completion of HIV prevention trials, particularly interventions that require longer-term evaluations such as microbicides and PrEP. Indeed, almost one in ten (7.3%) women in our study were ineligible to initiate or complete (5.4%) the three-dose HPV vaccine series offered as part of the YWHS, due to pregnancy within the past six months [39]. These risk-related dropouts potentially bias study samples, impacting generalizability and, in the long term, the efficacy of related future interventions. Given the high burden of unintended pregnancy and low use of hormonal contraceptives among FESW in Cambodia (and elsewhere), there is a need to explore the potential of offering hormonal contraceptives to FESW not desiring pregnancy as part of future HIV prevention interventions.

Our analysis has several limitations. Firstly, the small sample size (and small number of incident pregnancies) may have limited the power of our multivariable analysis and the precision of our estimates. However, the use of multiple responses per participant in this longitudinal

Table 3 Multivariable Extended Cox analysis of correlates of incident pregnancy among 204 Female and Entertainment Sex workers (799 observations), working in Phnom Penh, Cambodia enrolled in the YWHS-II study

Characteristic	Unadjusted Hazard Ratio (HR)	Adjusted Hazard Ratio (AHR) MODEL 1 (FULL)	Adjusted Hazard Ratio (AHR) MODEL 2 (sig p < 0.05)
Socio-demographics, biological individual factors			
Age (years)			
16–18	1.00 (0.02–4.31)	1.59 (0.36–7.11)	1.37 (0.31–6.00)
19–24	2.28 (1.22–4.27)*	3.30 (1.57–6.96)[†]	2.56 (1.35–4.87)[†]
25–29 years	REF	REF	REF
Income, last month ($USD)			
≤ 150	2.29 (0.96–5.44)*	2.63 (1.02–6.77)[†]	–
> 150	REF	REF	–
Education			
No schooling	1.38 (0.40–4.70)	1.39 (0.38–5.12)	–
1–6 years	2.43 (0.86–6.89)*	1.87 (0.64–5.50)	–
7+ years	REF	REF	–
Marital status			
Legally married	2.09 (0.49–8.99)	1.42 (0.28–7.07)	1.76 (0.40–7.66)
Living together, not legally married	2.05 (1.09–3.84)[†]	1.92 (0.23–15.9)	1.95 (1.03–4.71)[†]
Single, widowed, divorced or separated	REF	REF	REF
Number of previous children	0.76 (0.56–1.03) [†]	0.67 (0.38–1.17)	–
HIV positive	0.36 (0.11–1.16) [†]	0.47 (0.13–1.63)	–
Days drank alcohol, last month	0.77 (0.51–1.18)	–	–
ATS use, last 3 months (self-report)	0.79 (0.35–1.78)	–	–
Condom self-efficacy‡	0.92 (0.85–0.99)[†]	0.89 (0.81–0.98)[†]	0.92 (0.84–0.99)[†]
Hormonal contraceptive use, last 3 months‡	5.63 (0.78–41.0)*	0.17 (0.02–1.27)	–
Interpersonal factors			
Condom use, last sex (yes)	0.45(0.23–0.88)[†]	0.57 (0.28–1.13)	–
Condom use, last client (yes)	0.74 (0.09–5.81)	–	–
Condom use, non-paying partner (yes)	0.53 (0.13–2.26)	–	–
Number of sexual partners, last month	1.11 (0.51–2.41)	–	–
Client physical or sexual violence, last year	1.88 (0.73–4.85)	–	–
Intimate partner physical or sexual violence, last year	0.96 (0.23–3.98)	–	–
Sex work factors			
Entertainment venue-based sex work, last month	0.67 (0.34–1.31)	–	–
Non- entertainment venue-based sex work, last month	REF	–	–
Had a manager	0.65 (0.35–1.21)	–	–

*p < 0.10
† p < 0.05
‡ at baseline
All variables (except condom self-efficacy) are time-updated to refer to occurrences in the past three months

analysis increased the number of observations, tempering this bias. While the observational nature of this study precludes temporal inference (compared to an experimental study), the longitudinal design serves to strengthen the validity of these findings. Secondly, many of the variables in this analysis (including our pregnancy outcome) were self-reported and may be subject to social desirability bias. Despite this potential limitation, which would bias our results towards the null, significant associations with our outcome remained. Thirdly, we were unable to assess whether the incident pregnancies measured were intended or unintended. Future investigations into the pregnancy intentions/fertility desires of Cambodian FESW are needed. Fourthly, condom self-efficacy and contraceptive usage were only measured at baseline, and thus we were not able to account for changes in these variables over the follow-up period. Fifth, since the aim of the study was to examine pregnancy among women in entertainment and sex work venues with high sexual risk patterns, we did not collect data on nor were able to separate female sex workers from entertainment workers with high sexual risk in this analysis. Finally, the clandestine nature of sex work made systematic or probabilistic sampling a challenge, thus limiting the study's generalizability to all young FESW in Cambodia. Despite this drawback, the current sample was able to capture a wide range of FESW working in a variety of sex work settings across Phnom Penh.

Conclusions

Our results highlight a high incidence of pregnancy and unmet reproductive health need among FESW, with younger age, lower income and low condom-self efficacy associated with reduced time to the occurrence of pregnancy. These findings suggest a need for combined interventions to increase access to SRH services. To be successful, such interventions would need to be supported by legislative and policy shifts that permit FESW to work in safer, more supportive formal indoor settings [29, 33]. Finally, the high level of pregnancy among FESW observed in the current study has important implications for the SRH rights of FESWs and the recruitment, retention and the success of HIV prevention trials targeting FESW. There is a need to offer SRH information and services to potential HIV prevention trials participants not desiring pregnancy. Access to SRH services may improve trial recruitment and retention and, more importantly, help support the unmet reproductive rights of FESWs.

Abbreviations
ATS: Amphetamine-type stimulants; CWDA: Cambodian Women's Development Association; FESW: Female and Entertainment Sex Workers; HIV: Human Immunodeficiency Virus; HIV/AIDS: Human Immunodeficiency Virus/ Acquired immunodeficiency syndrome; HPV: Human papillomavirus; NCHADS: the National Center for HIV/AIDS, Dermatology and STD; SRH: Sexual and Reproductive Health; STI: Sexually Transmitted Infections; UCSF: the University of California, San Francisco; UNSW: University of New South Wales; YWHS: Young Women's Health Study

Acknowledgments
The authors would like to thank the women who participated in the study and generously shared their expertise with us. The authors would also like to acknowledge the expert leadership and collaboration from partners who were at the Cambodia National Center for HIV/AIDS, Dermatology and STDs at the time this work was conducted, especially Dr. Neth SanSothy, who provided study management and coordination. We also acknowledge our collaborators at the Cambodian Women's Development Agency, especially Keo Sichan. We are also grateful to Cindy Feng, Sabina Dobrer and Melissa Braschel for providing guidance with the statistical analyses for this study.

Funding
The Young Women's Health Study-2 was supported by an award R01NR010995 from the U.S. National Institutes of Health, National Institute of Nursing Research. Professors Lisa Maher and John Kaldor are supported by Australian National Health and Medical Research Council (NHMRC) Research Fellowships. The Kirby Institute is affiliated with the Faculty of Medicine, University of New South Wales and is funded by the Australian Government Department of Health and Ageing. The content is solely the responsibility of the authors and does not necessarily represent the official views of the National Institutes of Health, nor the Australian Government.

Authors' contributions
K.P and E.S.S designed the YWHS prospective study and contributed to data acquisition. P.D. and L.M designed the analysis, with input from K.P, E.S.S. and J.L.E. J.L.E. prepared the dataset and advised on statistical analysis. P.D. conducted the statistical analysis, wrote the first draft of the manuscript and incorporated comments and suggestions from all authors. All authors reviewed, provided substantial input and approved the final version of the manuscript.

Competing interests
The authors have no conflicts of interest to declare.

Author details
[1]British Columbia Centre for Excellence in HIV/AIDS, St. Paul's Hospital, 608-1081 Burrard Street, Vancouver, BC, Canada. [2]Department of Medicine, University of British Columbia, St. Paul's Hospital, 608-1081 Burrard Street, Vancouver, BC, Canada. [3]Institute for Global Health, Department of Epidemiology, University of California-San Francisco, San Francisco, California, USA. [4]Division of Epidemiology, Biostatistics and Preventive Medicine, Department of Internal Medicine, University of New Mexico Health Sciences Center, Albuquerque, NM, USA. [5]Kirby Institute for Infection and Immunity (formerly the National Centre in HIV Epidemiology and Clinical Research), UNSW Australia I, Wallace Wurth Building, Sydney, NSW 2052, Australia. [6]Cambodian Women's Development Association (CWDA, No. 19, Street 242, Boeung Prolit, Khan 7 Makara, Phnom Penh, Cambodia. [7]Department of Medicine, University of California San Francisco, 513 Parnassus Ave; UCSF, San Francisco, CA, USA. [8]National Center for HIV/AIDS, Dermatology and STDs (NCHADS), #245H, Street 6A, Phum Kean Khlang, Sangkat Prekleap Russey Keo, Phnom Penh, Cambodia.

References
1. Becker M, Ramanaik S, Halli S, Blanchard JF, Raghavendra T, Bhattacharjee P, Moses S, Avery L, Mishra S. The intersection between sex work and reproductive health in northern Karnataka, India: identifying gaps and opportunities in the context of HIV prevention. AIDS research and treatment. 2012;2012:–842576.
2. Bautista CT, Mejía A, Leal L, Ayala C, Sanchez JL, Montano SM. Prevalence of lifetime abortion and methods of contraception among female sex workers in Bogota, Colombia. Contraception. 2008;77(3):209–13.
3. Elmore-Meegan M, Conroy RM, Agala CB. Sex workers in Kenya, numbers of clients and associated risks: an exploratory survey. Reprod Health Matters. 2004;12(23):50–7.
4. Duff P, Shoveller J. High lifetime pregnancy and low contraceptive usage among sex workers who use drugs-an unmet reproductive health need. BMC Pregnancy Childbirth. 2011;11:61.
5. Feldblum PJ, Nasution MD, Hoke TH, Van Damme K, Turner AN, Gmach R, Wong EL, Behets F. Pregnancy among sex workers participating in a condom intervention trial highlights the need for dual protection. Contraception. 2007;76(2):105–10.
6. Yam EA, Mnisi Z, Sithole B, Kennedy C, Kerrigan D, Tsui A, Baral S. Association between condom use and use of other contraceptive methods among female sex Workers in Swaziland: a relationship-level analysis of condom and contraceptive use. Sex Transm Dis. 2013;40(5):406–12.
7. Todd CS, Alibayeva G, Sanchez JL, Bautista CT, Carr JK, Earhart KC. Utilization of contraception and abortion and its relationship to HIV infection among female sex workers in Tashkent, Uzbekistan. Contraception. 2006;74(4):318–23.
8. Delvaux T, Crabbe F, Seng S, Laga M. The need for family planning and safe abortion services among women sex workers seeking STI care in Cambodia. Reprod Health Matters. 2003;11(21):88–95.
9. Beckham SW, Shembilu Cr Fau - Brahmbhatt H, Brahmbhatt H Fau - Winch PJ, Winch Pj Fau - Beyrer C, Beyrer C Fau - Kerrigan DL, Kerrigan DL: Female

sex workers' experiences with intended pregnancy and antenatal care services in southern Tanzania. (0039–3665 (Print)).

10. Duff P, Shoveller J, Feng C, Ogilvie G, Montaner J, Shannon K: Pregnancy intentions among female sex workers: recognising their rights and wants as mothers. (2045–2098 (Electronic)).

11. Schwartz S, Papworth E Fau - Thiam-Niangoin M, Thiam-Niangoin M Fau - Abo K, Abo K Fau - Drame F, Drame F Fau - Diouf D, Diouf D Fau - Bamba A, Bamba A Fau - Ezouatchi R, Ezouatchi R Fau - Tety J, Tety J Fau - Grover E, Grover E Fau - Baral S et al: An urgent need for integration of family planning services into HIV care: the high burden of unplanned pregnancy, termination of pregnancy, and limited contraception use among female sex workers in Cote d'Ivoire. (1944–7884 (Electronic)).

12. Zhang XD, Kennedy E Fau - Temmerman M, Temmerman M Fau - Li Y, Li Y Fau - Zhang W-H, Zhang Wh Fau - Luchters S, Luchters S: High rates of abortion and low levels of contraceptive use among adolescent female sex workers in Kunming, China: a cross-sectional analysis. (1473–0782 (Electronic)).

13. Swain SN, Saggurti N, Battala M, Verma RK, Jain AK. Experience of violence and adverse reproductive health outcomes, HIV risks among mobile female sex workers in India. BMC Public Health. 2011;11:357.

14. Weldegebreal R, Melaku YA, Alemayehu M, Gebrehiwot TG: Unintended pregnancy among female sex workers in Mekelle city, northern Ethiopia: a cross-sectional study. (1471–2458 (Electronic)).

15. Page K, Stein E, Sansothy N, Evans J, Couture MC, Sichan K, Cockroft M, Mooney-Somers J, Phlong P, Kaldor J, et al. Sex work and HIV in Cambodia: trajectories of risk and disease in two cohorts of high-risk young women in Phnom Penh, Cambodia. BMJ Open. 2013;3(9):e003095.

16. Maher L, Dixon T, Phlong P, Mooney-Somers J, Stein E, Page K. Conflicting rights: how the prohibition of human trafficking and sexual exploitation infringes the right to health of female sex Workers in Phnom Penh, Cambodia. Health Hum Rights. 2015;17(1):E102–13.

17. UNAIDS: More women in Cambodia turning to sex trade amid financial crisis. In.; 2009.

18. United Nations Development Program. Sex work and the law in Asia and the Pacific. Bangkok: UNDP; 2012.

19. Francis C: HIV prevention and anti-trafficking in conflict? The public health consequences of Cambodia's fight against trafficking. In.: FHI (in collaboration with PSI, Care, UNAIDS); 2008.

20. Nemoto T, Iwamoto M, Colby D, Witt S, Pishori A, Le MN, Vinh DT, Giang Le T. HIV-related risk behaviors among female sex workers in ho chi Minh City, Vietnam. AIDS Educ Prev. 2008;20(5):435–53.

21. Decker MR, Pearson E, Illangasekare SL, Clark E, Sherman SG. Violence against women in sex work and HIV risk implications differ qualitatively by perpetrator. BMC Public Health. 2013;13(1):876.

22. Deering KN, Amin A, Shoveller J, Nesbitt A, Garcia-Moreno C, Duff P, Argento E, Shannon K. A systematic review of the correlates of violence against sex workers. Am J Public Health. 2014;104(5):e42–54.

23. National Institutes of Statistics. Cambodia demographic health survey, 2014: key indicators report. Phnom Penh: National Institutes of Statistics; 2015.

24. Morineau G, Neilsen G, Heng S, Phimpachan C, Mustiakawati D. Falling through the cracks: contraceptive needs of female sex workers in Cambodia and Laos. Contraception. 2011;84:194–8.

25. National Institue of Statistics. Directorate General for Health, Macro I: Cambodia Demographic and Health Survey, 2010. Phnom Penh, Cambodia and Calverton, Maryland: National Institute of Statistics, Directorate General for Health, and ICF Macro; 2011.

26. Delvaux T, Crabbé F, Seng S, Laga M. The need for family planning and safe abortion services among women sex workers seeking STI care in Cambodia. Reproductive Health Matters. 2003;11(21):88–95.

27. Maher L, Mooney-Somers J, Phlong P, Couture M-C, Stein E, Evans J, Cockroft M, Sansothy N, Nemoto T, Page K. Selling sex in unsafe spaces: sex work risk environments in Phnom Penh, Cambodia. Harm reduction journal. 2011;8(1):30.

28. Krüsi A, Chettiar J, Ridgway A, Abbott J, Sa S, Shannon K. Negotiating safety and sexual risk reduction with clients in unsanctioned safer indoor sex work environments: a qualitative study. Am J Public Health. 2012;102(6):1154–9.

29. Shannon K, Sa S, Goldenberg SM, Duff P, Mwangi P, Rusakova M, Reza-Paul S, Lau J, Deering K, Pickles MR, et al. Global epidemiology of HIV among female sex workers: influence of structural determinants. Lancet. 2014;6736(14)

30. Goldenberg SM, Duff P, Krusi A. Work environments and HIV prevention: a qualitative review and meta-synthesis of sex worker narratives. BMC Public Health. 2015;15:1241.

31. Tan SY, Melendez-Torres GJ. A systematic review and metasynthesis of barriers and facilitators to negotiating consistent condom use among sex workers in Asia. Cult Health Sex. 2015:1–16.

32. Andrews CH, Faxelid E, Sychaerun V, Phrasisombath K. Determinants of consistent condom use among female sex workers in Savannakhet, Lao PDR. BMC Womens Health. 2015;15:63.

33. Duff P, Shoveller J, Dobrer S, Ogilvie G, Montaner J, Chettiar J, Shannon K: The relationship between social, policy and physical venue features and social cohesion on condom use for pregnancy prevention among sex workers: a safer indoor work environment scale. (1470–2738 (Electronic)).

34. Couture M-C, Sansothy N, Sapphon V, Phal S, Sichan K, Stein E, Evans J, Maher L, Kaldor J, Vun MC, et al. Young women engaged in sex work in Phnom Penh, Cambodia, have high incidence of HIV and sexually transmitted infections, and amphetamine-type stimulant use: new challenges to HIV prevention and risk. Sex Transm Dis. 2011;38(1):33–9.

35. UNAIDS: Cambodia Country Progress Report: Monitoring the Progress towards the Implementation of the Declaration of Commitment on HIV and AIDS. In.: Prepared by National AIDS Authority for United Nations General Assembly Special Session (UNGASS); Reporting period: January 2010–2011.

36. Chen Y, Li X, Zhou Y, Wen X, Wu D: AIDS Care : Psychological and Socio-medical Aspects of AIDS/HIV Perceived peer engagement in HIV-related sexual risk behaviors and self-reported risk-taking among female sex workers in Guangxi, China. 2013(March):37–41.

37. Dworkin SL, Blankenship K. Microfinance and HIV/AIDS prevention: assessing its promise and limitations. AIDS Behav. 2009;13(3):462–9.

38. Witte SS, Aira T, Tsai LC, Riedel M, Offringa R, Chang M, El-Bassel N, Ssewamala F. Efficacy of a savings-led microfinance intervention to reduce sexual risk for HIV among women engaged in sex work: a randomized clinical trial. Am J Public Health. 2015;105(3):e95–102.

39. Wadhera P, Evans JL, Stein E, Gandhi M, Couture MC, Sansothy N, Sichan K, Maher L, Kaldor J, Page K, et al. Human papillomavirus knowledge, vaccine acceptance, and vaccine series completion among female entertainment and sex workers in Phnom Penh, Cambodia: the young Women's health study. Int J STD AIDS. 2015;26(12):893–902.

Reference intervals for hemoglobin A1c (HbA1c) in healthy Mexican pregnant women

Cristina M. Sánchez-González[1,8], Alfredo Castillo-Mora[2], Itzel N. Alvarado-Maldonado[1], Carlos Ortega-González[2], Nayeli Martínez-Cruz[2], Lidia Arce-Sánchez[2], Mabel Ramos-Valencia[2], Anayansi Molina-Hernández[3], Guadalupe Estrada-Gutierrez[4], Salvador Espino Y. Sosa[5], Yesenia Recio-López[1,8], Ruth Hernández-Sánchez[7] and Enrique Reyes-Muñoz[6]* ⓘ

Abstract

Background: The reference intervals for hemoglobin A1c (HbA1c) in pregnant Mexican women without diabetes are not well defined. The study aims to determine the reference intervals for HbA1c at each trimester in healthy Mexican pregnant women.

Methods: This cross-sectional study included healthy Mexican pregnant women in trimester 1 (T1), 6–13.6 weeks of gestation (WG), trimester 2 (T2), 14–27 WG, and trimester 3 (T3), ≥27–36 WG, with a maternal age > 18 years, and pregestational body mass index (BMI) ranging between 18.5–24.9 kg/m^2. Women with gestational diabetes mellitus, pregestational diabetes, anemia, a pregestational BMI < 18.5 or ≥ 25 kg/m^2, and any hematologic, hepatic, immunological, renal, or cardiac disease were excluded. HbA1c was measured using high-performance liquid chromatography based on the National Glycohemoglobin Standardization Program-certified PDQ Primus guidelines. The HbA1c reference intervals were calculated in terms of the 2.5th to the 97.5th percentiles.

Results: We analyzed the HbA1c values of 725 women (T1 $n = 84$, T2 $n = 448$, and T3 $n = 193$). The characteristics of the participants were expressed as mean ± standard deviation and included: maternal age (28.2 ± 6.7 years), pregestational weight (54.8 ± 5.9 Kg), pregestational BMI (22.2 ± 1.7 Kg/m^2), and glucose values using a 75 g-2 h oral glucose tolerance test; fasting 4.5 ± 0.3 mmol/L (81.5 ± 5.5 mg/dL), 1 h 6.4 ± 1.5 mmol/L (115.3 ± 26.6 mg/dL), and 2 h 5.7 ± 1.1 mmol/L (103.5 ± 19.6 mg/dL). Reference intervals for HbA1c, expressed as median and 2.5th to 97.5th percentile for each trimester were: T1: 5.1 (4.5–5.6%), T2: 5.0 (4.4–5.5%), and T3: 5.1 (4.5–5.6%).

Conclusions: The reference range of HbA1C in healthy Mexican pregnant women during pregnancy was 4.4% to 5.6%. We suggest as upper limits of HbA1c value ≤5.6%, 5.5%, and 5.7% for T1, T2, and T3, respectively among Mexican pregnant women.

Keywords: Glycated hemoglobin, HbA1c, Pregnancy, Healthy pregnancy, Reference intervals, Gestational diabetes

* Correspondence: dr.enriquereyes@gmail.com
[6]Division of Obstetrics and Gynecology, Hospital Regional Universitario de Colima, Colima, Mexico
Full list of author information is available at the end of the article

Background

Pregestational diabetes refers to any type of diabetes diagnosed before a pregnancy. Gestational diabetes mellitus (GDM) refers to diabetes diagnosed in the second trimester (T2) or third trimester (T3) of pregnancy that is not clearly overt diabetes [1]. The International Diabetes Federation estimated a global prevalence of 16.9% for hyperglycemia in pregnancy in 2013 [2].

During pregnancy, diabetes increases the risk of adverse perinatal outcomes, such as congenital malformations, macrosomia, preeclampsia, large fetus for gestational age, cesarean birth, and neonatal morbidity [3, 4]. The Hyperglycemia and Adverse Pregnancy Outcomes (HAPO) study reported associations between maternal glucose levels and increased birth weight, cesarean rate, and increased serum levels of C-peptide in the umbilical cord [5]. Several studies have shown that tight control of blood glucose levels during pregnancy may decrease the risk of adverse perinatal outcomes [6–8]. Good glycemic control is the first target of treatment for women with GDM [4, 8, 9].

According to the American Diabetes Association (ADA), health care providers and patients can use two techniques to evaluate the efficacy of glycemic control treatment: blood glucose self-monitoring (BGS) and hemoglobin A1c (HbA1c) [9]. An HbA1c target value ranging between 6 and 6.5% (42–48 mmol/mol) is recommended; however, an HbA1c of 6% (42 mmol/mol) may be optimal as a woman's pregnancy progresses [9].

Some physiological changes in HbA1c during pregnancy should be considered to determine its optimal value for glycemic control. Erythrocytes half-life decreases during pregnancy, which is reflected in a decrease in HbA1c [10]. In addition, it has been shown that red cell turnover increases in a normal pregnancy, which contributes to a decrease in HbA1c [11]. These assertions suggest that, in order to ensure optimal glycemic control in pregnant woman with diabetes, it is necessary to use HbA1c reference values specific for each trimester [9–11]. The decrease in HbA1c levels in the first trimester (T1) is known to be caused by lower pre- and postprandial mean blood glucose values and an increase in young erythrocytes, which causes a decrease in the percentage of HbA1c [10]. The increase in HbA1c in T3 is caused by an increase in the mean postprandial blood glucose values [12].

Recent evidence has also shown that, despite optimal preconception control and unplanned pregnancies with good glycemic control in early pregnancy with optimal HbA1c levels, the development of complications associated with diabetes cannot always be prevented [13, 14].

These considerations highlight the need to carefully review glycemic control goals during pregnancy. Although HbA1c reference intervals for the general population are well established, they are not clearly defined in Mexican pregnant women. Therefore, the present study aimed to determine the reference intervals of HbA1c in each trimester of pregnancy in healthy Mexican pregnant women.

Methods

Design and participants

This cross-sectional study was approved by the Ethic and Research Internal Review Board of the Instituto Nacional de Perinatología in Mexico City, Mexico (register number 212250–42081). All the participants provided written informed consent. We included pregnant women who receive prenatal care at our institution from January 1, 2010 to April 30, 2011. Each of the women had a single pregnancy. Their maternal age was > 18 years old, and their pregestational body mass index (BMI) ranged between 18.5 kg/m^2 and 24.9 kg/m^2. We excluded women with gestational diabetes mellitus (GDM) diagnosed using a 75 g-2 h oral glucose tolerance test (OGTT) with one or more of the following glucose cut-off points: fasting ≥5.1 mmol/L (92 mg/dL), 1 h ≥ 10 mmol/L (180 mg/dL), and 2 h ≥ 8.5 mmol/L (153 mg/dL) according to ADA criteria [1]. Women with pregestational diabetes mellitus diagnosed using a 75 g-2 h OGTT, defined by fasting ≥7 mmol/L (126 mg/dL) or 2 h ≥11.1 mmol/L (200 mg/dL), women with a pregestational BMI < 18.5 kg/m^2 or ≥ 25 kg/m^2, women with anemia defined by total hemoglobin concentration < 11 g/dL according to World Health Organization criteria [15], a multiple pregnancy, or any hematological, hepatic, immunological, renal, or cardiac disease were also excluded. Participants were divided into three groups based on the trimester (T) of pregnancy: T1: 6–13.6 weeks of gestation (WG), T2: 14–27.6 WG, and T3: 28–36 WG. Each participant fasted for 8 to 12 h prior to perform a 75 g-2 h OGTT as part of the universal 1-step screening method for GDM at first prenatal visit. Blood samples for measuring HbA1c level and fasting of OGTT were taken at the same time.

Study variables

HbA1c was determined in plasma based on the National Glycohemoglobin Standardization Program–certified PDQ Primus guidelines (Primus Diagnostics, Kansas City, MO, USA) using high performance liquid chromatography (inter-assay CVs < 2%).

Glucose was measured using the Vitros DT60 II chemistry system (OrthoClinical Diagnostics, Tilburg, The Netherlands), according to the manufacturer's instructions. The system has a sensitivity of 20 mg/dL (1.11 mmol/L) and a coefficient of variation of 1.4–1.8%.

The pregestational BMI was self-reported by each of the participants when the OGTT was conducted, and it was calculated using the following formula: weight in Kg /height in m^2.

Sample size

According to the International Federation of Clinical Chemistry (IFCC) [16, 17] recommendation on estimation of reference intervals the sample size must consist of a minimum of 40 participants in each group. Thus, we decided to include all the participants that met the study's inclusion criteria.

Statistical analysis

Descriptive statistics were used to characterize the three groups. The central tendency and/or frequency and percentage were measured, based on the type and distribution of each variable. An ANOVA test with Bonferroni correction was performed to compare the quantitative variables in each trimester. To determine the reference intervals, the median and 2.5th to 97.5th percentile were calculated according to the recommendations of the IFCC [16]. Statistical analysis was performed with the Statistical Package for the Social Sciences for Windows version 15.

Results

During the study period, there were 2209 women assessed for eligibility at the study institution, 1014 of which were eligible to participate. Of these women, 725 met the inclusion criteria T1 ($n = 84$), T2 ($n = 448$), and T3 ($n = 193$); 289 were excluded because of GDM ($n = 181$), pregestational diabetes ($n = 2$), uncomplete OGTT ($n = 4$), declined enrollment ($n = 4$), anemia ($n = 42$), or some additional pathology ($n = 56$). Figure 1 shows the flow chart of the study participants.

Figure 2 shows the reference intervals for HbA1c for T1 expressed as median and percentile (2.5th to 97.5th), which were: T1: 5.1% (4.5–5.6%), T2: 5.0% (4.4–5.5%)

T3: 5.1% (4.5–5.6%). A statistically significant decrease was found between the T1 and T2 groups ($p = 0.0001$), and a statistically significant increase was found between the T2 and T3 groups ($p = 0.0001$). No statistically significant differences were found between the T1 and T3 groups.

The general characteristics of the 725 participants were expressed as mean ± standard deviation and included: maternal age (28.2 ± 6.7 years), pregestational weight (54.8 ± 5.9 Kg), pregestational BMI (22.2 ± 1.7 Kg/m^2), maternal hemoglobin (13.2 ± 1.0 g/dL), and glucose values using a 75 g-2 h oral glucose tolerance test; fasting 4.5 ± 0.3 mmol/L (81.5 ± 5.5 mg/dL), 1 h 6.4 ± 1.5 mmol/L (115.3 ± 26.6 mg/dL), and 2 h 5.7 ± 1.1 mmol/L (103.5 ± 19.6 mg/dL).

Table 1 shows the characteristics of the participants at admission to the study. The weeks gestation at determination of HbA1c were 12.3 ± 1.6, 20.1 ± 3.6 and 30.4 ± 2.4 for T1, T2 and T3 groups, respectively. Maternal age was significantly higher in the T1 group than the T2 and T3 groups; however, pregestational BMI was similar in all three groups. Maternal hemoglobin was significantly higher in the T1 group (13.7 ± 1.1 g/dL) than the T2 (13.2 ± 0.96) and T3 groups (13. ± 1.01 g/dL). No statistically significant difference in glucose values obtained from the 75 g-2 h OGTT were observed for the T1 group in comparison to the T2 and T3 groups. The glucose values in OGTT were significantly higher in the T3 group than the T2 group.

Discussion

In our study, we found that the HbA1c reference interval in healthy Mexican pregnant women in the 97.5th percentile for the T1, T2, and T3 groups was ≤5.6%, 5.5%, and 5.6%, respectively. Our findings are important

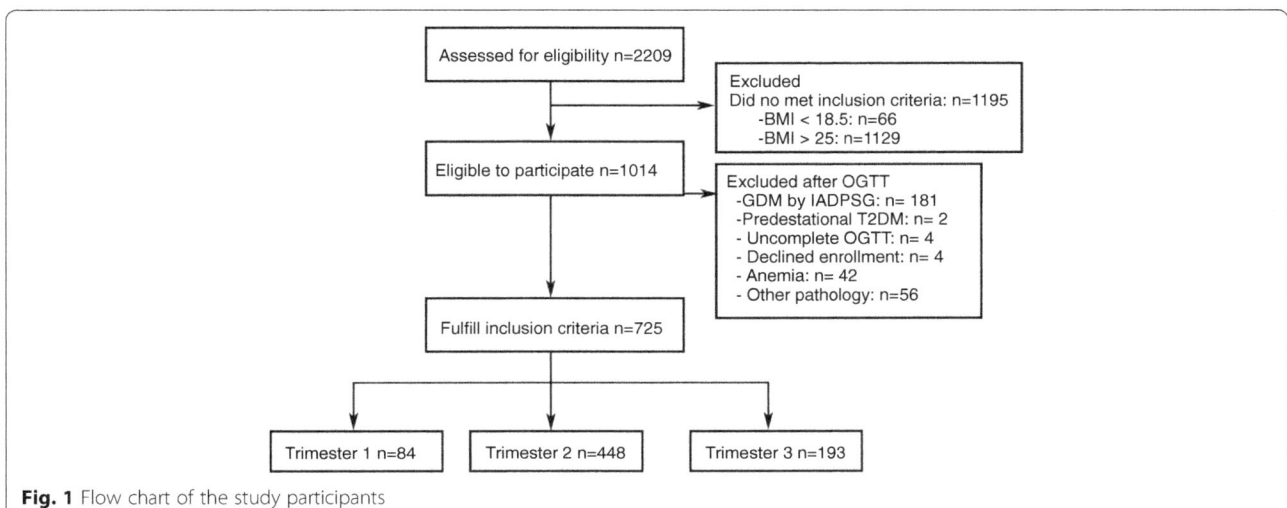

Fig. 1 Flow chart of the study participants

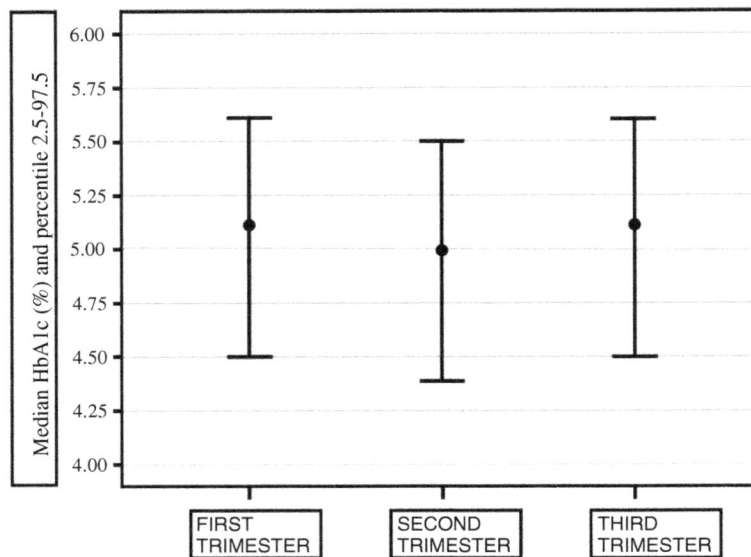

Fig. 2 Median and percentile (2.5th to 97.5th) for HbA1c for Mexican women for each trimester

because this is the first study to evaluate HbA1c levels in healthy Mexican pregnant women.

While HbA1c levels have been reported to be lower in healthy pregnant women in comparison to non-pregnant women [14], there is controversy regarding whether there are differences in HbA1c reference intervals at each trimester of pregnancy. Worth et al. [18] reported a significant increase among T1, T2, and T3 groups. Versantvoort et al. [19] reported a small decrease in HbA1c levels during T1 (5.4%), compared with T2 (5.5%), and T3 (5.8%). They also suggested a correlation between HbA1c levels during T1 and T2 and the birth weight percentile [19]. However, Hartland et al. [20], O'Kane et al. [21], Hanson et al. [22], and Günter et al. [23], Hiramatsu et al. [24] reported a significant decrease in HbA1c in T2, which is similar to our findings.

Evers et al. [25] conducted a nationwide study in the Netherlands on the risk of complications in pregnant women with type 1 diabetes mellitus (DM1). They reported that the incidence of all congenital malformations in women with HbA1c levels of 6.3% during T1 was twice that of the population without DM1. They also reported that the incidence of congenital malformations was 12.9% in women with HbA1c levels > 7%; they concluded that maintaining HbA1c < 7% does not decrease the risk of congenital malformations [25]. Another study on this same population reported that the incidence of macrosomia was very high (48%) despite the fact that 84% of women with DM1 had good glycemic control (HbA1c < 7%) [26].

Radder et al. [27] suggested that to prevent congenital malformations and macrosomia in diabetic and pregnant

Table 1 Characteristics per trimester of pregnancy of 725 healthy pregnant Mexican women

Characteristics	Group T1 $n = 84$	Group T2 $n = 448$	*p T1 vs T2	Group T3 $n = 193$	*p T1 vs T3
Maternal age (years)	30.1 ± 5.9	28.1 ± 6.7	0.04	27.5 ± 7.0	0.01
Pregestacional BMI (Kg/m^2)	22.4 ± 1.6	22.3 ± 1.7	0.98	22.1 ± 1.6	0.78
Hemoglobin (g/dL)	13.7 ± 1.1	13.2 ± 0.96	0.0001	13.0 ± 1.0	0.0001
Hemoglobin HbA1c (%)	5.12 ± 0.2	5.0 ± 0.2	0.0001	5.1 ± 0.2**	0.98
Glucose values in OGTT (mmol/L)					
Fasting	4.56 ± 0.3	4.52 ± 0.3	0.74	4.52 ± 0.31	0.78
1-h	6.51 ± 1.6	6.2 ± 1.43	0.23	6.82 ± 1.45**	0.28
2-h	5.76 ± 1.2	5.65 ± 1.05	0.98	6.0 ± 1.08 **	0.22

*ANOVA Test
**$p < 0.0001$ for the comparison T2 Vs T3
BMI Body mass index, OGTT Oral glucose tolerance test

women, HbA1c levels should be < 5% in T1 and less than 6% in T3. Mosca et al. [28] reported a lower level of HbA1c in 445 Italian pregnant women (median 4.8% and the 2.5th to 97.5th percentile [4–5.5%]) in comparison to 384 control women without pregnancy (median 5.6 and the 2.5th to 97.5th percentile (4.8–6.2%). While Mosca et al. [28] did not report the BMI or the age of the women in their study, the reference interval for HbA1c was similar to the interval in our study.

Our study had several limitations. Due to the study's design, HbA1c was determined for different women in each trimester. The pregestational BMI was self-reported by the participants, so it could be less exact than pregestational BMI that is documented by a clinician. The study results are only applicable to Mexican women and, potentially, Latin women. Future prospective and multi-center studies are needed to corroborate our findings.

Our study also has several strengths. It is the first study to evaluate HbA1c in healthy Mexican woman; pregestational and gestational diabetic women were excluded using OGTT, and the sample size included women in each trimester.

Diabetes in pregnancy involves an additional risk for both the mother and the fetus and it is directly related to glycemic control, which is evaluated using the HbA1C value. This correlation highlights the importance of accurate measurement as well as correct interpretation of and comparison with the appropriate reference values. HbA1c reference values per trimester of pregnancy are necessary in order to ensure better management of women with pregnancies complicated by diabetes because strict glycemic control is essential in order to minimize maternal and fetal morbidity [26, 29]. Several authors have demonstrated that the measurement of HbA1c is a useful parameter in glycemic control [20, 21, 30]; Therefore, we suggest that these results be considered when determining treatment goals in Mexican women with diabetes during pregnancy, however studies among diabetic women using this reference value for HbA1c are needed.

Conclusions

The HbA1C reference range for healthy Mexican pregnant women during pregnancy is 4.4% to 5.6%. Based on our results, we suggest as upper limits of HbA1c value ≤5.6%, 5.5%, and 5.6% for T1, T2, and T3, respectively among Mexican pregnant women.

Abbreviations
ADA: American Diabetes Association; BMI: Body mass index; DM1: Diabetes Mellitus Type 1; DM2: Diabetes Mellitus Type 2; GDM: Gestational Diabetes Mellitus; HbA1C: Glycated hemoglobin; WG: Weeks of gestation

Acknowledgements
The authors thank the Instituto Nacional de Perinatología, Mexico City.

Funding
The present study was supported by the Instituto Nacional de Perinatología in Mexico City. Register number 212250–42081. The funding body/bodies did not have a role in the design of the study and collection, analysis, and interpretation of data and in writing the manuscript.

Authors' contributions
ERM, CMSG and ACM, conceived and designed the study, analysed the data, and wrote the paper. NMC, LAS, COG, AMH, GEG and SES, analysed the data, and reviewed the paper. ACM, INAM, MRV, YRL and RHS acquired the data, and reviewed the paper. All authors read and approved the final version of the manuscript.

Competing interests
SES and ERM are speakers for Nestle Mexico.
CMSG, ACM, NMC, INAM, COG, NMC, LAS, MRV, AMH, GEG, YRL, RHS declare that they have no competing interests.

Author details
[1]Division of Reproductive Medicine, Instituto Nacional de Perinatología Isidro Espinosa de los Reyes, Mexico City, Mexico. [2]Department of Endocrinology, Instituto Nacional de Perinatología Isidro Espinosa de los Reyes, Mexico City, Mexico. [3]Departament of Physiology and Cellular Development, Instituto Nacional de Perinatología Isidro Espinosa de los Reyes, Mexico City, Mexico. [4]Direction of Research, Instituto Nacional de Perinatología Isidro Espinosa de los Reyes, Mexico City, Mexico. [5]Division of Clinical Research, Instituto Nacional de Perinatología Isidro Espinosa de los Reyes, Mexico City, Mexico. [6]Division of Obstetrics and Gynecology, Hospital Regional Universitario de Colima, Colima, Mexico. [7]Department of Gynecological and Perinatal Endocrinology, Instituto Nacional de Perinatología Isidro Espinosa de los Reyes, Montes Urales 800, Lomas Virreyes, Miguel Hidalgo, CP 11000 Mexico City, DF, Mexico. [8]Programa de Maestría en Ciencias Médicas de la Universidad Anáhuac Norte, Mexico City, Mexico.

References
1. American Diabetes Association. Classification and Diagnosis of Diabetes. Diabetes Care. 2016;39(Suppl) 1):S13–22.
2. Guariguata L, Linnenkamp U, Beagley J, Whiting DR, Cho NH. Global estimates of the prevalence of hyperglycaemia in pregnancy. Diabetes Res Clin Pract. 2014;103(2):176–85.
3. National Institute for Health and Care Excellence. Diabetes in pregnancy: management of diabetes and its complications from preconception to the postnatal period. Clinical guidelines. London: National Collaborating Centre for Women's and Children's Health (UK); 2015.
4. Committee on Practice Bulletins-Obstetrics. Practice Bulletin No. 137: Gestational diabetes mellitus. Obstet Gynecol. 2013;122(2 Pt 1):406–16.
5. HAPO Study Cooperative Research Group, Metzger BE, Lowe LP, Dyer AR, Trimble ER, Chaovarindr U, et al. Hyperglycemia and adverse pregnancy outcomes. N Engl J Med. 2008;358(19):1991–2002.
6. Nathan DM. The diabetes control and complications trial/epidemiology of diabetes interventions and complications study at 30 years: overview. Diabetes Care. 2014;37(1):9–16.
7. Ray JG, O'Brien TE, Chan WS. Preconception care and the risk of congenital anomalies in the offspring of women with diabetes mellitus: a meta-analysis. QJM. 2001;94(8):435–44.
8. Willhoite MB, Bennert HW, Palomaky GE, Zaremba MMH, WH WJ. The impact of preconception counselling on pregnancy outcomes. The experience of the Maine diabetes in pregnancy program. Diabetes Care. 1993;16:450–5.
9. American Diabetes Association. 13. Management of Diabetes in Pregnancy. Diabetes Care. 2017;40(Suppl 1):S114-S119.
10. Lurie S, Blickstein I. Age distribution of erythrocyte population in late pregnancy. Gynecol Obstet Investig. 1993;36(3):163–5.
11. Lurie S, Danon D. Life span of erythrocytes in late pregnancy. Obstet Gynecol. 1992;80(1):123–6.

12. Cousins L, Rigg L, Hollingsworth D, Brink G, Aurand JYS. The 24-hour excursion and diurnal rhythm of glucose, insulin, and C-peptide in normalpregnancy. Am J Obstet Gynecol. 1980;136(4):483–8.

13. Penney GC, Mair G, Pearson DW. Scottish diabetes in pregnancy group. Outcomes of pregnancies in women with type 1 diabetes in Scotland: a national population-based study. BJOG. 2003;110(3):315–8.

14. Boulot P, Chabbert-Buffet N, d'Ercole C, Floriot M, Fontaine P, Fournier A, Diabetes and Pregnancy group France. French multicenter survey of outcome of pregnancy in women with pregestational diabetes. Diabetes Care. 2003;26(11):2990–3.

15. World Health Organization, Vitamin and Mineral Nutrition Information System, WHO, Geneva, 2011 (WHO/NMH/NHD/MNM/11.1). http://www.who.int/vmnis/indicators. Accessed 8 Sept 2018.

16. Solberg HE. The IFCC recommendation on estimation of reference intervals. The RefVal program. Clin Chem Lab Med. 2004;42(7):710–4.

17. Solberg HE. International Federation of Clinical Chemistry, expert panel on theory of reference values, and International Committee for Standardization in Haematology, standing committee on reference values. Approved recommendation (1987) on the theory of reference values. Part 5. Statistical treatment of collected reference values. Determination of reference limits. J Clin Chem Clin Biochem. 1987;25(9):645–56.

18. Worth R, Potter JM, Drury J, Fraser RB, Cullen DR. Glycosylated haemoglobin in normal pregnancy; a longitudinal study with two independent methods. Diabetologia. 1985;28(2):76–9.

19. Versantvoort AR, van Roosmalen J, Radder JK. Course of HbA1c in non-diabetic pregnancy related to birth weight. Neth J Med. 2013;71(1):22–5.

20. Hartland AJ, Smith JM, Clark PM, Webber J, Chowdhury TDF. Establishing trimester- and ethnic group-related reference changes for fructosamine and HbA1c in non-diabetic pregnant women. Ann Clin Biochem. 1999;36(2):235–7.

21. O'Kane MJ, Lynch PL, Moles KW, Magee SE. Determination of a diabetes control and complications trial – aligned HbA(1c) reference range in pregnancy. Clin Chim Acta. 2001;311(2):157–9.

22. Hanson U, Hagenfeldt L, Hagenfeldt K. Glycosylated hemoglobins in normal pregnancy; sequential changes and relation to birth weight. Obstet Gynecol. 1983;62(6):741–4.

23. Günter HH, Ritter C, Reinhardt W, Strahl B, Niesert SMH. Influence of non-diabetic pregnancy on fructosamine and HbA1c concentration. Z Geburtshilfe Neonatol. 1995;199(4):148–55.

24. Hiramatsu Y, Shimizu I, Omori Y, Nakabayashi M. Determination of reference intervals of glycated albumin and hemoglobin A1c in healthy pregnant Japanese women and analysis of their time courses and influencing factors during pregnancy. Endocr J. 2012;59(2):145–51.

25. Evers IM, de Valk HWVG. Risk of complications of pregnancy in women with type 1 diabetes: nationwide prospective study in the Netherlands. BMJ. 2004;328(7445):915–8.

26. Evers IM, de Valk HW, Mol BW, ter Braak EW, Visser GH. Macrosomia despite good glycaemic control in type 1 diabetic pregnancy; results of a nationwide study in the Netherlands. Diabetologia. 2002;45(11):1484–9.

27. Radder JK, van Roosmalen J. HbA1c in healthy, pregnant women. Neth J Med. 2005;63(7):256–9.

28. Mosca A, Paleari R, Dalfrà MG, Di Cianni G, Cuccuru I, Pellegrini G, et al. Reference intervals for hemoglobin A1c in pregnant women: data from an Italian multicenter study. Clin Chem. 2006;52(6):1138–43.

29. Nielsen LR, Ekbom P, Damm P, Glümer C, Frandsen MM, Jensen DM, et al. HbA1c levels are significantly lower in early and late pregnancy. Diabetes Care. 2004;27(5):1200–1.

30. Kilpatrick ES. Glycated haemoglobin in the year 2000. J Clin Pathol. 2000; 53(5):335–9.

15

Uptake of antiretroviral therapy in HIV-positive women ever enrolled into 'prevention of mother to child transmission' programme, Mandalay, Myanmar

Khine Wut Yee Kyaw[1,8]*(iD), Srinath Satyanarayana[2], Khaing Hnin Phyo[3], Nang Thu Thu Kyaw[1], Aye Aye Mon[3], Than Than Lwin[4], Thet Ko Aung[3], Myo Minn Oo[1], Zaw Zaw Aung[4], Thurain Htun[5], Nang Seng Noon Kham[4], Theingi Mya[6], Ajay M. V. Kumar[2,7] and Htun Nyunt Oo[4]

Abstract

Background: Early initiation and longer duration of anti-retroviral therapy either as prophylaxis (pARV) or lifelong treatment (ART) in HIV-positive pregnant women prior to delivery has a huge impact in reducing mother to child transmission (MTCT) of HIV, maternal morbidity, mortality and increasing retention in care. In this study, we aimed to determine the following in a 'prevention of mother-to-child transmission' (PMTCT) programme in Central Women Hospital, Mandalay, Myanmar: i) uptake of ART and factors associated with the uptake ii) duration of ART/ pARV received by HIV-positive pregnant women prior to delivery, iii) factors associated with ART/ pARV initiation after delivery and iv) factors associated with shorter duration of ART/ pARV (≤ 8 weeks prior to delivery).

Method: This was a retrospective cohort study using routinely collected data from PMTCT programme. We used multivariable Cox proportional Hazard model or log binomial models to assess the association between socio-demographic and clinical factors with a) uptake of ART/pARV, b) initiation of ART/pARV after delivery, c) shorter (≤8 weeks) duration of ART/PARV prior to delivery.

Results: Of the 670 ART naïve HIV-positive women enrolled to PMTCT programme between March 2011 and December 2016, 588 (88%) were initiated on ART/pARV. In adjusted analysis, only pregnancy stage at enrolment was significantly associated with initiation of ART/pARV. Of 585 who had delivered babies on or before the censor date, 522 (89%) were on ART/pARV. Women who lived outside Mandalay were more likely to be initiated on ART after delivery (i.e., delayed ART initiation in those on ART). Among women who were initiated on ART/pARV before delivery (n = 468), only 59% got ART/pARV for > 8 weeks before delivery. Women whose spouses' HIV status was not recorded had 40% higher risk of short duration of ART/pARV.

(Continued on next page)

* Correspondence: dr.khinewutyeekyaw2015@gmail.com
[1]Department of Operational Research, International Union Against Tuberculosis and Lung Disease (The Union), Mandalay, Myanmar
[8]Department of Operational Research, International Union Against Tuberculosis and Lung Disease (The Union), Mandalay, Myanmar
Full list of author information is available at the end of the article

(Continued from previous page)

Conclusions: This study shows high uptake of ART/pARV among those enrolled into the PMTCT programme. However, about one in eight pregnant women did not receive ART before delivery. Among those initiated on ART/pARV before delivery, nearly half of them received ART/pARV for less than 8 weeks prior to delivery. These aspects need to be improved in order to eliminate mother-to-child transmission of HIV.

Keywords: PMTCT, Myanmar, Operational research, ART, pARV

Background

In pregnant women infected with human immunodeficiency virus (HIV), early diagnosis and antiretroviral therapy either as prophylaxis (pARV) or as lifelong treatment (ART) has several benefits such as prevention of opportunistic infections, reduction of morbidity and mortality and high retention on ART care in the long run in addition to reducing mother-to-child transmission (MTCT) of HIV [1–3]. Therefore, World Health Organization (WHO) recommends provider-initiated counselling and HIV testing to pregnant women attending antenatal care clinics in low-HIV prevalence setting as a key component of elimination of MTCT [4]. In addition to antenatal care, in high prevalence settings, provider-initiated counselling and HIV testing is also recommended at childbirth, postpartum and pediatric care setting to diagnose patients that may have been missed earlier or to identify women who have acquired new infections during this time period [4].

In Myanmar, HIV prevalence among adult population aged ≥15 years was estimated at 0.59% in 2015, a substantial decline compared to 0.94% in 2000 [5, 6]. UNAIDS estimated that there were 5100 pregnant women living with HIV in 2015 in Myanmar [7]. Myanmar has also set a target of reducing MTCT to < 5% by 2020 from the baseline of 15% in 2015 [8] and eliminating mother-to-child transmission of HIV by 2025. In order to achieve this, the National AIDS Programme has set 90–90-90 targets for HIV testing of pregnant women, provision of ART to HIV-positive pregnant women and provision of anti-retroviral prophylaxis to exposed babies [8]. The gaps in the provision of ART to HIV-positive pregnant mothers and antiretroviral (ARV) prophylaxis to exposed babies are largely unknown. HIV prevalence among pregnant women in Mandalay region of Myanmar was estimated at 0.81, 0.89 and 0.69% with testing rate of 41.4, 40.5 and 70.5% in 2012, 2013 and 2015 respectively [9].

In HIV-positive women who enrolled into 'Prevention of mother-to-child transmission' (PMTCT) programme in Central Women Hospital, Mandalay, the MTCT transmission rate was 2% [10]. However, the rates of transmission among HIV-positive pregnant women who failed to get enrolled into PMTCT services are unknown. In addition to early ART initiation, previous studies have shown that longer duration of ART can suppresses maternal viral load and each additional week of ART during antenatal period can reduce MTCT of HIV by 20% [11–13]. In Mandalay region, information on some of these programmatically relevant issues such as ART initiation, duration of ART before delivery, the factors associated with shorter duration of ART in HIV-positive pregnant women have not yet been studied and this information can help in improving the performance of the PMTCT programme.

In this study, we aimed to determine the following in pregnant women enrolled into the PMTCT programme in Mandalay, Myanmar: a) uptake of ART/pARV and factors associated with the uptake; b) duration of ART/pARV received by HIV-positive pregnant women prior to delivery; c) factors associated with ART initiation after delivery and d) factors associated with shorter duration of ART/pARV (≤ 8 weeks prior to delivery).

Methods
Study design

This was a retrospective cohort study involving secondary analysis of routinely collected data as part of the PMTCT programme of Central Women Hospital, Mandalay.

Setting

Myanmar is one of the South-East Asian countries with a population of 51 million (in 2014) with 30% of population living in urban areas [14]. Mandalay region has 3rd largest population in the country (6.2 million) where the study was conducted [14].

Prevention of mother to child transmission programme in central women hospital

Central Women Hospital is a 500-bedded public hospital providing maternal and child health care services in Mandalay. The International Union Against Tuberculosis and Lung Disease (The Union), an international non-governmental organization, has been implementing a PMTCT programme in Central Women Hospital in Mandalay in collaboration with National AIDS Programme (NAP), public hospitals and clinics under the Ministry of Health and Sports (MoHS) since 2011. The pregnant women attending antenatal care clinics at the public hospitals (central women hospital or township health departments) are offered HIV testing and referred to PMTCT clinic if they are tested HIV-positive. HIV testing at antenatal clinics is performed using a rapid, point-of-care, finger-prick test and is offered free of charge. HIV-positive pregnant women and post-partum women along with their exposed babies are referred and enrolled into PMTCT programme. Comprehensive PMTCT services are provided by a team of obstetricians and neonatologists from the Central Women Hospital, physicians from the Mandalay General Hospital, medical officers employed by The Union and People Living with HIV (PLHIV) network. HIV-positive women who were eligible for treatment were offered ART for life if their CD4 count was lower than cutoff point (350 cells/mm^3 before 2015, 500 cells/mm^3 from 2015 to 2016) and regardless of CD4 count after 2016. Women with CD4 count higher than cutoff point were given pARV as per the protocols of different time periods:

1. PMTCT option A (prior to 2013): women received Zidovudine (AZT) only.
2. PMTCT option B (from 2011 to 2014): women received triple ART during pregnancy, delivery and discontinued one week after breast feeding was stopped.
3. PMTCT option B+ (2014 to 2016): women received triple ART during pregnancy, delivery and continued for life [15, 16].

The management of HIV-positive women during post-partum period and exposed infants at central women hospital are described in detail elsewhere [10]. In brief, after delivery, mother and infant are followed-up until 18 months post-partum. Hence the follow up visit schedule depends on the infant feeding practices, the health status of mother and infant, availability of the attending physician and distance of patients' residence from the hospital. The infants are tested for HIV, first at the age of 4–6 weeks and then at the age of 9 months. Infants tested positive for HIV antibodies are confirmed by another test between 9 and 18 months of age. All HIV-positive infants are transferred out to nearest pediatric integrated HIV Care clinic for ART initiation and continuation of care. All PMTCT services provided by the hospital are free of charge to the pregnant women and exposed infants.

Study population

The study population includes ART-naïve HIV-positive women enrolled in Central Women Hospital's PMTCT programme between March 2011 and December 2016. The HIV-positive women who were already on ART at the time of enrolment to PMTCT programme were excluded from the study analysis.

Sources of data, data variables

Data of each study participant are collected in a structured proforma and entered into an electronic database of PMTCT programme routinely. We extracted data on the following variables: age, occupation, literacy, spouse's HIV status, patient's resident township, baseline CD4 count, baseline WHO clinical staging, baseline haemoglobin level, Hepatitis B, Hepatitis C, history of previous ART before enrolment, date of HIV diagnosis, date of ART initiation, ART regimen, and date of delivery.

Statistical analysis

The data from the electronic database of the PMTCT programme was extracted and imported into STATA version 14.2 (College Station, TX). The uptake of ART and delivery status was assessed as of 31st March 2017 (censor date) or outcome date whichever date was earlier. To study the socio-demographic factors associated with uptake of ART/pARV, we used Cox proportional Hazards model. Hazards ratios (HR) and 95% confidence intervals (CI) were calculated. Among those initiated on ART/pARV, we used Log-binomial model to assess the factors associated with a) shorter duration of ART/pARV (duration of ART/pARV ≤8 weeks among who initiated on ART/pARV before delivery) and b) ART/pARV after delivery among HIV-positive mothers who had delivery record. A P-value of less than 0.05 was considered statistically significant for all analyses. The pregnancy stage at enrolment into PMTCT programme was categorized into before delivery, during delivery and post-partum periods.

Results

There were 792 HIV-positive pregnant women enrolled into PMTCT programme between March 2011 and December 2016. The median age (interquartile range - IQR) and median CD4 cell count (IQR) at enrolment were 29 (25–33) years and 357 (218–511) cells/mm^3 respectively. Among them, 122 (15%) had been initiated on ART before enrolment to PMTCT programme and were excluded for further analysis. The flowchart of HIV-positive women in PMTCT programme with ART status is described in Fig. 1.

Of 670 ART naïve HIV-positive pregnant women enrolled into PMTCT programme, 588 (88%) were initiated on ART/pARV and 82 (12%) were not initiated on ART/pARV. The uptake of ART under option A or option B was 42% and under option B+ was 58%. Among 588 women, 234 (39%) were initiated ART/pARV on the first day of enrollment and 433 (74%) were initiated within two weeks of enrolment into the PMTCT programme. Among those who were initiated on ART/pARV, the median (IQR) duration between enrolment into PMTCT programme and ART/pARV

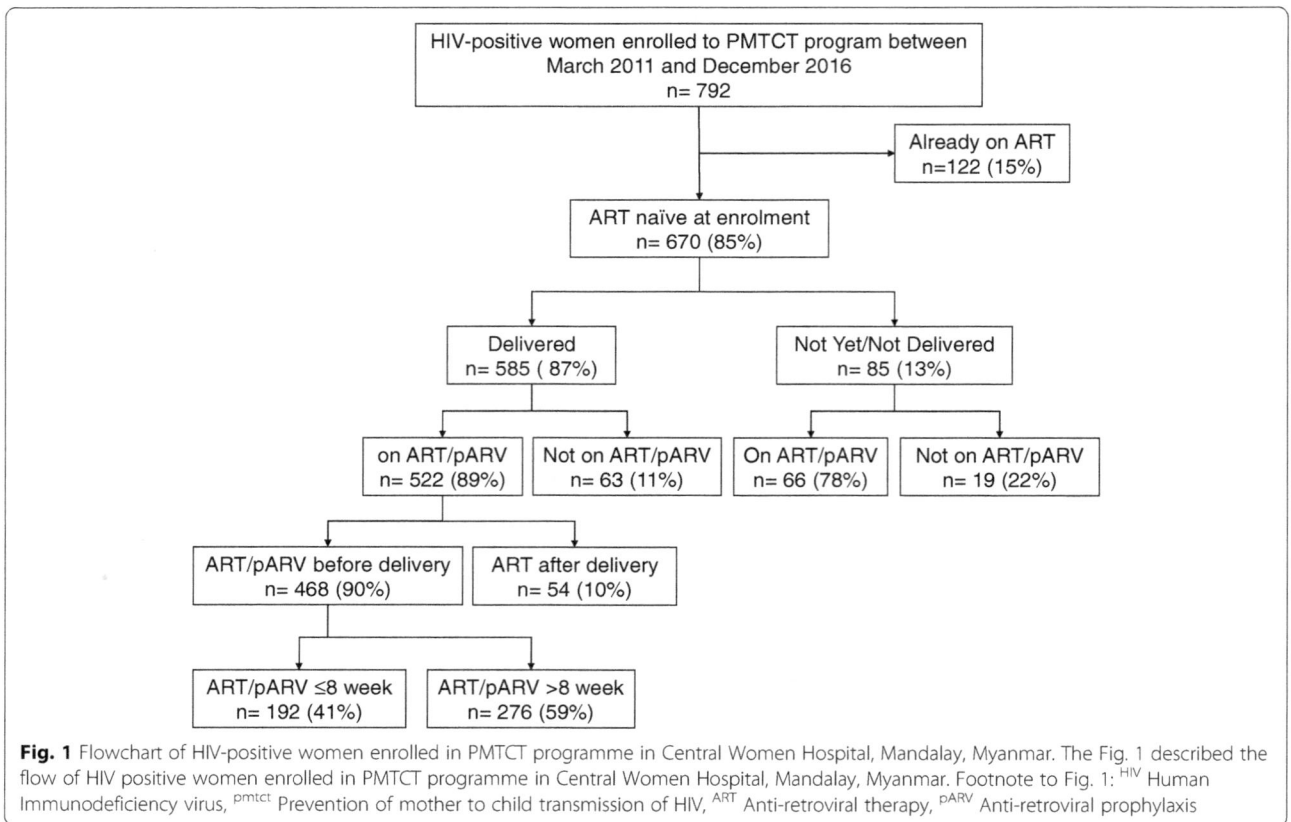

Fig. 1 Flowchart of HIV-positive women enrolled in PMTCT programme in Central Women Hospital, Mandalay, Myanmar. The Fig. 1 described the flow of HIV positive women enrolled in PMTCT programme in Central Women Hospital, Mandalay, Myanmar. Footnote to Fig. 1: [HIV] Human Immunodeficiency virus, [pmtct] Prevention of mother to child transmission of HIV, [ART] Anti-retroviral therapy, [pARV] Anti-retroviral prophylaxis

initiation was 7 (0–21) days and 485/588 (82%) were initiated on triple ART (option B or B+). Half (41 out of 82) of the women who were not initiated ART/pARV were lost to follow up (missed appointment more than three months from the last appointment day).

In unadjusted analysis, women whose spouse's HIV status was recorded (either positive or negative), women with hemoglobin < 11 g% at enrollment and women who were enrolled in the programme during antenatal period were more likely to have been initiated on ART/pARV as shown in Table 1. We included factors with p value less than 0.15 in unadjusted analysis (spouse HIV status, baseline CD4 count, baseline hemoglobin level, literacy status and pregnancy stage at enrolment) in the multivariable model to obtain the adjusted hazard ratios. After adjustment, only 'pregnancy stage at enrolment' was significantly associated with initiation of ART [adjusted HR 4.4 (95% CI 3.2–6.1)] as shown in Table 1. The occupation, hepatitis B and Hepatitis C status were not significantly associated with initiation of ART (data not shown in Table 1).

Of 670 HIV-positive women, 585 (87%) women had delivered their babies before censor date. Of the 85/670 (13%) who did not have a delivery record until censor date of 31st March 2017, 10/85 (12%) had died, 35/85 (41%) were lost to follow-up, 34/85 (40%) were

transferred out to other ART centres before delivery and 6/85 (7%) were on regular follow-up. The median (IQR) follow up time for those 6 women on regular follow up was 20 (15–24) weeks.

Of 585 HIV-positive women who delivered babies, 522 (89%) were initiated on ART/pARV. Among them, 54/522(10%) were initiated on ART after delivery. Living outside Mandalay was significantly associated with initiation of ART after delivery with the adjusted risk ratio (95% CI) of 2.8 (1.7–4.6).

The duration of ART/pARV before delivery was calculated for 468 HIV-positive women who were initiated on ART/pARV before delivery and the median (IQR) duration of ART before delivery was 10 (5–14) weeks. About 192 (41%) women received ART/pARV for ≤8 weeks before delivery. Women whose spouse's HIV status was unknown (i.e., not recorded) had 40% higher risk of shorter duration of ART [adjusted risk ratio (95% CI) 1.4 (1.2–1.8)].

Of the 585 children that were born, HIV test results were recorded for 410 children, and of those tested, 9 children were HIV positive (transmission rate of ~ 2.2%).

Discussion

In this study, we found that 9 out of 10 women enrolled into the PMTCT Programme were initiated on ART/

Table 1 Characteristics and factors associated with initiation of ART/pARV in Central Women Hospital, Mandalay, Myanmar

Characteristics	Total n	ART or pARV initiation, n (%)	ART initiation rate (100 person-month-follow-up)	cHR (95% CI)	P value	aHR* (95% CI)	P value
Total	670	588 (88)	54				
Age (in years)							
<=30	400	348 (87)	48	1			
> 30	270	240 (89)	63	1.1 (0.9–1.3)	0.27		
Patients' residence							
Outside MDY	159	139 (87)	61	1 (0.8–1.1)	0.55		
MDY	511	449 (88)	51	1			
Spouse HIV status recorded							
No	223	177 (79)	34	1		1	
Yes	447	411 (92)	72	1.3 (1.1–1.6)[§]	< 0.01	1.1 (0.9–1.4)	0.18
Baseline CD4 count (cells/mm3)							
<=350	311	297 (95)	93	1.2 (1–1.4)	0.06	1.1 (0.9–1.3)	0.28
> 350	302	271 (90)	42	1		1	
missing	57	20 (35)					
Baseline WHO staging							
I & II	311	272 (87)	50	1			
III & IV	359	316 (88)	57	1 (0.8–1.2)	0.75		
Baseline Haemoglobin level							
< 11 g%	372	357 (96)	97	1.2 (1.0–1.5)[§]	< 0.05	1.0 (0.8–1.2)	0.95
≥11 g%	234	205 (88)	36	1		1	
missing	64	26 (41)					
Literacy status							
Literate	622	553 (89)	53	1.5 (1–2.2)	0.05	1.4 (0.9–2.2)	0.11
Illiterate	36	25 (69)	44	1		1	
Missing	12	10 (83)					
Pregnancy stage at enrolment							
Before delivery	566	539 (95)	102	4.7 (3.5–6.4)[§]	< 0.001	4.4 (3.2–6.1)[§]	< 0.001
During deivery/Post-partum	104	49 (47)	9	1		1	

ART Anti-retroviral therapy, pARV Anti-retroviral prophylaxis, cHR crude Hazard Ratio, aHR Adjusted Hazard Ratio, p p value, 95% CI 95% confident interval, MDY Mandalay
[§]Statistically significant
*Characteristics with p < 0.15 in unadjusted analysis were included in adjusted analysis

pARV with the rate of 54 per 100 person-months of follow-up. More than 70% were initiated on ART/pARV within 2 weeks of enrolment with 39% initiated on the date of enrollment to PMTCT programme. The proportion of HIV-positive women initiated on ART/pARV reported in our study was higher than global data on pregnant women living with HIV receiving medicines to prevent MTCT of HIV in 2016 (76%), in China (71%), in Cape town (46%), in Malawi where 63% in ART integrated model (HIV testing, ART provision integrated to antenatal care) and 51% in non-ART integrated model (only HIV testing integrated to antenatal care) [17–20].

We also found that women with anemia, women whose spouses had their HIV status ascertained and women who were enrolled into to PMTCT program before delivery were more likely to be initiated on ART/pARV. Anemia in HIV-positive pregnancy was usually associated with advanced HIV stage which might have led the clinician to initiate ART early for those with low hemoglobin levels [21]. Women whose spouses knew their HIV status might indicate better disclosure between the partners and better spouse support, which may be a facilitator for uptake of ART/pARV and longer duration of ART. This is similar to findings in other studies that show that involvement of spouse in care and disclosure of HIV status to partners enable initiation of ART, adherence to ART, and for minimizing fear, stigma and discrimination [22]. Our finding on lower rate of

ART/pARV initiation among intrapartum/ post-partum women at enrolment may be due to the fact that clinician might give priority to pregnant women compared to those who have already delivered.

The major reason of non-ART/pARV was lost to follow-up and most of these happened within four weeks from enrolled date. This might be related to deficiencies in counselling on the importance of regular follow-up to clinic and importance of ART. In our setting, the counselling is being done predominantly to the pregnant women and this could be insufficient to bring them back to our clinic regularly as they may be dependent on other family members to come to the PMTCT clinic. In addition, there could be several other reasons for not initiating ART/pARV (as shown in other studies) such as patient's refusal to get on to ART due to stigma, costs involved in accessing ART clinics (e.g., transportation cost), treatment seeking decision being made by husband, unwillingness to disclose HIV serostatus, long waiting time at the clinic and patient-unfriendly health care worker attitudes [22–24]. We did not explore these reasons in our study and therefore this is a potential area for further research.

Among HIV-positive mothers who delivered the babies and initiated on ART/pARV, 10% were initiated on ART after delivery and this proportion was relatively lower than a study conducted in Cape Town [2]. The delay in initiating ART was higher among HIV-positive women who lived outside Mandalay in our study. Patients living outside Mandalay might face several challenges in reaching our hospital such as financial constraints, inadequate transportation facilities, transportation cost, fear of stigma or discrimination and inadequate family support, similar to the reasons reported in other studies [22, 24, 25].

WHO recommends early ART in HIV-positive women (as soon as possible) well before delivery to be more effective in reducing mother to child transmission of HIV and studies show that at least 4–13 weeks of ART is required to achieve viral suppression at the time of delivery [26, 27]. About 40% of the women, who were initiated on ART, in our study were on ART for less than 8 weeks prior to delivery. We did not measure viral loads at the time of delivery and therefore what proportion of women in our study had low/suppressed viral loads at the time of delivery is unknown.

Strengths
This is the first study conducted in Myanmar on the ART/pARV initiation and the delays involved in HIV-positive women enrolled under PMTCT programme. We used data that is collected by this programme under routine conditions and therefore this is likely to reflect ground realities. The findings of the study therefore have direct relevance to the hospital based PMTCT care setting. In addition, there is a system of routine data quality assurance in our programme and the data quality is regularly checked and corrected. Therefore, data errors, if any are likely to be minimal.

Limitations
First, The PMTCT programme does not collect data on variables such as socio-economic status, last menstrual period or gestational week at enrolment and other factors shown to be associated in other studies [2, 22, 26]. Therefore, we were unable to study the association between these factors and ART initiation. Second, there was some missing data and we have tried to address this issue by creating a category for missing values and by not excluding such cases. We are not sure how this has affected the estimates used to study the associations in our study.

Recommendations for strengthening the PMTCT programme and future research
First, an assessment should be conducted to know what proportion of eligible pregnant women are enrolled into PMTCT programme, the timing of their first antenatal care visit and time taken to enroll HIV-positive pregnant women into the PMTCT programme from the date of this first antenatal care visit. Second, qualitative studies to assess health seeking behavior among pregnant women, the reasons of late antenatal care presentation, delays in enrolment to PMTCT programme and barriers in ART initiation are required.

Third, recording and reporting of programme data should be strengthened and integrated with the hospital data to get full information on some important variables such as gestational week at HIV diagnosis and at enrolment to PMTCT programme, presence or absence of co-morbidities such as TB. Fourth, mechanisms to expand PMTCT care services to the decentralized ART centers should be strengthened so that the services are more accessible to all HIV-positive women (living outside Mandalay) and can result in earlier initiation of ART.

Fifth, lost to follow-up tracing should be strengthened and reasons for lost to follow-up must be periodically assessed and addressed. Lastly, effort must be made to increase spouse HIV testing and family support to HIV-positive pregnant women by raising awareness about it during antenatal care, PMTCT clinic and in community.

Conclusion
This study shows high uptake of ART/pARV among HIV-positive women enrolled into the PMTCT programme in Myanmar. However, about 13% did not

receive ART before delivery. Among those initiated on ART/pARV before delivery, nearly half of them did not receive ART/pARV for more than 8 weeks prior to delivery. These aspects need to be improved, if we are to eliminate mother to child transmission of HIV in Myanmar.

Abbreviations
AIDS: Acquired Immune Deficiency Syndrome; aRR: Adjusted Risk Ratio; ART: Antiretroviral therapy; ARV: Antiretroviral drugs; CI: Confidence interval; HIV: Human Immunodeficiency Virus; HR: Hazard Ratio; IQR: Interquartile range; MDY: Mandalay; MTCT: Mother to child transmission; NAP: National AIDS Programme; PMTCT: Prevention of mother to child transmission; RR: Risk Ratio; UNAIDS: Joint United Nations Programme on HIV/AIDS; WHO: World Health Organization

Acknowledgments
We gratefully acknowledge the support of National AIDS Programme (NAP), HIV unit (The Union), Central Women Hospital and PLHIV network and all the PLHIV participated in this study.

Author contributions
KWYK: Principal Investigator and corresponding author, conception and design of the protocol, acquisition of data, data analysis, interpretation, drafted the first and final version of the manuscript to be published. SS, KHP, AAM, NTTK, TTL: Conception, design of the protocol, data analysis, interpretation of results, critically reviewing the paper, giving approval for the final version to be published. TKA, TH, MMO, NSNK, ZZA, TM, AKM: Design of the protocol, acquisition of data, critically reviewing the paper, giving approval for the final version to be published. HNO: role of senior investigator during conception, design, acquisition of data, data analysis, interpretation, critically reviewing the paper, giving approval for the final version to be published.

Funding
We thank the Department for International Development (DFD), UK for funding the Global Operational Research Fellowship Programme at the International Union Against Tuberculosis and Lung Disease (The Union), Paris, France in which the first author works as an operational research fellow.

Competing interest
The authors declare that they have no competing interests.

Author details
[1]Department of Operational Research, International Union Against Tuberculosis and Lung Disease (The Union), Mandalay, Myanmar. [2]Center for Operational Research, International Union Against Tuberculosis and Lung disease (The Union), Paris, France. [3]HIV unit, International Union Against Tuberculosis and Lung Disease (The Union), Mandalay, Myanmar. [4]National AIDS Programme, Department of Public Health, Ministry of Health and Sports, Nay Pyi Taw, Myanmar. [5]Monitoring, Evaluation, Accountability and Learning Unit, HIV, International Union Against Tuberculosis and Lung Disease (The Union), Mandalay, Myanmar. [6]Department of Obstetrics and Gynecology, Central Women Hospital, Mandalay, Myanmar. [7]Department of Operational Research, International Union Against Tuberculosis and Lung Disease (The Union), Delhi, India. [8]Department of Operational Research, International Union Against Tuberculosis and Lung Disease (The Union), Mandalay, Myanmar.

References
1. Meyers K, Qian H, Wu Y, Lao Y, Chen Q, Dong X, et al. Early initiation of ARV during pregnancy to move towards virtual elimination of motherto-child-transmission of HIV-1 in Yunnan, China. PLoS One. 2015;10:e0138104.
2. Myer L, Zulliger R, Bekker L-G, Abrams E. Systemic delays in the initiation of antiretroviral therapy during pregnancy do not improve outcomes of HIV-positive mothers: a cohort study. BMC pregnancy and childbirth. BMC Pregnancy and Childbirth. 2012;12:94.
3. Phillips T, Thebus E, Bekker L-G, Mcintyre J, Abrams EJ, Myer L. Disengagement of HIV-positive pregnant and postpartum women from antiretroviral therapy services: a cohort study. J Int AIDS Soc. 2014;17:1–10.
4. World Health Organization (WHO). Consolidated guidelines on HIV testing services 2015. Geneva: World Health Organization; 2015.
5. National AIDS Programme. Global AIDS Response Progress Report Myanmar. Nay Pyi Taw; 2015.
6. National AIDS Programme. Global AIDS Response Progress Report Myanmar. Nay Pyi Taw; 2014.
7. Joint United Nations Programme on HIV/AIDS (UNAIDS). Prevention GAP Report. Geneva; 2016.
8. National AIDS Programme. National Strategic Plan on HIV and AIDS Myanmar (2016-2020). Nay Pyi Taw: National AIDS Programme; 2017.
9. Mon MM, Htut KM, Oo HN, Lwin SM, Aung MY. Assessment on Cascade of Prevention of Mother-to-Child Transmission Services Received by HIV positive Mothers during 2012 and 2014, Myanmar. Dep Med Res UNICEF:2016.
10. Kyaw KWY, Oo MM, Kyaw NTT, Phyo KH, Aung TK, Mya T, et al. Low mother-to-child HIV transmission rate but high loss-to-follow-up among mothers and babies in Mandalay , Myanmar ; a cohort study. PLoS One. 2017;12: e0184426.
11. Patel D, Cortina-Borja M, Thorne C, Newell M-L. Time to undetectable viral load after highly active antiretroviral therapy initiation among HIV-infected pregnant women. Clin Infect Dis. 2007;44:1647–56.
12. Townsend CL, Cortina-Borja M, Peckham CS, de Ruiter A, Lyall H, Tookey PA. Low rates of mother-to-child transmission of HIV following effective pregnancy interventions in the United Kingdom and Ireland, 2000-2006. AIDS. 2008;22:973–81.
13. Fitzgerald FC, Bekker LG, Kaplan R, Myer L, Lawn SD, Wood R. Mother-to-child transmission of HIV in a community-based antiretroviral clinic in South Africa. S Afr Med J. 2010;100:827–31.
14. Department of Population. The 2014 Myanmar population and housing census. Nay Pyi Taw; 2015.
15. World Health Organization (WHO). Consolidated guidelines on the use of antiretroviral drugs for treating and preventing HIV infection: recommendations for a public health approach. Geneva: World Health Organization; 2013.
16. World Health Organization (WHO). Consolidated guidelines on the use of antiretroviral drugs for treating and preventing HIV infection: recommendations for a public health approach. 2nd ed. Geneva: World Health Organization; 2016.
17. Stinson K, Jennings K, Myer L. Integration of antiretroviral therapy services into antenatal care increases treatment initiation during Pregnancy : a cohort study. PLoS One. 2013;8:e63328.
18. Chan AK, Kanike E, Bedell R, Mayuni I, Manyera R, Mlotha W, et al. Same day HIV diagnosis and antiretroviral therapy initiation affects retention in option B+ prevention of mother-to-child transmission services at antenatal care in Zomba District, Malawi. J Int AIDS Soc. 2016;19:20672.
19. World Heath Organization (WHO). HIV/AIDS; Data and statistics. World Health Organization; 2016. http://www.who.int/hiv/data/en/. Accessed 20 Sept 2017.
20. Huang Z, Jin M, Zhou H, Dong Z, Zhang S, Han J, et al. The uptake of prevention of mother-to-child HIV transmission programs in China: a systematic review and meta-analysis. PLoS One. 2015;10:e0135068.
21. Langford SE, Ananworanich J, Cooper DA. Predictors of disease progression in HIV infection: a review. BioMed Central. 2007:11:11.
22. Hodgson I, Plummer ML, Konopka SN, Colvin CJ, Jonas E, Albertini J, et al. A systematic review of individual and contextual factors affecting ART initiation, adherence, and retention for HIV-infected pregnant and postpartum women. PLoS One. 2014;9:e111421.

23. Buregyeya E, Naigino R, Mukose A, Makumbi F, Esiru G, Arinaitwe J, et al. Facilitators and barriers to uptake and adherence to lifelong antiretroviral therapy among HIV infected pregnant women in Uganda: a qualitative study. BMC Pregnancy Childbirth. 2017;17:1–9.

24. Duff P, Kipp W, Wild TC, Rubaale T, Okech-Ojony J. Barriers to accessing highly active antiretroviral therapy by HIV-positive women attending an antenatal clinic in a regional hospital in western Uganda. J Int AIDS Soc. 2010;13:37.

25. O'Gorman DA, Nyirenda LJ, Theobald SJ. Prevention of mother-to-child transmission of HIV infection: views and perceptions about swallowing nevirapine in rural Lilongwe, Malawi. BMC Public Health. 2010;10:1–8.

26. Chintu N, Mulindwa J, Benjamin J, Chi BH, Stringer JSA. Optimal time on HAART for prevention of Motherto-child transmission of HIV. NIH Public Access. 2013;58:224–8.

27. World Health Organization (WHO). Antiretroviral Drugs for Treating Pregnant Women and Preventing HIV Infection in Infants. Geneva: World Health Organization; 2010.

16

Valuing breastfeeding: a qualitative study of women's experiences of a financial incentive scheme for breastfeeding

Maxine Johnson[1]* ⓘ, Barbara Whelan[1], Clare Relton[1], Kate Thomas[1], Mark Strong[1], Elaine Scott[1] and Mary J. Renfrew[2]

Abstract

Background: A cluster randomised controlled trial of a financial incentive for breastfeeding conducted in areas with low breastfeeding rates in the UK reported a statistically significant increase in breastfeeding at 6–8 weeks. In this paper we report an analysis of interviews with women eligible for the scheme, exploring their experiences and perceptions of the scheme and its impact on breastfeeding to support the interpretation of the results of the trial.

Methods: Semi-structured interviews were carried out with 35 women eligible for the scheme during the feasibility and trial stages. All interviews were recorded and verbatim transcripts analysed using a Framework Analysis approach.

Results: Women reported that their decisions about infant feeding were influenced by the behaviours and beliefs of their family and friends, socio-cultural norms and by health and practical considerations.
They were generally positive about the scheme, and felt valued for the effort involved in breastfeeding. The vouchers were frequently described as a reward, a bonus and something to look forward to, and helping women keep going with their breastfeeding. They were often perceived as compensation for the difficulties women encountered during breastfeeding. The scheme was not thought to make a difference to mothers who were strongly against breastfeeding. However, women did believe the scheme would help normalise breastfeeding, influence those who were undecided and help women to keep going with breastfeeding and reach key milestones e.g. 6 weeks or 3 months.

Conclusions: The scheme was acceptable to women, who perceived it as rewarding and valuing them for breastfeeding. Women reported that the scheme could raise awareness of breastfeeding and encourage its normalisation. This provides a possible mechanism of action to explain the results of the trial.

Keywords: Financial incentives, Breastfeeding, Qualitative

Background

The World Health Organisation recommends exclusive breastfeeding for the first 6 months of an infant's life, followed by continued breastfeeding alongside solid foods until at least 2 years of age [1]. There are a range of risks associated with not breastfeeding [2], including increased morbidity [3] and related healthcare and treatment costs [4]. Despite all four UK Departments of Health endorsing the WHO recommendations, and multiple initiatives to improve breastfeeding rates, the average 6–8 week prevalence in England during 2015/2016 was below 46% [5].

Financial incentives have previously been used in public health to motivate behaviour change, for example smoking cessation in pregnancy [6]. One small-scale, peer-support led, gift based incentive for breastfeeding was generally positively received by participating women and peer supporters [7]. However, authors of a systematic review of non-financial incentives to improve breastfeeding rates were not able to determine the overall effectiveness of incentives due to the heterogeneity of the studies identified [8].

* Correspondence: m.johnson@sheffield.ac.uk
[1]School of Health and Related Research (ScHARR), University of Sheffield, Sheffield, UK

The Nourishing Start for Health (NOSH) research project developed and tested the effectiveness of a financial incentive scheme in the form of vouchers which were exchangeable at supermarkets and other retail shops with no restriction on allowable purchases. The scheme was initially developed with midwives, health visitors, healthcare commissioners, breastfeeding peer support workers and local women [9], resulting in offered vouchers worth £200 paid in five £40 instalments at time points based on infant age: 2 days, 10 days, 6–8 weeks, 3 months and 6 months. Receipt of vouchers was conditional on mothers and healthcare professionals (HCPs) signing and countersigning a form stating that exclusive or partial breastfeeding was taking place. HCPs had the option of confidentially notifying the research team if they had a concern that an infant whose mother was claiming was not receiving breast milk, without those claims being jeopardised.

Women and HCPs were interviewed at each of the three stages of the NOSH project. Responses from the first stage (development) were used to inform the study design [9] which was tested in the second (feasibility) stage [10]. The purpose of this paper is to help interpret the results of the full trial (details [11] and findings [12] are published elsewhere). The trial reported a significant increase in breastfeeding at 6–8 weeks for those clusters where the NOSH Scheme was offered [12]. Findings from interviews with HCPs during the trial stage have been submitted for publication (Whelan B, Relton C, Johnson M, Strong M, Thomas K, Umney D, Renfrew MJ. Healthcare professionals' experiences of an area level conditional cash transfer scheme for breastfeeding. Forthcoming). This paper reports on interviews with women eligible for participation in the second and third stages of the project.

Methods
Aim, design and setting
Interviews were conducted in order to identify, through women's reports, influences on infant feeding decisions, (dis) satisfaction with (non) participation in the scheme, and the ways in which participation might impact on breastfeeding. A qualitative design was used for this part of the study, utilising semi-structured interviews, to provide rich data rather than responses to, for example, a survey tool. Pilot interview schedules were developed and shared with the research team for feedback. The final versions were piloted and adapted following discussion with the team.

We report qualitative data collected from single interviews with 35 women during the pre-trial feasibility and the cluster randomised controlled trial stages (see Table 1 for participant characteristics). All women lived in electoral wards with breastfeeding rates < 40% at 6–8 weeks

Table 1 Characteristics of women interviewed

Age	(n)	Previous children	
18–24	6	Yes	19
25–29	8	No	16
30–34	15		
35–40	6	Applied to participate in NOSH	
		Yes	31
District		No	4
Sheffield	5		
Rotherham	12	No of claims for NOSH Scheme voucher at time of interview	
Chesterfield	5	No of claims	No of women
N. Derbyshire	5	0	7 (5 did not participate)
Bassetlaw	6	1	2
Doncaster	2	2	2
		3	9
Ethnicity		4	5
White British	33	5	10 (this includes double claim for twins)
White other	2		

(the primary endpoint for the trial). The mean area-level deprivation scores were higher (more deprived) than the average mean for England [12]. The pre-trial feasibility stage assessed the acceptability and deliverability of the NOSH scheme in three areas of Sheffield, Rotherham (South Yorkshire) and Chesterfield (North Derbyshire). The cluster trial stage was conducted across a wider area that also included Doncaster, Bassetlaw and an extended region of North Derbyshire. The same financial incentive scheme was offered during both the feasibility and trial stages thus we considered it appropriate to analyse both sets of data together.

Recruitment and participants
Women were recruited for interview by health visitors either by postal invitation or in health visitor clinics in Children's centres. Researchers developed a sampling frame in order to purposively sample women with a mix of characteristics (for example, age, electoral ward) who were willing to be interviewed, This included women who were eligible for the scheme regardless of whether or not they had or had not participated in the scheme. Women who expressed an interest in being interviewed were sent an information sheet about the study and contacted by the researchers (BW, PvC and MJ) by telephone or e-mail to organise a telephone or in-person interview. Women were given the opportunity to ask questions about the study prior to signing a consent form.

The ages of the interviewees ranged between 18 and 40, and all but two (who described themselves as British Other) described themselves as British White. Just over half of the women were feeding their first baby. Five interviewees had not participated in the NOSH scheme, or had applied but not claimed vouchers because they did not breastfeed. A further two women had not claimed vouchers by the time they were interviewed. The remaining interviewees had claimed between one and five vouchers prior to interview.

Data collection

All individual and group interviews were carried out by BW, MJ or PvC between 2015 and 2016, prior to the results of the trial being known. All three interviewers were female researchers with PhD qualifications and experience of carrying out qualitative research. Two had health visiting and nursing backgrounds and two had personal experience of infant feeding. Interview schedules were developed for women participating and not participating in the scheme by the study team and piloted during the first interviews with participants and non-participants of the feasibility phase (see Additional file 1).

Women mainly took part in one individual interview each (n = 33), though one group interview was also carried out (n = 2). Interviews were carried out in women's homes and lasted between 30 and 70 min, depending on the participants' available time. Interviews were audio-recorded and transcribed verbatim with written consent from the participants. Field notes were made following interviews of any details that might help with transcribing or analysis, for example, interruptions by babies or small children. We stopped making new participant contacts when no new accounts were emerging in interviews.

Data analysis

Analysis of the data was carried out using the Framework approach [13], a method which was developed for systematically analysing qualitative data. The approach consists of five phases including familiarisation with data, the construction of a thematic framework, indexing the data and reviewing and summarising data. An initial framework was developed by BW and MJ following independent reading and joint discussion of the data. Themes were shared and discussed with CR and KJT prior to summarising in the Framework matrices (see Additional file 2).

At this point we (BW MJ CR KJT) knew the results of the NOSH trial, and were particularly interested in answering the question 'How did the intervention increase breastfeeding rates?' This article focusses on the themes from the data that relate to this question. A narrative structure (presented in the following section) was developed that included the final themes. NVivo 10 [14] software was used to enable data organisation and retrieval. The findings were not shared with participants as they represent an interpretation of the synthesis of women's views and do not necessarily reflect the views of each participant [15].

Results

In this section we present themes identified from analysed data that help to interpret the NOSH trial results and provide explanations for intervention mechanisms. The themes represent women's experiences of infant feeding, participating in the NOSH scheme, and impact of the NOSH scheme.

Deciding whether or not to breast feed

When asked about their initial infant feeding plans, women spoke of the influences that informed them, and how their initial plans developed or changed over time. Only one interviewee openly stated that she was influenced by the prospect of receiving vouchers. Rather, a range of influences were described including health-related information, practicalities such as preparing bottles, support from peers and health care professionals and their own past experiences.

Family and friends

Women reported being influenced by the attitudes and actions of their family and friends and the prevailing culture in their home area or country of origin. For some women, breastfeeding was the norm among their family and peers, whilst for others formula feeding was presented as the norm or the easier option, and breastfeeding as "*weird*" or "*disgusting*",

> "*I can think of two friends who think it's a bit weird and disgusting and why would you get your breasts out and let your baby suck...*" (F17)

Other women reported times when family members were quick to suggest turning to formula feeding when they were struggling to breastfeed. In some cases they were able to provide reasons to override suggestions to stop breastfeeding:

> "*But, I had a lot of people say to me, like family members, why don't you just give her a bottle, you know even my other half, who was supportive when he saw me really upset and struggling he, why don't you just give her a bottle, and that wasn't the answer, you know the answer, he was, it wasn't just, it's not just about feeding, it's about that bonding, and me feeling that's what I wanted to give her*" (T7)

There were suggestions that social norms have oscillated through generations, with younger (and some middle aged) women now holding less positive attitudes to breastfeeding:

"breastfeeding is kind of like, it died out didn't it, I know I weren't breastfed. And it's kind of come full circle again and we're trying to get it back in, we're realising what a positive thing it is but I think people of a certain generation don't kind of see the benefits of it" (T8)

Past experience
Another important influence on women's feeding decisions was their own previous experience. Breastfeeding was reported to be a greater challenge with first born babies due to an initial lack of knowledge, skill and confidence. Many of those who had previous experience of breastfeeding and made the decision to breastfeed with subsequent births, reporting these experiences as more relaxed. Women were either put off from breastfeeding by difficult experiences or more determined to breastfeed, feeling that they had somehow failed the first time:

"when I had her I was more determined, because I think that's when my baby blues set in when I'd finished feeding him because I knew it was my fault, I'd messed up" (T5)

Reported negative past experiences also included lack of support to breastfeed in public spaces:

"I changed me mind when I got kicked out of [restaurant name] for breastfeeding me daughter yeah cause someone complained and they told me to stop or get out so I got up and walked out so that put me off so I didn't do it after that" (F10)

This particular experience influenced the decision not to breastfeed her second child and not to apply for the NOSH scheme.

Health care professionals
Many women discussed how midwives, health visitors and infant feeding support workers encouraged breastfeeding from pregnancy onward. Such encouragement could sway the decision to breastfeed, and discussions about the NOSH scheme may have contributed to women's perceptions of breastfeeding regardless of the financial incentive. Conversely, over-encouragement to breastfeed could foster annoyance:

"Oh gosh yeah, all way through my pregnancy, every time I saw the midwife they discussed it....it's just like

you think (sigh) for goodness sake, I've made my own decision, let me, at the end of the day it's my choice so let me make that choice." (F13)

Support from HCPs to initiate (or continue) breastfeeding post birth was inconsistent across different women's reported experiences and sometimes women reported less support from hospital staff (often attributed to busy wards) than from community midwives and health visitors.

Changing from initial decision
Occasionally, women reported changing their decision about how to feed their baby after the birth. These changes were evident for both breastfeeding and formula feeding women. For example, one woman who did not breastfeed her first baby and did not intend to do so for her second, put her baby to the breast once at home:

"I bottle fed him for the first two days then that night, I don't know what it was I think it was just, I picked him up and I thought 'your boobs feel like they need emptying anyway don't they', put him to me breast and I thought I'll breastfeed him tonight and that were it then" (F5)

She subsequently applied for the scheme and received vouchers, reporting that although this felt rewarding, it did not influence her decision to change. Another woman reported changing to breastfeeding because of the inconvenience of preparing bottles and formula.

Decisions to breastfeed were also subject to change following the birth. Reasons for such change were that the actual experience of breastfeeding did not match expectations. For example, one woman felt less positive toward breastfeeding in practice than she had during pregnancy. For another woman, insufficient milk was produced to nourish the baby, which led her to report that the decision not to breastfeed had been made against her will:

"Well I wasn't, you know it wasn't my, it really wasn't my decision, it's my body you know made the decision for me but like I say I wanted to do it, that was the plan.." (T4)

Whilst disappointment was reported when expectations changed, many women also showed awareness, usually from past experience, that their pre-birth feeding plans to breastfeed can change due to a number of unpredictable factors. In practice the factors reported for stopping breastfeeding included traumatic or premature birth, the baby not latching on, uncertainty regarding how much milk the baby was receiving, feeding becoming too frequent, infection and cracked skin, hospitalisation of mother or baby and perceived lack of support.

Experiences of the NOSH scheme
Participants in the scheme
Participating women interviewed were generally positive about their experience of the process of applying to the NOSH scheme, claiming vouchers and their participation in the scheme. The following quotation is a typical response:

"When I got the information booklet it was very straightforward after that. It explained everything to me so I knew, sort of each stage and then my health visitor filled in the rest but if I had any questions when she came out, she asked about it every time... how I was getting on and about it, so yeah, it's very, very clear to us" (T11)

Women reported spending their vouchers on the weekly shopping, food, nappies, and children's clothes.

Non-participants in the scheme
Seven interviewees did not participate in the scheme. There were several reasons for not participating. One did not apply because she felt too busy at the time of the birth:

"It was just that busy and that hectic that I never would have never even thought to get the paper work out or fill any information in" (F15).

Two expressed uncertainty about the criteria for claiming vouchers, for example, for mixed feeding or for only 2 or 10 days of breastfeeding. Three women expressed their frustration about not being able to breastfeed and one of these reported less positive views about the scheme:

"if it's all about benefitting your baby, I don't think high street vouchers are perhaps the right thing, I think it should have been something like I don't know, like passes to toddler groups or vouchers for perhaps you know like kiddi care or something" (F14)

These views highlight the importance of accurate information for eligible women and also that women who plan to breastfeed can feel disappointed when this does not happen, not merely because they could not apply for the scheme, but because their expectations regarding feeding their infant were not fulfilled.

Perceived impact of the NOSH scheme
As part of the analysis, and in the light of positive trial results, we wanted to explore the impact of the NOSH scheme on infant feeding. This included the impact on decision making and the impact on breastfeeding continuation.

Impact on decision making
A view that had been expressed in the press was that the NOSH financial incentive amounted to "bribery" [16, 17] for breastfeeding. None of the participants in this study put forward the view (though the interviewers did not raise this topic – see Additional File A). Conversely, many interviewees reported that they had already decided to breastfeed before hearing about the scheme and women generally thought that vouchers would not make a difference for mothers who had strong opinions against breastfeeding, or for whom breastfeeding was not regarded as the norm or perceived as distasteful or even taboo:

"if someone's of the definitely of the other mind set, that they're just not going to breast feed, I'm not sure that something like that would sway them, to be honest" (T10)

However, some women suggested that participating in the scheme could provide a platform from which to raise the topic of, and normalise breastfeeding in social spheres, rejecting the social norms and negative discourses around breastfeeding (i.e. breastfeeding as "abnormal") that they might encounter. This could eventually erode the idea that breastfeeding is no longer an option worth considering and open up more choices:

"But, I think, what surprised me, like I don't know with regards to my brother's partner, I didn't think that she'd breast feed at all and I don't know whether me talking about it, and having sort of a positive experience of breast feeding, whether that's influenced her in to have a go herself as well".

None of the interviewees reported financial difficulty as a reason for taking up the offer of the scheme, although many appreciated the impact that vouchers had on their monthly income at a time when expenses were increasing:

"We still couldn't believe that we got, money for, you know what I mean for food and everything, it really helped with the shopping. It really was amazing, it really, really was" (T11)

Only one participant described having been at least partially influenced by the NOSH scheme to initiate breastfeeding:

"It gave me that little extra incentive to at least try it and I kept, on that day when it felt like I couldn't carry on I did keep pushing and pushing myself but in the end I was just like, couldn't do it" (T6)

The trial results show that rather than breastfeeding initiation being increased in intervention areas (which could be expected if women felt they were being "bribed" to breastfeed), it was the breastfeeding data at 6–8 weeks that showed a statistically significant increase. The following section describes how women described the impact of the scheme on breastfeeding continuation.

Help to keep going, reaching milestones

The timing of offered vouchers (2 days, 10 days, 6–8 weeks, 3 months and 6 months) was viewed positively by participating women. The anticipation of receiving vouchers, either as an extrinsic reward in the form of a "treat" or intrinsic reward such as a sense of feeling valued, was reported as an incentive to continue breastfeeding through difficult stages:

"I wanted to breastfeed anyway but I think it has helped me with the various stages, I think I struggled at nine ten weeks and then knowing that I could keep going to twelve weeks it did encourage me. I don't know so much if it was the vouchers that were coming I think it was just more the, you know the kind of three more weeks to go and it's twelve weeks..." (F18)

"it does give you a little bit of extra incentive and when you reach each sort of milestone it does make you feel, sort of good about yourself, you've got to the next one" (T11)

This was particularly pertinent at times when women were facing the wide range of physical, practical and socio-cultural challenges described in this article. Women reported that their early experiences of multiple feeds during the night were especially dispiriting and that the prospect of receiving vouchers would encourage them to continue and feel more positive than they might otherwise have done.

Compensating efforts: "Reward, bonus and boost"

For women who had already made a decision to breastfeed prior to becoming involved in the scheme, receiving vouchers was described in terms of "reward", "bonus", "boost", a way of feeling valued and recognised for doing something positive for their baby.

"It was like a little extra boost to think, you know what I mean, you're doing something good, you're doing the right thing and it's helping. So, I appreciated that" (T10)

Despite having strong preferences to breastfeed, a number of women described their experiences as anything but straightforward. Choosing to formula feed might have lessened the physical problems they faced, but receiving vouchers went some way toward compensating women when they managed to overcome difficulties, and gave them something to look forward to.

"I think you feel almost like valued that you're breastfeeding I think is how it felt and encouraged. I think the vouchers do then help as well." (F18)

These accounts highlight the complex and shifting decisions and experiences that women face regarding infant feeding, and the positive impact of the financial incentive in encouraging the continuation of breastfeeding once initiated.

Discussion

These interviews need to be interpreted in the light of the NOSH trial results where there was evidence that the scheme was both acceptable (46% of all eligible mother-infant dyads were signed up for the scheme, and 34% claimed vouchers) and effective in increasing breastfeeding rates at 6–8 weeks in areas with low breastfeeding rates [12]. In this study, both participants and non-participants in the NOSH scheme described their experiences as mainly positive. However, non-participants reported a lack of clarity regarding eligibility for the scheme or not being able to apply for the scheme due to early problems.

Data from interviews suggest that although offering vouchers might (hypothetically) incentivise breastfeeding initiation, women generally attributed their initial infant feeding decisions to other influences. These findings support the idea that practical and health related factors are taken into account when weighing up feeding options prior to the birth [18]. They are also in line with evidence that pre and post birth decisions regarding infant feeding are influenced by a range of historical, socio-economic, cultural and individual factors [3]. Our findings show that decisions tend to be made in response to past experiences and support from others, as well as to social norms, although some women are able to overcome strong influences from well-meaning friends and family members if they are keen to breastfeed. Equally, women remain susceptible to the unpredictable effects of physical problems, lack of support and their own changing attitude to feeding following the birth. Giving up breastfeeding due to these effects can lead to feelings of guilt for women if they are not supported in having realistic expectations [19].

For women who decide to breastfeed, national statistics for England illustrate a steep decline in rates from initiation (73.8%) to breastfeeding rates at 6–8 weeks (45.2%) in the first quarter of 2015–2016 [5], suggesting that it is the continuation of breastfeeding that women find challenging. Continuation is reported to be more likely where women intend to breastfeed and are positive about breastfeeding [20]. Our findings show that even when women are positive about breastfeeding, they often face a range of difficulties that can discourage them from continuing. Financial incentives did seem to help women to work through some of the more personal difficulties associated with breastfeeding and also to motivate them to continue to breastfeed to reach the more general milestones at which the vouchers were offered. Women who received vouchers regarded them as a reward, a bonus and a boost for the challenges they faced during breastfeeding and felt valued for their efforts:

"it added the incentive to carry on and it sort of gives you a little boost of help, especially in the early months it's very important to have enough money to eat well" (T11)

These findings resonate with those of Thomson et al. [7] who reported that women who breastfed felt rewarded by the gift they received from an incentive scheme.

Women in our study also suggested ways that the scheme might indirectly impact on future infant feeding decisions, including changing the social norm around breastfeeding. A number of women associated low breastfeeding rates with cultural and social circumstances, and negative discourses of breastfeeding. Raising awareness of breastfeeding and treating it as "normal" was one way that they thought the scheme might help to break through these discourses and gradually increase breastfeeding rates. The concept of 'normalcy' derived from breastfeeding support has previously been identified where mothers faced embarrassment and isolation in a culture that demeaned breastfeeding, particularly in public [21]. Rollins et al. [3] support the need for positive messages around breastfeeding in society, as well as practical changes that enable women to breastfeed without disadvantage and stigma, for example, ensuring that maternity leave and public space policies are breastfeeding friendly.

Strengths and limitations
This is the first study of women's experiences of being offered a financial incentive to breastfeed. It was conducted alongside a large cluster randomised controlled trial of the financial incentive (details [11] and findings [12] are published elsewhere) to explore acceptability of the scheme in practice and to contextualise the trial findings [22].

All attempts were made to include women with a range of perspectives by targeting first time and experienced mothers from different age groups living in a range of IMD (Index of Multiple Deprivation) profiles. Despite these efforts the findings may not be fully representative of all women who took part in the NOSH scheme. Women who came forward to be interviewed were mostly older and from the least deprived areas. It could be argued that older and more affluent women might be more likely to breastfeed [23] and to participate in interviews. Women were also of white ethnicity and nearly all were British, which limits generalisation of the findings to diverse populations. However, non-white women are generally associated with higher rates of breastfeeding [23] and therefore the study was not specifically examining the influence of ethnicity on breastfeeding or participation in the scheme.

New mothers are busy and occasionally had to cancel interviews. Nevertheless, the views presented here are helpful in determining how the scheme was received, the perceived impact of the intervention and some potential ways that the scheme might impact on decision-making. We consider that the experiential backgrounds of the interviewers helped them to conduct the interviews in a sensitive yet conversational style whilst adhering to the research objectives.

Conclusions
A range of practical and socio-cultural factors influence infant feeding decisions at important stages in the process. Talking about the scheme with others provided a channel through which negative beliefs about breastfeeding could be rejected. Women described the vouchers as a 'reward' which incentivised continued feeding. These suggest possible mechanisms of action for the statistically significant increase in breastfeeding at 6–8 weeks reported in the trial of the NOSH Scheme.

These interviews with participants gave no credence to initial media-reported claims that a financial incentive scheme amounted to "bribery" to breastfeed [16, 17]. These interviews appear to support the trial findings that the scheme had a greater impact on the decision to continue breastfeeding for longer, rather than on the decision to initiate breastfeeding.

Abbreviations
HCP: Health Care Professional; IMD: Index of Multiple Deprivation; NOSH: Nourishing Start for Health; PhD: Doctor of Philosophy; UK: United Kingdom; WHO: World Health Organization

Acknowledgments

We would like to thank the women who gave their time for the interviews. Thanks are also extended to Patrice van Cleemput (PvC) on the NOSH team who carried out a number of interviews for the feasibility study. Also to Zoe Furniss and Kathryn Mackellar, who facilitated transcribing the interviews and Darren Umney who provided feedback on the draft manuscript. The Nourishing Start for Health research team acknowledges the support of the National Institute for Health Research through the Comprehensive Research Network (NIHR CRN Portfolio ID number: 15385).

Funding

Medical Research Council (MR/J000434/1) via the National Prevention Research Initiative Phase 4 Award. Funding for the costs of the intervention (shopping vouchers) for the trial was supported by Public Health England.

Authors' contributions

CR, MS, KJT and MJR, conceived of and were involved in designing the original randomised controlled trial of the NOSH scheme. ES provided managerial support for the study as well as critical feedback on the paper. BW and MJ conducted individual and group interviews, read the transcripts, developed the analytical framework and analysed the data. BW, MJ, CR, KJT and MJR contributed to the interpretation of the analysis. MJ drafted the manuscript and all authors critically reviewed and approved the final content.

Competing interests

The authors declare that they have no competing interests.

Author details

[1]School of Health and Related Research (ScHARR), University of Sheffield, Sheffield, UK. [2]Mother and Infant Research Unit, School of Nursing and Health Sciences, University of Dundee, Dundee, UK.

References

1. World Health Organisation. Health topics: breastfeeding. 2017.
2. Victora CG, Bahl R, Barros AJ, et al. Breastfeeding in the 21st century: epidemiology, mechanisms, and lifelong effect. Lancet. 2016;387(10017):475–90.
3. Rollins NC, Bhandari N, Hajeebhoy N, et al. Why invest, and what it will take to improve breastfeeding practices? Lancet. 2016;387(10017):491–504.
4. UK U. Preventing disease and saving resources: the potential contribution of increasing breastfeeding rates in the UK. UNICEF: UK; 2012.
5. NHS England. Statistical Release Breastfeeding Initiation & Breastfeeding Prevalence 6–8 weeks quarter 1 2015/16. 2017.
6. Tappin D, Bauld L, Purves D, et al. Financial incentives for smoking cessation in pregnancy: randomised controlled trial. BMJ. 2015;350:h134.
7. Thomson G, Dykes F, Hurley M, et al. Incentives as connectors: insights into a breastfeeding incentive intervention in a disadvantaged area of north-West England. BMC Pregnancy Childbirth. 2012; https://doi.org/10.1186/1471-2393-12-22.
8. Moran VH, Morgan H, Rothnie K, et al. Incentives to promote breastfeeding: A systematic review. Pediatrics 2015:peds. 2014–221.
9. Whitford H, Whelan B, van Cleemput P, et al. Encouraging breastfeeding: financial incentives. Practising Midwife. 2015;18(2):18–21. published Online First: 2015/09/04
10. Whelan B, Thomas KJ, Van Cleemput P, et al. Healthcare providers' views on the acceptability of financial incentives for breastfeeding: a qualitative study. BMC Pregnancy Childbirth. 2014;14(1):355.
11. Relton C, Strong M, Renfrew MJ, et al. Cluster randomised controlled trial of a financial incentive for mothers to improve breast feeding in areas with low breastfeeding rates: the NOSH study protocol. BMJ Open. 2016;6(4):e010158.
12. Relton C, Strong M, Thomas K, et al. Do conditional cash transfers improve 6-8 week breastfeeding prevalence? The NOurishing start for health (NOSH) trial, an area-based cluster randomised controlled trial in England. JAMA Pediatr. 2017; https://doi.org/10.1001/jamapediatrics.2017.4523.
13. Ritchie J, Lewis J. Qualitative Research Practice: A Guide for Social Science Students and Researchers 2003.
14. QSR International. NVivo 10 for windows. 2012.
15. Mays N, Pope C. Quality in Qualitative Health Research. In: Mays N, Pope C, editors. Qualitative Research in Health Care. 3rd ed. Oxford: Blackwell; 2006. p. 82–101.
16. Ellen B. Breastfeeding bribes? What a grubby little idea. The Guardian 2013.
17. Donnelly L, Holehouse M. Mothers might not breastfeed after taking £200 NHS bribe, MP warns. The Telegraph 2017.
18. Roll CL, Cheater F. Expectant parents' views of factors influencing infant feeding decisions in the antenatal period: a systematic review. Int J Nurs Stud. 2016;60:145–55.
19. Fox R, McMullen S, Newburn M. UK women's experiences of breastfeeding and additional breastfeeding support: a qualitative study of baby Café services. BMC Pregnancy Childbirth. 2015;15(147):1–12. https://doi.org/10.1186/s12884-015-0581-5.
20. Lamontagne C, Hamelin A-M, St-Pierre M. The breastfeeding experience of women with major difficulties who use the services of a breastfeeding clinic: a descriptive study. Int Breastfeed J 2008;3(17) https://doi.org/10.1186/1746-4358-3-17.
21. Leahy-Warren P, Creedon M, Mahoney A, et al. Normalising breastfeeding within a formula feeding culture: an Irish qualitative study. Women Birth. 2017;30:e103–e10.
22. O' Cathain A, Thomas KJ, Drabble SJ, et al. What can qualitative research do for randomised controlled trials? A systematic mapping review. BMJ Open. 2013;3:e002889. https://doi.org/10.1136/bmjopen-2013-002889.
23. Oakley LL, Renfrew MJ, Kurinczuk JJ, et al. Factors associated with breastfeeding in England: an analysis by primary care trust. BMJ Open. 2013; 3(6):e002765.

17

Do pregnancies reduce iron overload in *HFE* hemochromatosis women?

Virginie Scotet[1][*][†], Philippe Saliou[1,2][†], Marianne Uguen[1], Carine L'Hostis[1], Marie-Christine Merour[3], Céline Triponey[3], Brigitte Chanu[3], Jean-Baptiste Nousbaum[1,4], Gerald Le Gac[1,5] and Claude Ferec[1,3,5]

Abstract

Background: *HFE* hemochromatosis is an inborn error of iron metabolism linked to a defect in the regulation of hepcidin synthesis. This autosomal recessive disease typically manifests later in women than men. Although it is commonly stated that pregnancy is, with menses, one of the factors that offsets iron accumulation in women, no epidemiological study has yet supported this hypothesis. The aim of our study was to evaluate the influence of pregnancy on expression of the predominant *HFE* p.[Cys282Tyr];[Cys282Tyr] genotype.

Methods: One hundred and forty p.Cys282Tyr homozygous women enrolled in a phlebotomy program between 2004 and 2011 at a blood centre in western Brittany (France) were included in the study. After checking whether the disease expression was delayed in women than in men in our study, the association between pregnancy and iron overload was assessed using multivariable regression analysis.

Results: Our study confirms that women with *HFE* hemochromatosis were diagnosed later than men cared for during the same period (52.6 vs. 47.4 y., $P < 0.001$). Compared to no pregnancy, having at least one pregnancy was not associated with lower iron markers. In contrast, the amount of iron removed by phlebotomies appeared significantly higher in women who had at least one pregnancy ($e^\beta = 1.50$, $P = 0.047$). This relationship disappeared after adjustment for confounding factors ($e^\beta = 1.35$, $P = 0.088$).

Conclusions: Our study shows that pregnancy status has no impact on iron markers level, and is not in favour of pregnancy being a protective factor in progressive iron accumulation. Our results are consistent with recent experimental data suggesting that the difference in disease expression observed between men and women may be explained by other factors such as hormones.

Keywords: Genetic hemochromatosis, Iron overload, Phenotype, Pregnancy

Background

HFE-related hemochromatosis (or type 1 hemochromatosis; OMIM #235200) is an inborn iron metabolism disorder that is particularly common in Caucasian populations [1, 2]. This genetic disease is characterised by an inappropriate high iron absorption from enterocytes and by an excessive iron release from macrophages. It is due to a defective regulation of the synthesis of hepcidin, the key regulator of iron homeostasis [3–5]. As human body is not capable of eliminating the excess of iron, this will gradually affect various organs and may result in serious damages, e.g. cirrhosis, hepatocellular carcinoma or cardiomyopathy [6].

HFE hemochromatosis is inherited as an autosomal recessive trait and is mainly associated with the *HFE* p.[Cys282Tyr];[Cys282Tyr] genotype [7]. The penetrance of this genotype is clearly incomplete [8–10], and its expression is influenced by genetic and environmental factors that may increase or reduce the iron burden [8, 11, 12].

This expression of this genetic disorder is delayed in women than in men. Moreover, *HFE* hemochromatosis women present with a less severe clinical profile, notably

---

* Correspondence: virginie.scotet@univ-brest.fr; virginie.scotet@inserm.fr
[†]Equal contributors
[1]UMR1078 "Génétique, Génomique Fonctionnelle et Biotechnologies", Inserm, EFS, Université de Brest, ISBAM, 22 avenue Camille Desmoulins, 29200 Brest, France

a lower prevalence of liver injury [13, 14]. This difference between genders has classically been attributed to the protective effects mediated by iron losses related to menses and pregnancy [15–17].

During pregnancy, maternal iron requirements increase substantially to allow for the physiological expansion of the haemoglobin mass, to promote formation of the foetus and placenta, and to cope with blood losses at delivery [18]. While it is commonly stated in the literature that these pregnancy-associated iron losses are one of the factors that offset the lifelong iron accumulation in women [15–17], this assertion has not been supported by any epidemiological studies in humans.

As recent literature has shown that other factors such as hormones may explain the differences observed according to gender [19, 20], we sought to investigate the association between pregnancy and the phenotypic expression of the predominant HFE p.[Cys282Tyr];[Cys282Tyr] genotype.

Methods
Study design and participants
This work evaluated a cohort of 140 consecutive p.Cys282Tyr homozygous hemochromatosis women who started phlebotomies between January 1st, 2004 and December 31st, 2011 at a blood centre in western Brittany (Brest, France) where this disease is particularly common [21, 22].

Included patients presented elevated iron markers (with transferrin saturation (TS) > 45% and serum ferritin (SF) > 200 µg/L) and were referred by general practitioners or gastroenterologists to the blood centre for phlebotomy.

Questionnaire
This study relied on data obtained using a clinical questionnaire that was filled out upon admission to the phlebotomy program. As previously described [22], this questionnaire, which was completed by a referral physician, collected information on socio-demographic characteristics (gender, age at diagnosis, etc.), lifestyle factors (height, weight, alcohol intake, etc.) and biological parameters (including transferrin saturation and serum ferritin).

It also recorded data on reproductive functions, on the presence (and number if any) of pregnancies prior to the beginning of the treatment (excluding miscarriages and abortions occurring in the first trimester), as well as on the menopausal status at admission to the phlebotomy program. Patients were also asked if they were regular blood donors, if they had chronic bleedings (including gastrointestinal bleedings, chronic hematuria, bleedings due to parasitic infections) and if they received blood transfusions (and how many if any), all this prior to admission to the phlebotomy program.

At the end of the depletion stage, treatment-related data (i.e. the number and average volume of the phlebotomies) were recorded. These data enable estimation of the amount of iron removed (AIR; in grams) to normalise patient's iron stores (i.e. to reach SF < 100 µg/L). This calculation was performed assuming that 1 L of blood contains 0.5 g of iron [23].

Statistical analysis
Statistical analysis was carried out using the SAS software (version 9.4; SAS Institute Inc., Cary, NC). All tests were performed two-sided, and the significance level was set at 5% for all analyses.

First, we described the baseline characteristics of the studied population. Continuous variables were described in means and standard deviation (SD), and were compared using Student's t test or Anova. When these variables were not normally distributed, they were described by median and interquartile range (IQR), and compared by the Mann-Whitney test. Categorical variables were summarised in percentages, and were compared using χ^2 test or Fisher's exact test when appropriate.

Before assessing the influence of pregnancy, we explored the impact of gender on disease expression. For this, we compared the age at diagnosis of women in the study to that observed in the men cared for during the same period in our blood centre ($n = 161$) (using Student's t test). We also evaluated whether the proportion of diagnosed female patients increased with the age at diagnosis i.e. if the sex ratio $_{(M/F)}$ decreased with the age at diagnosis (using a linear trend χ^2 test).

In a second time, we compared women characteristics according to their pregnancy status (number of previous pregnancies). We then investigated the association between pregnancy and the degree of iron overload (assessed by SF and AIR) using linear regression analysis. As the distributions of these quantitative dependant variables were highly skewed (Kolmogorov-Smirnov test), we performed logarithmic (ln) transformations to normalise them. With such a transformation, the exponential of the estimated regression coefficient (e^β) indicates how many times the outcome variable varies for each unit increment in the explanatory variable. This means, in other words, that each unit increment in the explanatory variable multiplies the expected value of Y by e^β. We then tested the association between the iron parameters and potential confounding factors such as age at diagnosis, alcohol intake (whose hepatotoxic effect increases the disease severity) [24, 25]) and menopausal status. We thereafter fitted a multivariable model to enable adjustment for confounders. All explanatory variables associated with the outcome variables at a conservative threshold of $P < 0.20$ in the univariable analysis were included in this multivariable analysis.

In the present study, excessive alcohol intake was defined, in accordance with the World Health Organization definition, as daily consumption exceeding two glasses per day (i.e. 14 glasses per week) for women. Overweight status was defined as a body mass index (BMI) ≥ 25 kg/m^2.

Results

Baseline characteristics of the study population

During the study period, 140 p.Cys282Tyr homozygous hemochromatosis women were enrolled into a phlebotomy program at the blood centre of Brest. The "pregnancy" variable was documented for 137 (97.9%) women and 127 of them (92.7%) completed the depletion phase during the study. The baseline characteristics of the women included in the study and for whom data on pregnancies was available are presented in Table 1. These women were diagnosed in mean at the age of 52.5 years ($\pm$ 14.0). Among them, 29.8% were overweight (BMI ≥ 25 kg/m^2) and 4.5% declared having excessive alcohol consumption. More than 60% of the women were menopausal at entry into the

phlebotomy program, with a mean age at menopause of 49.2 y. ($\pm$ 4.3).

Analysis of the gender difference in expression of the p.[Cys282Tyr];[Cys282Tyr] genotype

Our study confirmed that the age at diagnosis was delayed in women in comparison to the men cared for during the same period (52.6 vs. 47.4 y.; $P < 0.001$). As illustrated in Table 2, the sex ratio decreased significantly with the age at diagnosis, especially after the age of 50 years ($\chi^2_{linear\ trend}$: 10.5; $P = 0.001$). Thus, women represented about 38% of the p.Cys282Tyr homozygous patients diagnosed before the age of 50 (sex ratio = 1.64), 47.3% of patients diagnosed between 50 and 59 years (sex ratio = 1.12), and 64.6% of patients diagnosed after the age of 60 (sex ratio = 0.55).

Baseline characteristics of women according to the pregnancy status

The number of pregnancies of the 137 p.Cys282Tyr homozygous hemochromatosis women ranged from zero to six, with an average of 2.4 pregnancies per woman ($\pm$

Table 1 Baseline characteristics of the p.Cys282Tyr homozygous hemochromatosis women according to the number of pregnancies that women had prior to entry into the phlebotomy program

Variables	All women		Number of pregnancies: 0		Number of pregnancies: 1 or 2		Number of pregnancies: ≥ 3		P^*
	n	%	n	%	n	%	n	%	
Number of women	137		14		65		58		
Age at diagnosis (n = 137)									
≥ 60 y^a	41	29.9%	2	14.3%	16	24.6%	23	39.7%	0.077
< 60 y.	96	70.1%	12	85.7%	49	75.4%	35	60.3%	
Body mass index (n = 131)									
≥ 25 kg/m^2	39	29.8%	2	14.3%	19	30.6%	18	32.7%	0.395
< 25 kg/m^2	92	70.2%	12	85.7%	43	69.4%	37	67.3%	
Alcohol intake (n = 134)									
Excessive^b	6	4.5%	0	0.0%	2	3.1%	4	7.0%	0.418
Non excessive	128	95.5%	13	100.0%	62	96.9%	53	93.0%	
Menopause (n = 126)									
Yes	80	63.5%	3	21.4%	36	66.7%	41	70.7%	0.002
No	46	36.5%	11	78.6%	18	33.3%	17	29.3%	
Regular blood donations (n = 136)									
Yes	37	27.2%	5	35.7%	15	23.1%	17	29.8%	0.530
No	99	72.8%	9	64.3%	50	76.9%	40	70.2%	
Chronic bleedings (n = 135)									
Yes	4	3.0%	2	14.3%	0	0.0%	2	3.4%	0.313
No	131	97.0%	12	85.7%	63	100.0%	56	96.6%	
Blood transfusions (n = 134)									
Yes	15	11.2%	1	7.1%	6	9.7%	8	13.8%	0.681
No	119	88.8%	13	92.9%	56	90.3%	50	86.2%	

^{a}Classical cut-off for describing the beginning of the expression of *HFE* hemochromatosis in women
^{b}Daily consumption ≥2 glasses/day or 14 glasses/week in women (World Health Organization definition)
$^*\chi^2$ or Fisher exact test

Table 2 Distribution of men and women by age at diagnosis

Age at diagnosis	Total	Men		Women		Sex ratio
		n	%	n	%	
< 40 y.	68	42	61.8%	26	38.2%	1.62
[40–50[y.	77	48	62.3%	29	37.7%	1.66
[50–60[y.	91	48	52.7%	43	47.3%	1.12
≥ 60 y.	65	23	35.4%	42	64.6%	0.55
Total	301	161	53.5%	140	46.5%	1.15

1.3). Nearly 90% of the women in our sample ($n = 123$) had at least one pregnancy before entering the phlebotomy program, with the majority of women having had two (42.3%; $n = 58$) or three (27.0%; $n = 37$) pregnancies. Approximately 15% of the women had four pregnancies or more (15.3%; $n = 21$).

The baseline characteristics and the biological markers of women according to the number of pregnancies (categorised in three groups) are summarised in Tables 1 and 3. As illustrated in Table 1, the age at diagnosis, the proportion of overweight patients and the frequency of alcohol abusers did not differ significantly between the three groups. Similar results were observed for the proportion of patients with previous regular blood donations, chronic bleedings or blood transfusions. At the opposite, a significant association was observed between the number of pregnancies and the proportion of postmenopausal women ($P = 0.002$). Table 3 shows that there was no significant difference in iron markers according to the number of pregnancies.

Association between pregnancy and iron markers

The results of linear regression modelling the association between pregnancy and iron markers (SF and AIR, respectively) are summarised in Tables 4 and 5. Unlike what one might expect, women having had at least one pregnancy did not present lower iron markers than women with no pregnancy. Indeed, the univariable analysis showed that, in comparison to

women with no pregnancy, the SF concentration was not different in women who had one or two pregnancies ($P = 0.288$) nor in women who had three or more pregnancies ($P = 0.126$). Combination of these two modalities provided similar findings ($e^{\beta}_{\geq 1 \text{ vs. 0 pregnancy}} = 1.32$; 95% confidence interval [CI]: 0.88–1.97; $P = 0.177$). Adjustment for potential confounders such as age at diagnosis, alcohol intake and menopausal status did not change the observed trends, whatever the coding used.

Similar findings were obtained for the second iron marker: AIR (Table 5). The univariable analysis revealed no significant association between pregnancy and AIR. When comparing women who had at least one pregnancy to women with no pregnancy, AIR was even significantly higher (i.e. 1.5 time higher) in women who had at least one pregnancy ($e^{\beta}_{\geq 1 \text{ vs. 0 pregnancy}} = 1.50$; 95% CI: 1.01–2.23, $P = 0.047$). However, this relationship became non-significant after adjustment for potential confounders ($e^{\beta}_{\geq 1 \text{ vs. 0 pregnancy}} = 1.35$; 95% CI: 0.96–1.90, $P = 0.088$). The results remained still at the limit of significance after adjustment for age at diagnosis, alcohol consumption, menopausal status and baseline SF level, when comparing women having one or two pregnancies to women having no pregnancy ($P = 0.058$).

Discussion

Pregnancy has been suggested to be one potential factor responsible for the later manifestation of *HFE* hemochromatosis in women [15–17]. Yet, our work is the first epidemiological study entirely devoted to the analysis of the association between pregnancy and the phenotypic expression of the main *HFE* genotype in humans. Our study confirms that p.Cys282Tyr homozygous women are diagnosed at a later age than men, and thus corroborates the existence of a difference in the expression of this genotype between men and

Table 3 Biological parameters of the p.Cys282Tyr homozygous hemochromatosis women according to the number of pregnancies that women had prior to entry into the phlebotomy program

Biological parameters	Number of pregnancies: 0		Number of pregnancies: 1 or 2		Number of pregnancies: ≥ 3		P‡
	Median	IQRᵃ	Median	IQR	Median	IQR	
Transferrin saturation (%) *(n = 137)*							
	81	[72–89]	78	[65–88]	83	[67–97]	0.998
Serum ferritin (µg/L) *(n = 137)*							
	298	[236–529]	414	[279–693]	412	[297–770]	0.293
Amount of iron removed (g) *(n = 127)*							
	1.3	[1.1–2.0]	2.5	1.4–4.0]	2.3	[1.6–3.6]	0.140
Hemoglobin (g/dL) *(n = 108)*							
	13.6	[13.3–14.6]	14.0	[13.6–14.5]	13.9	[13.4–14.4]	0.815

ᵃInterquartile range ([Quartile 1 – Quartile 3])
‡Mann-Whitney test

Table 4 Results of the linear regression analysis modelling the association between pregnancies and serum ferritin

Variables	Univariable analysis			Multivariable analysis		
	e β	95% CI	P	e β	95% CI	P
No. of pregnancies						
0	1.00			1.00		
1 or 2	1.25	[0.82–1.91]	0.288	1.03	[0.67–1.57]	0.902
≥ 3	1.39	[0.91–2.13]	0.126	1.02	[0.66–1.57]	0.944
Age at diagnosis						
< 60 y.[a]	1.00			1.00		
≥ 60 y.	1.35	[1.04–1.73]	0.026	1.20	[0.89–1.62]	0.230
Body mass index						
< 25 kg/m²	1.00					
≥ 25 kg/m²	1.13	[0.86–1.48]	0.387	–		
Alcohol intake						
Non excessive	1.00			1.00		
Excessive[b]	2.38	[1.34–4.20]	0.003	2.06	[1.11–3.85]	0.023
Menopause						
No	1.00			1.00		
Yes	1.55	[1.20–2.00]	< 0.001	1.39	[1.03–1.87]	0.032
Regular blood donations						
No	1.00					
Yes	0.84	[0.64–1.11]	0.219	–		
Chronic bleedings						
No	1.00					
Yes	0.96	[0.46–1.99]	0.904	–		
Blood transfusions						
No	1.00					
Yes	1.02	[0.69–1.50]	0.938	–		

[a]Classical cut-off for describing the beginning of the expression of *HFE* hemochromatosis in women
[b]Daily consumption ≥ 2 glasses/day or 14 glasses/week in women (World Health Organization definition)
Univariable analysis for pregnancy: global *P*-value = 0.293

Table 5 Results of the linear regression analysis modelling the association between pregnancies and the amount of iron removed by phlebotomies

Variables	Univariable analysis			Multivariable analysis		
	e β	95% CI	P	e β	95% CI	P
No. of pregnancies						
0	1.00			1.00		
1 or 2	1.49	[0.98–2.26]	0.061	1.41	[0.99–2.02]	0.058
≥ 3	1.51	[0.99–2.31]	0.058	1.27	[0.89–1.83]	0.191
Age at diagnosis						
< 60 y.[a]	1.00			1.00		
≥ 60 y.	1.19	[0.90–1.56]	0.214	1.11	[0.86–1.43]	0.415
Body mass index						
< 25 kg/m²	1.00					
≥ 25 kg/m²	0.96	[0.72–1.27]	0.766	–		
Alcohol intake						
Non excessive	1.00			1.00		
Excessive[b]	2.29	[1.32–3.97]	0.004	1.32	[0.80–2.19]	0.279
Menopause						
No	1.00			1.00		
Yes	1.28	[0.97–1.71]	0.084	0.92	[0.72–1.19]	0.530
Regular blood donations						
No	1.00					
Yes	1.01	[0.76–1.34]	0.930	–		
Chronic bleedings						
No	1.00					
Yes	1.01	[0.50–2.05]	0.979	–		
Blood transfusions						
No	1.00					
Yes	0.98	[0.67–1.43]	0.924	–		
Baseline ferritin	1.00	[1.00–1.00]	< 0.001	1.00	[1.00–1.00]	< 0.001

[a]Classical cut-off for describing the beginning of the expression of *HFE* hemochromatosis in women
[b]Daily consumption ≥2 glasses/day or 14 glasses/week in women (World Health Organization definition)
Univariable analysis for pregnancy: global *P*-value = 0.140

women. Nevertheless, these results do not confirm the protective effect typically attributed to pregnancy to explain the slower iron accumulation in women.

Our study was subject to little selection bias for several reasons. First, it was a cohort study that included prospectively almost all of the p.Cys282Tyr homozygous hemochromatosis women enrolled in a phlebotomy program at our centre over the study period. Second, the rate of missing values for the main explanatory variable (pregnancy) was very low (~ 2.0%), making our sample fully representative of the p.Cys282Tyr homozygous women who come to medical attention in our area. Finally, we also ensured that the baseline characteristics of women excluded from the multivariable analysis (due to missing values) did not differ from those of included women.

Moreover, iron burden was measured using SF but also AIR, which is the reference method to assess body iron stores [26]. AIR is a more reliable marker than SF, which may also be increased beyond the real degree of iron burden by secondary causes of hyperferritinaemia as excessive alcohol intake or metabolic or inflammatory syndromes [27].

Our study was also able to take into account major confounders, as alcohol intake or menopausal status at entry into the phlebotomy program. Nevertheless, we did not have information on the presence of some other factors susceptible to modify the iron burden (iron supplementation during pregnancy, blood losses from labor and delivery, postpartum hemorrhage, pregnancy complications (pre-eclampsia, abruption, placenta previa), importance of menstrual blood losses, ...) [28]. However, most of these data are not easy to quantify precisely. Some of them may also only have a small effect on iron status, as maternal breastfeeding because its duration (with its consecutive amenorrhea) is in average relatively short and because very little iron is transferred to the milk. We are also aware that it would have been ideal to know the delay between various pregnancies, as well as between the last pregnancy and the beginning of the treatment.

To the best of our knowledge, no epidemiological study has so far been exclusively devoted to the study of the relationship between pregnancy and iron overload in *HFE* hemochromatosis in humans. Some studies have nevertheless shown interest to pregnancy. In a study comparing clinical features of 176 women and 176 matched men [14], Deugnier et al. mentioned that they found no significant correlation between the number of pregnancies and the hepatic iron concentration or the AIR, but no data were presented. They also observed, through a population-based screening study [13], that the number of pregnancies did not differ between 23 expressive and 19 non expressive women. More recently, the same team explored pregnancy as a potential confounder in a model assessing the relationship between body mass index and iron burden in *HFE* hemochromatosis [29]. They found no significant association between the number of pregnancies and AIR ($\geq$ 6 g or < 6 g) in univariable analysis. All these data are consistent with our results.

Our findings seem quite plausible in the current context of fertility. Given the 2016 French fertility rate estimated at 1.93 children per woman [30], it is not surprising that iron losses resulting from an average of two pregnancies per woman are not sufficient to protect against this disease. This situation was most likely different in the past when the fertility rate was higher.

During pregnancy, the daily requirements for absorbed iron markedly increase, from approximately 0.8 mg/day in the first trimester to ~ 8 mg/day in the third trimester [18, 31–33]. Globally, for a singleton pregnancy, a woman needs up to one gram of iron to ensure the balance of iron (depending on iron stores at the beginning of gestation). This corresponds to ~ 500 mg for the physiological expansion of haemoglobin mass, ~ 315 mg for the constitution of foetal tissue and placenta and ~ 250 mg for basal losses [32, 34, 35]. Blood losses at delivery also account to about 150 to 250 mg iron. These additional needs are drawn from the reserves of the mother and are transported to the foetus via the placenta. To cope with extra needs and to replenish the maternal stores, intestinal iron absorption also increases during pregnancy (about approximately 25%) [36]. A part of iron is also made available from the stopping of menses (although this is not sufficient) and from prophylactic iron supplementation that is usually recommended.

It would have been interesting to compare the amount of iron lost during pregnancy to that lost during menses. For example, it has been shown that healthy women with normal menses lose an average of 26 to 65 mL of blood per cycle [37–39], which corresponds at most to a loss of 1 mg iron per cycle (according to the recent assays performed by Napolitano et al.) (20) [38]. Therefore, if we consider that the entire childbearing period lasts average of 40 years (from the mean age at menarche (~ 12 y.) until the mean age at menopause (51 y.)), the total quantity of iron lost due to menses over a lifetime is approximately 520 mg (assuming 13 cycles of 28 days per year). This quantity appears lower than that lost during one pregnancy.

Our findings are also consistent with the results of an experimental study in a mouse model [20] showing that multiple pregnancies do not reduce body iron stores in $Hfe^{-/-}$ mice. This study found that all relevant clinical parameters of hemochromatosis (except TS) were not significantly decreased (or even increased) in multiparous females compared with nulliparous females. The hepatic expression of hepcidin [40] and its regulator (BMP6) [41] was reduced in multiparous females, suggesting that the inhibition of intestinal iron absorption was inactivated in response to pregnancy.

Current experimental data suggest that other factors such as hormonal factors may explain the difference in disease expression observed between men and women. Recent findings revealed that the gender difference observed in diseases associated with altered hepcidin expression such as *HFE* hemochromatosis may be explained by the negative regulation of hepcidin transcription by testosterone [19]. Latour et al. showed that testosterone inhibits hepcidin transcription in mice, via enhancement of epidermal growth factor (EGF) receptors signalling in the liver (knowing that EGF was recently shown to inhibit liver hepcidin synthesis [42]). The authors stated that the selective inhibition of EGF receptor in male mice stops testosterone-induced repression and clearly increases hepcidin expression. Moreover, castration of male mice enhances hepcidin expression thus lowers iron overload. Therefore this work highlights that testosterone should be one major hormone responsible for the observed gender difference in regulation of iron metabolism.

Conclusions

Our work challenges an old and well-established, yet unproven, hypothesis that pregnancy slows iron accumulation in women with *HFE* hemochromatosis. Combined with recent experimental data from the literature, our findings clearly show that the effect of pregnancy is not as important as initially announced and that the search for the factors responsible for the gender difference should continue.

Acknowledgements
The authors are grateful to Pascal Trouvé (Inserm UMR 1078, Brest, France) and to Zarrin Alavi (EA3878, Inserm, CIC 1412, Brest, France) for reviewing the manuscript.

Funding
This study was supported by a grant from the Etablissement Français du Sang. The funding had no role in the study design, in the collection, analysis, and interpretation of data, in the writing of the manuscript, or in the decision to submit the manuscript for publication.

Authors' contributions
VS and CF conceived and designed the study. VS wrote the first draft of the manuscript. VS, PS and MU analysed and interpreted the data. CLH performed the additional analyses requested by the reviewers and interpreted the data. CT and BC were responsible for patients' inclusion and data acquisition. MCM managed the data. GLG helped in interpreting findings and in drafting the manuscript. JBN helped in interpreting findings and critically revised the manuscript for important intellectual content. All authors revised the manuscript and approved the final manuscript.

Competing interests
The authors declare that they have no competing interests.

Author details
[1]UMR1078 "Génétique, Génomique Fonctionnelle et Biotechnologies", Inserm, EFS, Université de Brest, ISBAM, 22 avenue Camille Desmoulins, 29200 Brest, France. [2]Laboratoire d'Hygiene et de Sante Publique, Hopital Morvan, Brest, France. [3]Etablissement Français du Sang – Bretagne, Site de Brest, Brest, France. [4]Service d'Hepato-Gastroenterologie, Hopital La Cavale Blanche, Brest, France. [5]Laboratoire de Genetique Moleculaire et d'Histocompatibilite, Hopital Morvan, Brest, France.

References
1. EASL clinical practice guidelines for HFE hemochromatosis. European Association For The Study Of The Liver. J Hepatol. 2010;53:3–22.
2. Adams P, Brissot P, Powell LW. EASL international consensus conference on haemochromatosis. J Hepatol. 2000;33:485–504.
3. Anderson GJ, McLaren GD. Iron physiology and pathophysiology in humans. New York: Humana Press; 2012. p. 697.
4. Bridle KR, Frazer DM, Wilkins SJ, Dixon JL, Purdie DM, Crawford DH, et al. Disrupted hepcidin regulation in HFE-associated haemochromatosis and the liver as a regulator of body iron homoeostasis. Lancet. 2003;361:669–73.
5. Nemeth E, Tuttle MS, Powelson J, Vaughn MB, Donovan A, Ward DM, et al. Hepcidin regulates cellular iron efflux by binding to ferroportin and inducing its internalization. Science. 2004;306:2090–3.
6. Pietrangelo A. Hemochromatosis: an endocrine liver disease. Hepatology. 2007;46:1291–301.
7. Feder JN, Gnirke A, Thomas W, Tsuchihashi Z, Ruddy DA, Basava A, et al. A novel MHC class I-like gene is mutated in patients with hereditary haemochromatosis. Nat Genet. 1996;13:399–408.
8. Bacon BR, Britton RS. Clinical penetrance of hereditary hemochromatosis. N Engl J Med. 2008;358:291–2.
9. Beutler E, Felitti VJ, Koziol JA, Ho NJ, Gelbart T. Penetrance of 845G>a (C282Y) HFE hereditary haemochromatosis mutation in the USA. Lancet. 2002;359:211–8.
10. McCune A, Worwood M. Penetrance in hereditary hemochromatosis. Blood. 2003;102:2696.
11. Allen KJ, Gurrin LC, Constantine CC, Osborne NJ, Delatycki MB, Nicoll AJ, et al. Iron-overload-related disease in HFE hereditary hemochromatosis. N Engl J Med. 2008;358:221–30.
12. Rochette J, Le Gac G, Lassoued K, Ferec C, Robson KJ. Factors influencing disease phenotype and penetrance in HFE haemochromatosis. Hum Genet. 2010;128:233–48.
13. Deugnier Y, Jouanolle AM, Chaperon J, Moirand R, Pithois C, Meyer JF, et al. Gender-specific phenotypic expression and screening strategies in C282Y-linked haemochromatosis: a study of 9396 French people. Br J Haematol. 2002;118:1170–8.
14. Moirand R, Adams PC, Bicheler V, Brissot P, Deugnier Y. Clinical features of genetic hemochromatosis in women compared with men. Ann Intern Med. 1997;127:105–10.
15. Bacon BR, Adams PC, Kowdley KV, Powell LW, Tavill AS. Diagnosis and management of hemochromatosis: 2011 practice guideline by the American Association for the Study of Liver Diseases. Hepatology. 2011;54:328–43.
16. Hanson EH, Imperatore G, Burke W. HFE gene and hereditary hemochromatosis: a HuGE review. Human genome epidemiology. Am J Epidemiol. 2001;154:193–206.
17. Wood MJ, Powell LW, Ramm GA. Environmental and genetic modifiers of the progression to fibrosis and cirrhosis in hemochromatosis. Blood. 2008;111:4456–62.
18. Milman N. Iron and pregnancy–a delicate balance. Ann Hematol. 2006; 85:559–65.
19. Latour C, Kautz L, Besson-Fournier C, Island ML, Canonne-Hergaux F, Loreal O, et al. Testosterone perturbs systemic iron balance through activation of epidermal growth factor receptor signaling in the liver and repression of hepcidin. Hepatology. 2014;59:683–94.
20. Neves JV, Olsson IA, Porto G, Rodrigues PN. Hemochromatosis and pregnancy: iron stores in the Hfe−/− mouse are not reduced by multiple pregnancies. Am J Physiol Gastrointest Liver Physiol. 2010;298:G525–9.
21. Jouanolle AM, Fergelot P, Raoul ML, Gandon G, Roussey M, Deugnier Y, et al. Prevalence of the C282Y mutation in Brittany: penetrance of genetic hemochromatosis? Ann Genet. 1998;41:195–8.
22. Saliou P, Le Gac G, Mercier AY, Chanu B, Gueguen P, Merour MC, et al. Evidence for the high importance of co-morbid factors in HFE C282Y/H63D patients cared by phlebotomies: results from an observational prospective study. PLoS One. 2013;8:e81128.
23. Haskins D, Stevens AR Jr, Finch S, Finch CA. Iron metabolism; iron stores in man as measured by phlebotomy. J Clin Invest. 1952;31:543–7.
24. Fletcher LM, Dixon JL, Purdie DM, Powell LW, Crawford DH. Excess alcohol greatly increases the prevalence of cirrhosis in hereditary hemochromatosis. Gastroenterology. 2002;122:281–9.
25. Scotet V, Merour MC, Mercier AY, Chanu B, Le Faou T, Raguenes O, et al. Hereditary hemochromatosis: effect of excessive alcohol consumption on disease expression in patients homozygous for the C282Y mutation. Am J Epidemiol. 2003;158:129–34.
26. Brissot P, Bourel M, Herry D, Verger JP, Messner M, Beaumont C, et al. Assessment of liver iron content in 271 patients: a reevaluation of direct and indirect methods. Gastroenterology. 1981;80:557–65.
27. Deugnier Y, Bardou-Jacquet E, Le Lan C, Brissot P. Hyperferritinemia not related to hemochromatosis. Gastroenterol Clin Biol. 2009;33:323–6.
28. Blanco-Rojo R, Toxqui L, Lopez-Parra AM, Baeza-Richer C, Perez-Granados AM, Arroyo-Pardo E, et al. Influence of diet, menstruation and genetic factors on iron status: a cross-sectional study in Spanish women of childbearing age. Int J Mol Sci. 2014;15:4077–87.
29. Desgrippes R, Laine F, Morcet J, Perrin M, Manet G, Jezequel C, et al. Decreased iron burden in overweight C282Y homozygous women: putative role of increased hepcidin production. Hepatology. 2013;57:1784–92.
30. https://www.insee.fr/fr/statistiques/2554860.
31. Viteri FE. The consequences of iron deficiency and anaemia in pregnancy on maternal health, the foetus and the infant. SCN News. 1994;11:14–8.
32. Leong WILB. Iron nutrition. In: Iron physiology and pathophysiology in humans. New York: Humana Press; 2012. p. 81–99.
33. Cao C, O'Brien KO. Pregnancy and iron homeostasis: an update. Nutr Rev. 2013;71:35–51.
34. Food and Nutrition Board, Institute of Medicine. Dietary reference intakes for vitamin a, vitamin K, arsenic, boron, chromium, copper, iodine, iron, manganese, molybdenum, nickel, silicon, vanadium, and zinc. Washington (DC): The National Academies Press; 2002. p. 290–393.
35. FAO/WHO. Requirements of vitamin a, iron, folate and vitamin B12. In: FAO food and nutrition series. Volume N°23. Rome: FAO; 2004. p. 246–78.
36. Millard KN, Frazer DM, Wilkins SJ, Anderson GJ. Changes in the expression of intestinal iron transport and hepatic regulatory molecules explain the enhanced iron absorption associated with pregnancy in the rat. Gut. 2004;53:655–60.

37. Harvey LJ, Armah CN, Dainty JR, Foxall RJ, John Lewis D, Langford NJ, et al. Impact of menstrual blood loss and diet on iron deficiency among women in the UK. Br J Nutr. 2005;94:557–64.
38. Napolitano M, Dolce A, Celenza G, Grandone E, Perilli MG, Siragusa S, et al. Iron-dependent erythropoiesis in women with excessive menstrual blood losses and women with normal menses. Ann Hematol. 2014;93:557–63.
39. Dasharathy SS, Mumford SL, Pollack AZ, Perkins NJ, Mattison DR, Wactawski-Wende J, et al. Menstrual bleeding patterns among regularly menstruating women. Am J Epidemiol. 2012;175:536–45.
40. Nicolas G, Viatte L, Lou DQ, Bennoun M, Beaumont C, Kahn A, et al. Constitutive hepcidin expression prevents iron overload in a mouse model of hemochromatosis. Nat Genet. 2003;34:97–101.
41. Andriopoulos B Jr, Corradini E, Xia Y, Faasse SA, Chen S, Grgurevic L, et al. BMP6 is a key endogenous regulator of hepcidin expression and iron metabolism. Nat Genet. 2009;41:482–7.
42. Goodnough JB, Ramos E, Nemeth E, Ganz T. Inhibition of hepcidin transcription by growth factors. Hepatology. 2012;56:291–9.

18

Births and induced abortions among women of Russian, Somali and Kurdish origin, and the general population in Finland

Satu Jokela[1]* iD, Eero Lilja[1], Tarja I. Kinnunen[2], Mika Gissler[3,4], Anu E. Castaneda[1] and Päivikki Koponen[5]

Abstract

Background: Since reproductive health is often considered a highly sensitive topic, underreporting in surveys and under coverage of register data occurs frequently. This may lead to inaccurate information about the reproductive health. This study compares the proportion of women having births and induced abortions among migrant women of Russian, Somali and Kurdish origin in Finland to women in the general Finnish population and examines the agreement between survey- and register-based data.

Methods: The survey data from the Migrant Health and Wellbeing Study conducted in 2010–2012 and data from the Health 2011 Survey with corresponding information on women in the general population were used in this study. The respondents were women aged 18–64: 341 Russian, 176 Somali and 228 Kurdish origin women and 630 women in the general population. The survey data were linked to the Finnish Medical Birth Register and the Register of Induced Abortions.

Results: In the combined (survey and register) data, migrant groups aged 30–64 had a higher proportion (89–96%) compared to the general population (69%) of women with at least one birth. Under-coverage of registered births was observed in all study groups. Among women aged 18–64, 36% of the Russian group and 24% of the Kurdish group reported more births in the survey than in the register data. In the combined data, the proportions of Russian origin (69%) and Kurdish origin (38%) women who have had at least one induced abortion in their lifetime are higher than in the general population (21%). Under-reporting of induced abortions in survey was observed among Somali origin women aged 18–29 (1% vs. 18%). The level of agreement between survey and register data was the lowest for induced abortions among the Somali and Russian groups (− 0.01 and 0.27).

Conclusion: Both survey- and register-based information are needed in studies on reproductive health, especially when comparing women with foreign origin with women in the general population. Culturally sensitive survey protocols need to be developed to reduce reporting bias.

Keywords: (5) reproductive health, Migrants, Women, Parturition, Induced abortion

* Correspondence: satu.jokela@thl.fi
[1]Department of Welfare, National Institute for Health and Welfare, Mannerheimintie 166, 00271 Helsinki, PL 30, Finland
Full list of author information is available at the end of the article

Background

Reproductive health is an important component of general health especially among women [1, 2]. It deals with the reproductive processes, functions and system at all stages of women's life [3]. Reproductive health and family planning services are available to all women in Finland. Most families are able to plan the number of children they desire as reliable methods of contraception are available to virtually everyone [4]. However, it has been found that it is more likely for women with only a basic education to have an abortion than it is for women with more education [5].

In 2015, the total fertility rate (births per women) in Finland was 1.65 [6, 7] and the number of induced abortions per thousand women aged 15–49 was 8.2 (13.3. in other Nordic countries). The number of induced abortions has decreased especially among women aged less than 20 years in all Nordic countries, being the lowest in Norway and in Finland [8]. The number of induced abortions among the other European countries was the highest in the area of former Soviet Union [6].

Some groups of migrant women and especially refugee women do not have equal access to health services nor access to reproductive health information neither in their home country nor their host country. Previous studies [9–12] have showed barriers to the use of health care services resulting from gender-related issues (such as patrilineal, patrilocal family systems), traditional values, norms and beliefs (such as perceptions of femininity, health beliefs and stigmatization), discrimination among health care providers, limited services for adolescents and unmarried women, as well as lack of adequate knowledge and information on sexual and reproductive health.

In Finland, a register-based study showed that the proportion of immigrant women among the women having an induced abortion had slightly increased between 1994 (4.6%) and 2002 (7.8%). The abortion rate increased particularly among young women of Somali and other African origin. The abortion rate among women of non-Western origin was lower than among Finnish women. Baltic, Chinese, Russian, Thai & Filipina, and African women aged 15–49 had more abortions per 1000 women than Finnish women in the same age group [13].

Also other European register-based studies [14, 15] and surveys [16, 17] show that abortion rates are higher among migrant women than in the general population and migrant women request abortion more often than women in the general population [14, 16]. Abortions have found to be associated with low education, weak social network, poverty, unemployment, and having limited access to healthcare [15, 16]. Immigrant women may thus be more vulnerable to abortions than women in the general population [15, 17].

Under-reporting of induced abortions in surveys is a generally recognized problem [18]. The usefulness of surveys in studying highly personal or sensitive individual characteristics, such as sexual reproductive health, has been questioned [19], but the usefulness of a survey depends on cultural issues as well as the data collection methods used. A study in the United States found that only 29% of actual induced abortions shown in Medicaid administrative data files were self-reported in a survey. The level of underreporting varied by ethnicity: white women reported about 71%, black women reported 24% and Hispanic women 34% of their actual abortions [20]. Under-reporting of induced abortions has been associated with socio-demographic characters, experiences in life (e.g. reproductive history) and the women's own and general attitudes on abortions and the context of the survey (for example the sex and training of interviewers) [20–25].

In this cross-sectional study we have examined the agreement between survey- and register –based data in comparing the proportions of women having births and induced abortions among migrant women of Russian, Somali and Kurdish origin to women in the general Finnish population. Previously very few studies have utilized both survey- and register data [18, 20, 21, 25].

The results can be utilized to improve estimates of fertility and unintended pregnancies, as well as to evaluate needs to improve access to services and use of contraceptives [18, 20, 24, 26].

Methods

Study population

The data on Russian, Somali and Kurdish origin migrant women living in Finland are from the Migrant Health and Wellbeing Study (Maamu) conducted by the National Institute of Health and Welfare (THL) between 2010 and 2012. The Maamu study is a comprehensive cross-sectional health interview and examination survey. The three groups of origin were selected to represent different types of migrants. Russian migrants are the largest migrant group in Finland with family and work as their main reasons for migration. Somali migrants are the largest refugee group, whereas Kurdish migrants coming from Iran or Iraq have been among the largest groups of quota refugees over the past decade. The survey data was collected by trained multilingual personnel. The study protocol included a face-to-face interview on health and wellbeing and a health examination [27]. A stratified random sample of 1000 Russian (622 women), 1000 Somali (531 women), and 1000 Kurdish (426 women) origin adults aged 18 to 64 and living in six Finnish municipalities (Helsinki, Espoo, Vantaa, Turku, Tampere and Vaasa) was selected from the National Population Register. Selection criteria for Russians were birthplace in the Former Soviet Union or Russia and mother tongue Russian or Finnish, for Somalis birthplace in Somalia, and for Kurdish birthplace in Iraq or Iran and mother tongue Kurdish Sorani. The invitees had a minimum one year of residence in Finland. In this study, we used the data that included the women who had participated in the interview. A total of 54.8% of invited Russian ($n = 341$), 36.0% of Somali ($n = 191$) and 54.0% of Kurdish ($n = 230$) origin women participated in the face-to-face interviews and answered questions on reproductive health.

The comparison group of the general Finnish population women is from the data of nationwide study, Health 2011 Survey. The study was conducted by THL in 2011–2012 [28]. Women aged between 18 to 64 and living in the same municipalities as in the Maamu study were included in the general population group ($n = 630$). The response rate in Health 2011 was 53%.

Both Maamu and Health 2011 surveys were approved by the Coordinating Ethical Committee of Helsinki and Uusimaa Hospital District. All participants gave written informed consent.

Data sources

Two data sets have been used in this study: 1) the survey data from two surveys: the Maamu and Health 2011 and 2) the register data from two registers: the Finnish Medical Birth Register (MBR) and the Register of Induced Abortions. Furthermore, we created combined data from these data sets by linking the self-reported survey data to the register data [8, 29].

The MBR contains data on all live births and stillbirths that have occurred in Finland since 1987. Furthermore the MBR includes information on the number of previous pregnancies, births and induced abortions that have been self-reported in maternity health services. If a woman has ever given birth in Finland, the MBR will also contain data on self-reported births and induced abortions in the woman's lifetime, including those that

had taken place before the register was set up and those that had been performed in other countries [29].

The Register of Induced Abortions contains information on all legally induced abortions in Finland. The register also includes information on the number of previous abortions that have been self-reported when seeking abortion/having the abortion as well as the number of previous pregnancies reported while in maternity care. The physician performing an abortion is required to report the case to THL. Data on induced abortions from 1983 onwards are available in electronic format [8]. In this study, the register data were limited to the time period before the person's participation in the interview. The coverage and validity of data on induced abortions in the Register of Induced Abortions [30] and on births in the MBR register [31] are good. Register linkages were made using the unique personal identity code given for all citizens and permanent residents living in Finland. Therefore it is possible to compare individual women's births and induced abortions between survey and register datasets (Table 1).

Definition of variables

In the Maamu study, the interviews were conducted in the native language of the participants mainly by female interviewers. The issue of births were addressed with the following question: "How many births have you had? Include all births, also Caesarean sections." The issue of induced abortions were addressed with following question: "Have you had any induced abortions and how many?" In the Health 2011 survey, questions on reproductive health were included in the interview for persons aged 29 to 64 while for young adults (aged 18 to 28) these questions were included in a self-administered postal questionnaire.

We found differences between the self-reported data and the register data regarding the amount of births and induced abortions. We created a variable on the maximum values of births/induced abortions by choosing whichever was the highest value, self-reported or

Table 1 Information on previous births and induced abortions in three data sets

The Maamu survey data	The Finnish Medical Birth Register	The Register of Induced Abortions
Self-reported births	Registered births (from year 1987)	Registered induced abortions (from year 1983)
Self-reported induced abortions	Self-reported previous births among those with given births in Finland since 1987	Self-reported previous induced abortions among those with induced abortions in Finland since 1983
	Self-reported previous induced abortions among those with given births in Finland since 1987	Self-reported previous births among those with induced abortions in Finland since 1983

Combined survey and register data

maximum number of births/induced abortions in survey or register

dichotomous variables for births/induced abortions: 1) no births/induced abortion, 2) at least one birth/induced abortion

categorized number of births: no births, 1–2 births and 3 or more births

categorized number of induced abortion: no induced abortions, one induced abortion and two or more induced abortions registered. These continuous variables were used for mean numbers of births and induced abortions.

Because of the observed differences between data sources, we also created dichotomous variables for births and induced abortions: 1) no births and 2) at least one birth and 1) no induced abortions and 2) at least one induced abortion. We also created variables on the number of births and induced abortions with three categories (no births, 1–2 births and 3 or more births and no induced abortions, one induced abortion and two or more induced abortions).

In order to highlight the differences between the age groups, the results of women aged 18–29 and 30–64 will be discussed separately.

We also present mean numbers of births among parous women and among all women and mean numbers of induced abortions among women who have had at least one induced abortion and among all women. Furthermore we present proportions of having 1–2 births and more than two births and mean number of births in lifetime among women aged 18–64 who have had their first birth after migration.

We used the aforementioned categorical variables when comparing the information from the survey data and the register data (more births/induced abortions in survey, similar reporting in survey and register data and more births/induced abortions in register data) and when examining the level of agreement between register- and survey- based data.

Statistical analyses

Inverse probability weights (IPW) based on the register information from the National Population Register on age, sex, marital status, migrant group and municipality were used to correct for the effects of non-response bias and different sampling probabilities in order to provide representative results with the survey and register data [32]. The population size being relatively small, a significant proportion of the total population was included in the sample of Maamu, and thus the finite population correction [33] was applied in all analyses.

Linear regression was applied to calculate age adjusted mean values for births and induced abortions. Logistic regression was applied to calculate model- adjusted estimates for having births or induced abortion and their 95% confidence interval (CI) for binary and multinomial variables. First age-adjusted and second age-, employment status-, marital status- and education adjusted proportions of women having births and induced abortions were estimated in each study group using predicted margins [34]. Weighted Cohen's kappa was used to examine the level of agreement between register and survey based data. The statistic was calculated for the three-category variables of births and induced abortions in each group

[35]. The statistical significances of the differences between groups were calculated using Satterthwaite adjusted F-statistic. A p-value of < 0.05 was considered statistically significant. SAS software (9.3) was used for constructing outcome variables and calculating crude values, whereas SUDAAN 11.0.1 was used for data analysis.

Results

Characteristics of the study population

The main characteristics of the women who answered the questions considering reproductive health are presented in Table 2. Somali and Kurdish women were younger than Russian and general population women. Most of the women were married or lived in a civil union. The proportion of women who had no formal education was highest in the Somali group (35%). Most migrant women had lived in Finland for at least five years. In the general population, more women (84%) were employed than in the Somali (37%), Kurdish (56%) and Russian (66%) groups.

Births

In the combined data Somali and Kurdish origin women aged 30–64 had more often had at least one birth in their lifetime (96%) than the other groups. (Table 3) In the general population, of women aged 18–29 9 % had given birth at least once in their lifetime. All migrant groups had significantly higher proportions of women aged 30–64 with at least one birth compared to the general population women. Somali origin women who had had their first birth before the migration were more likely to have three or more births compared to those who had had their first birth after the migration (91 and 69%).

The mean number of births was highest among Somali origin women; 5.9 among parous women aged 18–64 and 4.5 among all women aged 18–64. When adjusting for age, employment status, marital status and education there was still a significant difference between the proportion of women having at least one birth in Russian, Somali and Kurdish origin women and women in the general population.

Induced abortions

Based on the survey data, 1 % of Somali origin women aged 18–29 had gone through at least one induced abortion in their lifetime (Table 4), while based on the register data the proportion was much higher (18%). Instead, 66% of Russian origin women aged 30–64 had had at least one induced abortion in survey data but only 23% had had at least one induced abortion based on the register data.

In the combined data, higher proportions of Somali origin women aged 18–29 had had at least one induced abortion than women in the general population (19 and

Table 2 Characteristics of the study population

	General population (n = 630) %, 95 CI	Russian (n = 341) %, 95 CI	Somali (n = 176) %, 95 CI	Kurdish (n = 228) %, 95 CI
Marital status				
Unmarried/divorced/widow	39.1 (35.2–43.1)	43.6 (37.8–49.6)	32.3 (25.5–39.9)	33.7 (28.0–39.8)
Married/civil union	60.9 (56.9–64.8)	56.4 (50.4–62.2)	67.7 (60.1–74.5)	66.3 (60.2–72.0)
Education				
No formal education	0.0 (NA)	0.0 (NA)	35.3 (28.4–43.0)	19.4 (15.1–24.7)
Primary	27.7 (24.1–31.5)	15.5 (11.7–20.3)***	49.3 (41.4–57.3) ***	39.3 (33.5–45.5) ***
Secondary/higher	72.3 (68.5–75.9)	84.5 (97.7–88.3) ***	15.4 (10.6–21.8) ***	41.2 (35.4–47.3) ***
Employment status				
Working	83.7 (80.4–86.6)	65.8 (60.2–71.0) ***	37.3 (30.3–44.9) ***	56.2 (50.2–62.1) ***
Others	16.3 (13.4–19.6)	34.2 (29.0–39.8) ***	62.7 (55.1–69.7) ***	43.8 (37.9–49.8) ***
Moved to Finland (age yrs)				
≤18 yrs		38.4 (32.8–44.4)	46.2 (38.1–54.5)	41.4(34.9–48.2)
>18 yrs		61.6 (55.6–67.2)	53.8 (45.5–61.9)	58.6 (51.8–65.1)
Time lived in Finland				
≤5 yrs		23.0 (18.4–28.5)	20.6 (15.5–26.7)	16.6 (12.7–21.3)
6–14 yrs		37.6 (32.1–43.4)	38.9 (31.5–46.8)	56.0 (49.9–61.9)
≥15 yrs		39.4 (33.7–45.4)	40.6 (33.2–48.4)	27.5 (22.4–33.2)

Survey data:
Migrant Health and Wellbeing Study and the Health 2011 Survey
Statistically significant differences compared to the Finnish reference group (Satterthwaite adjusted F-statistic):
*p-value < 0.05
**p-value < 0.01
***p-value < 0.001
Age-adjusted
NA = Confidence interval not available

8%) whereas a higher proportion of general population women aged 30–64 had had at least one induced abortion compared to Somali origin women (21 and 10%). Russian and Kurdish origin women aged 30–64 had higher proportions of those with at least one induced abortion than general population women in the same age group. The mean number of induced abortions was the highest among Russian origin women; 2.3 among women with at least one induced abortion and 1.3 among all women.

When adjusting for age, employment status, marital status and education, significantly lower proportions of general population women had had induced abortions (18%) compared to Russian (60%) and Kurdish (35%) origin women. The number of Somali origin women who had had an induced abortion was too low to be adjusted for sociodemographic factors.

Comparison between data sets

When comparing the self-reported survey information to the register data, all study groups showed more births in the survey data than in the register data (Table 5). Among women aged 18–64, 36% of the Russian group and 24% of the Kurdish group reported more births in the survey compared to the register data. The level of agreement between self-reported survey information and register data for births was moderate or substantial among all women (kappa 0.46–0.74).

Only 1 % of Somali origin women reported more induced abortions in the survey than in the register data, while 12% of them had more induced abortions in the register data. In contrast, Russian origin women had more self-reported previous induced abortions than appeared in the register data (39 and 3%). Among Somali origin women, the level of agreement between self-reported survey information and register data for induced abortions was lower than the expected probability of agreement at random (kappa – 0.01) and among Russian origin women agreement was fair (kappa 0.27). The level of agreement was moderate among the Kurdish (0.56) and the general population (0.69) groups.

Discussion
Births and induced abortions
We compared the proportions of women having births and induced abortions among migrant women of Russian, Somali and Kurdish origin to women in the general Finnish population. In our study, Somali origin women had on

Table 3 The distribution of births in different data sets

	General population	Russian	Somali	Kurdish
18–29 years [a]	n = 182	n = 83	n = 70	n = 66
Survey data [1], women with at least one birth, %	8.5 (5.1–13.8)	17.0 (11.0–25.3)*	60.3 (48.1–71.3)***	41.2 (33.1–49.8)***
Register data [2], women with at least one birth, %	8.5 (5.1–13.8)	16.1 (10.3–24.4)*	54.5 (42.8–65.7)***	37.6 (30.0–46.0)***
Combined data [3], women with at least one birth, %	8.5 (5.1–13.8)	17.0 (11.0–25.3)*	60.3 (48.1–71.3)***	41.2 (33.1–49.8)***
30–64 years [b]	n = 448	n = 258	n = 104	n = 161
Survey data [1], women with at least one birth, %	69.2 (63.9–74.0)	89.0 (84.0–92.5)***	95.5 (89.9–98.1)***	95.7 (91.7–97.9)***
Register data [2], women with at least one birth, %	52.9 (47.6–58.1)	44.7 (38.4–51.1)*	67.5 (58.2–75.6)**	62.3 (55.3–68.8)*
Combined data [3], women with at least one birth, %	69.2 (63.9–74.1)	89.0 (84.0–92.5)***	95.5 (89.9–98.1)***	96.4 (92.6–98.3)***
18–64 years [c], Combined data [3]	n = 630	n = 341	n = 174	n = 227
Among all women				
no births, %	50.6 (46.9–54.2)	33.5 (29.0–38.3)***[5]	17.6 (13.1–23.3)***[5]	21.8 (17.8–26.5) ***[5]
1–2 births, %	36.8 (33.2–40.5)	58.6 (53.5–63.5)	18.5 (13.3–25.0)	36.4 (30.8–42.4)
≥3 births, %	12.6 (10.3–15.4)	7.9 (5.6–11.2)	63.9 (57.4–70.0)	41.8 (36.7–47.0)
Mean number of births among all women	1.0 (1.0–1.1)	1.0 (0.9–1.1)	4.5 (4.0–5.0)***	2.6 (2.3–2.8)***
Mean number of births among parous women	1.8 (1.7–2.0)	1.6 (1.4–1.7)**	5.9 (5.3–6.4)***	3.4 (3.1–3.7)***
Among women with first birth before migration		n = 179	n = 57	n = 117
1–2 births, %	NA	86.2 (80.2–90.6)	8.7 (3.7–19.3)	32.0 (24.5–40.5)
≥3 births, %	NA	13.8 (9.4–19.8)	91.3 (80.7–96.3)	68.0 (59.5–75.5)
mean	NA	1.6 (1.4–1.7)	7.2 (6.4–8.1)	3.8 (3.5–4.2)
Among women with first birth after migration †		n = 72	n = 50	n = 65
1–2 births, %	NA	92.7 (81.6–97.3)	30.8 (18.3–46.8)***	72.9 (60.1–82.7)***
≥3 births, %	NA	7.3 (2.7–18.4)	69.2 (53.2–81.7)***	27.1 (17.3–39.9)***
mean	NA	1.7 (1.5–2.0)	4.2 (3.6–4.73)***	2.4 (2.1–2.7)***
Women with at least one birth, model-adjusted [d] %	61.0 (56.3–65.6)	76.4 (72.0–80.3)***	85.7 (80.8–89.5)***	83.9 (80.2–87.1)***

[1]**Survey data:**
Migrant Health and Wellbeing Study and the Health 2011 Survey
Age-adjusted and weighted proportions
[a]18–29 years age adjusted
[b]30–64 years age adjusted
[2]**Register data:**
Medical Birth Register and the Register of Induced Abortions
Age-adjusted and weighted proportions
[3]**Combined survey and register data:**
Combined data from the surveys, Medical Birth Register and Register of Induced Abortions
Age-adjusted and weighted proportions
[c]18–64 years age adjusted
† Statistical differences in relation to migrant origin women whose first birth was before migration
NA = no observations
[d]Adjusted for age, work status, marital status and education
Statistically significant differences compared to the Finnish reference group (Satterthwaite adjusted F-statistic):* p-value < 0.05
**p-value < 0.01
***p-value < 0.001
[5]Overall p-value for the difference of the multinomial distribution between general population and the migrant group

average more births than the other groups. In the combined data, 96% of Somali origin women had had three or more births. The mean number of births among parous Somali origin women aged 18–64 was 5.9. Adjusting for age, employment status, marital status and education did not much impact the differences between our study groups. Even when adjusted for confounders migrant origin women still had significantly more often had at least one birth compared to the women in the general population.

Russian origin women had on average more induced abortions than the other groups. In the combined data, 32% of Russian origin women had had two or more induced abortions. The mean number of induced abortions among Russian origin women who had had at least one induced abortion was 2.3. Furthermore, when adjusted for confounders, Russian and Kurdish origin women had significantly more often had an induced abortion when compared to the general population

Table 4 The distribution of induced abortions in different data sets

	General population	Russian	Somali	Kurdish
18–29 years [a]	n = 181	n = 83	n = 65	n = 63
Survey data [1], women with at least one induced abortion, %	6.6 (3.6–11.8)	19.6 (11.4–31.5)**	0.7 (0.1–3.9)*	3.6 (1.0–11.8)
Register data [2], women with at least one induced abortion, %	7.0 (3.9–12.2)	12.5 (6.1–23.8)	17.6 (9.0–31.5)*	6.2 (2.6–14.2)
Combined data [3], women with at least one induced abortion %	7.7 (4.5–13.1)	20.0 (11.8–31.9)**	18.5 (9.8–32.1)*	7.8 (3.6–15.9)
30–64 years [b]	n = 447	n = 255	n = 99	n = 159
Survey data [1], women with at least one induced abortion, %	16.4 (13.1–20.3)	66.2 (59.7–72.1)***	1.1 (0.4–3.2)***	31.2 (24.6–38.6)***
Register data [2], women with at least one induced abortion, %	17.7 (14.2–21.8)	22.8 (17.6–29.1)	7.6 (3.6–15.0)*	21.8 (16.7–28.0)
Combined data [3], women with at least one induced abortion, %	20.8 (17.2–25.0)	68.9 (62.5–74.7)***	10.1 (5.2–18.7)*	37.8 (30.9–45.3)***
18–64 years [c], combined data [3]	n = 682	n = 308	n = 164	n = 222
no induced abortions, %	83.2 (80.0–85.9)	46.6 (41.2–52.0)***[5]	85.6 (77.6–91.1)	71.8 (66.2–76.9)***[5]
one induced abortion, %	13.5 (11.1–16.6)	21.3 (16.8–26.5)	8.4 (4.6–14.9)	14.9 (11.1–19.8)
≥2 induced abortions, %	3.3 (2.2–5.0)	32.2 (27.6–37.1)	6.0 (2.7–12.8)	13.2 (9.6–18.0)
Mean number of abortions				
among women who had at least one induced abortion	1.3 (1.1–1.4)	2.3 (2.1–2.6) ***	2.0(1.5–2.5)**	2.0 (1.6–2.2)***
among all women	0.2 (0.2–0.3)	1.3 (1.1–1.5)***	0.3 (0.2–0.4)	0.5 (0.4–0.7)***
Women with at least one induced abortion, model-adjusted [d] %	17.9 (14.7–21.6)	60.0 (54.4–65.4)***	NA	35.3 (28.8–42.5)***

[1]**Survey data:**
Migrant Health and Wellbeing Study and the Health 2011 Survey
Age-adjusted and weighted proportions
[a]18–29 years age adjusted
[b]30–64 years age adjusted
[2]**Register data:**
Medical Birth Register and the Register of Induced Abortions
Age-adjusted and weighted proportions
[3]**Combined survey and register data:**
Combined data from the surveys, Medical Birth Register and Register of Induced Abortions
Age-adjusted and weighted proportions
[c]18–64 years age adjusted
NA = Too few observations for statistical analysis
[d]Adjusted for age, work status, marital status and education
Statistically significant differences compared to the Finnish reference group (Satterthwaite adjusted F-statistic):
*p-value < 0.05
**p-value < 0.01
***p-value < 0.001
[5]Overall p-value for the difference of the multinomial distribution between general population and the migrant group

Table 5 Agreement between data sets: proportions of women (%) and Cohen's kappa values

	General population	Russian	Somali	Kurdish
Births				
more self-reported in survey, %	14.0 (11.6–16.8)	36.1 (30.7–41.9)	16.3 (11.7–22.3)	24.2 (19.4–29.7)
similar, %	85.3 (82.5–87.7)	63.8 (58.0–69.2)	82.9 (76.8–87.7)	74.9 (69.3–79.7)
more in register, %	0.7 (0.3–1.7)	0.0 (NA)	0.8 (NA)	0.9 (NA)
Cohen's kappa	0.75	0.46	0.69	0.56
Induced abortions				
more self-reported in survey, %	3.6 (2.4–5.3)	38.6 (33.0–44.4)	0.9 (0.4–2.1)	8.3 (5.4–12.5)
similar, %	92.3 (90.0–94.1)	58.5 (52.6–64.1)	87.2 (80.1–92.0)	83.9 (78.8–88.0)
more in register, %	4.1 (2.9–5.8)	3.0 (1.6–5.6)	11.9 (7.2–19.1)	7.8 (5.1–11.9)
Cohen's kappa	0.69	0.27	−0.01	0.56

Combined data from Maamu, Health 2011, MBR and Register of Induced Abortions
NA = Confidence interval not available

women. Although the numbers of respondents to the question about induced abortions are fairly low, the differences between migrant origin women and general population women are clearly significant.

There are many explanations for the differences in the proportions and mean numbers of births and induced abortions between migrant groups and women in the general population. Due to the heterogeneity of migrant women, there is no reason to assume that higher proportions of induced abortion in some groups of women are only due to their cultural background [16] or lower education. Previous studies have shown that there are many reasons for induced abortion, such as being a single mother, already having children and young age [17] as well as other reasons that are related to low socio-economic status. Also women with good socio-economic situation undergo induced abortions [36].

A previous study has shown that Russian origin women and the oldest Russian speaking Estonians had higher levels of self-reported induced abortions compared to other Estonian and Finnish women. High abortion rates were related to low contraceptive use [37].

Agreement between survey- and register data

We compared survey-based and register-based information to examine the level of agreement between the data sets. In this study, under-coverage of registered births was observed in all study groups. Among women aged 18–64, 36% of the Russian group and 24% of the Kurdish group reported more births in the survey compared to the register data. Somali origin women aged 18–29 under-reported induced abortions in survey compared to register data (1% vs. 18%). The level of agreement between survey and register data was lowest for induced abortions among the Somali and Russian groups.

In the general population women, the under-coverage of registered births is partly due to the births before year 1987 when the MBR was not in use. Furthermore, some general population women probably have given birth abroad. Most of the migrant women who reported more births in the survey have probably given birth elsewhere.

We observed substantial differences in the proportions of induced abortions between the two data sources. Especially Somali origin women under-reported their previous induced abortions, whereas Russian women had more self-reported abortions in the survey data. It is likely that the Russian women in our study had had induced abortions in Russia before they have moved to Finland or they might have travelled to Russia to get an induced abortion, leading to under-coverage of the register data.

The level of agreement between register- and survey-based data on induced abortions was the lowest among Somali origin women. Somali origin women might under-report induced abortions because termination of pregnancy is not culturally acceptable and there is a high level of social stigma related to induced abortions [18].The observed differences between self-reported and registered previous induced abortions among Somali and Kurdish origin women might be partly caused due to problems in the data collection process as well as the sensitive nature of these questions.

Meaning of the results

Our study clearly demonstrates the need for taking action in order to promote migrant women's reproductive health especially in family planning and abortion services. The high induced abortion levels among Russian origin women show a need to pay attention to the availability of contraceptives and family planning services. The high mean number of births among Somali origin women may reflect their personal wishes for larger families but there is also a need to make sure that there are no unnecessary barriers to use contraceptives, eg. their husbands' or their own beliefs and attitudes [38, 39].

Somali origin women who had had their first birth after migration, had less births, compared to Somali origin women who had had their first birth before moving to Finland. Part of the explanation might be that women who had given birth after migration where younger, but it might also reflect the fact that their fertility has decreased closer to the fertility of the majority of the population [40].

In order to maintain good reproductive health, women need to have access to information, prevention and treatment services [41]. Sexual education contributes to the use of contraception [42] but it should be noted that birth control is a complicated question in terms of cultural, religious and social norms [43] and therefore particular attention must be paid to women's ability to make their own decisions considering their sexual and reproductive health.

Health care professionals need more information on how to better take into account migrant origin women's special needs (such as information on family planning and trustable contraceptive methods). Depending on the country of origin, migrant women might also need information on women's rights and gender equality to improve their access and use of sexual and reproductive health care services [44, 45].

Strengths and limitations

The strength of our study is that it is based on a population-based survey among three major migrant groups in Finland. Moreover, Finland's population-based health registers have a high coverage of births and induced abortions in case a woman has given birth or had an induced abortion in Finland [30, 31]. The Health

2011 and Maamu -surveys had a relatively high participation rate, compared to most previous surveys among general populations [46], but especially when compared to response rates among migrant populations [47, 48].

Other strengths of this study are that the survey data were collected by trained fieldwork staff using standard protocols and questions to ensure comparability between the study groups. However, younger participants in the general population received the questionnaire by post and this may have affected their responses when compared to the face-to-face interviews.

All analyses were conducted using inverse probability weights to correct for the effects of non-response and different sampling probabilities. However, the small numbers of participants and selective non-response can cause some bias, especially in the Somali group which has the lowest response rate and low numbers of women reporting induced abortions.

In the Maamu study, the aim was that the questions on women's reproductive health would be asked by female interviewers with the same origin as the respondent whenever it was possible. It was assumed that sensitive questions (such as contraceptive use, births, miscarriages and abortions) were more culturally acceptable when asked by a same-sex interviewer. Unfortunately, e.g. due to absences of multilingual interviewers, these questions were in a few occasions asked by male interviewers. As the gender of the interviewer was not systematically recorded, we are not able to analyse whether this had an effect on the reporting.

Item non-response may have caused some bias for Somali and Kurdish origin women. Discussions with the interviewers revealed that a few interviewers had skipped the questions as they thought that it was inappropriate to ask questions about induced abortions and births when the interviewer was male, younger than the interviewee, or if the woman was unmarried. The low level of agreement between survey and register data on induced abortions among Somali origin women might be partly due to these problems in the data collection process. However, it is likely that abortions are underreported because they are not socially approved.

Because of the obvious inaccuracy of the numbers of births and induced abortions both self-reported and registered, we couldn't compare the exact numbers of births and induced abortions in the two data sets. Instead of examining the exact validity, we compared the agreement between these dataset using categorical variables.

Unfortunately, the number of women who had lived in Finland their whole reproductive age was low (less than 50 in each migrant group) and it was not possible to compare reporting of induced abortions and births among women who had moved to Finland when they were younger than 15 years old, compared to women who had moved to Finland when they were older.

Conclusions

Our study demonstrates that by using both survey- and register-based data it is possible to get more accurate information on women's reproductive health. Both survey- and register-based information, should be used when a study focuses on sensitive subject areas such as women's reproductive health, especially induced abortions. Attention should also be given to the training of survey interviewers and the need for same-sex interviewers as well as developing other methods to improve culturally sensitive survey protocols.

Acknowledgements
We would like to gratefully acknowledge all the study participants as well as field-work personnel and researchers involved in planning and collecting data for the Maamu study and Health 2011 Survey. Janina Hietala reviewed the English language.

Authors' contributions
SJ performed the literature search, conducted the statistical analyzes together with EL, and drafted the manuscript. PK, TK, MG and AC contributed to the design of the study, provided expertise for the Maamu and Health 2011 Survey data sets, selecting and defining variables and statistical models for the study as well as contributed significantly to the writing of the manuscript. All the authors reviewed and approved the final version of this manuscript before submission.

Competing interests
The authors declare that they have no competing interests.

Author details
[1]Department of Welfare, National Institute for Health and Welfare, Mannerheimintie 166, 00271 Helsinki, PL 30, Finland. [2]Faculty of Social Sciences, University of Tampere, PL 100, Arvo Ylpön katu 34, Tampere 33520, Finland. [3]Department of Information Services, National Institute for Health and Welfare, PL 30, Mannerheimintie 166, Helsinki 00271, Finland. [4]Department of Neurobiology, Care Sciences and Society, Division of Family Medicine, Karolinska Institute, Stockholm, Sweden. [5]Department of Public Health Solutions, National Institute for Health and Welfare, Mannerheimintie 166, 00271 Helsinki, PL 30, Finland.

References
1. UNFPA. Annual Report 2015: For People, Planet & Prosperity: United Nations Population Fund; 2016. ISBN: 978-0-89714-034-8 E/1,387/2016
2. World Health Organization. Dept. Of reproductive health and research. Developing sexual health programmes: a framework for action. Geneva: World Health Organization; 2010. http://www.who.int/iris/handle/10665/70501. Accessed 10 Nov 2016
3. Mishra G, Cooper R, Kuh D. A life course approach to reproductive health: theory and methods. Maturitas. 2010;65:92–7.
4. Ritamies M. The development of family planning in Finland from the 1960s to the 1990s. In: Finnish yearbook of population research; 36 Jan 2000. p. 29–45.
5. Väisänen H. The association between education and induced abortion for three cohorts of adults in Finland. Popul Stud (Camb). 2015;69:373–88.
6. Eurostat. Fertility Statistics ISSN 2443-8219. http://ec.europa.eu/eurostat/statistics explained/index.php/Fertility_statistics#Further_Eurostat_information. Accessed 31 May 2017.

7.   Official Statistics of Finland (OSF): Births. ISSN=1798-2413. Annual Review 2015. Helsinki: Statistics Finland. http://www.stat.fi/til/synt/2015/02/synt_2015_02_2016-12-08_tie_001_en.html. Accessed 29 Oct 2017.

8.   The Register of Induced Abortions. https://thl.fi/en/web/thlfi-en/statistics/information-on-statistics/registerdescriptions/register-of-induced-abortions Accessed 12 Jul 2017.

9.   Habersack M, Gerlich IA, Mand M. Migrant women in Austria: difficulties with access to health care services. Ethn Inequal Health Soc Care. 2011;4:6–15.

10. Delara M. Social determinants of immigrant Women's mental health. Advances in Public Health. 2016; https://doi.org/10.1155/2016/9730162.

11. Scheppers E, van Dongenb E, Dekkerc J, Geertzend J, Dekkere J. Potential barriers to the use of health services among ethnic minorities: a review. J Fam Pract. 2006;23:325–48.

12. Topa J, Neves S, Nogueira C. Immigration and health: women immigrants' (in) ability to access health care. Saude soc. 2013;22:328–41.

13. Malin M, Gissler M. Induced abortions among immigrant women in Finland. Finnish Journal of Ethnicity and Migration (FJEM). 2008;3:2–12.

14. Eskild A, Helgadottir LB, Jerve F, et al. Induced abortion among women with foreign cultural background in Oslo. Tidsskr Nor Laegeforen. 2002; 122:1355–7.

15. Zurriagaa O, Martínez-Beneitob MA, Galmés Truyolsc A, et al. Recourse to induced abortion in Spain: profiling of users and the influence of migrant populations. Gac Sanit. 2009;23:57–63.

16. Helstrom L, Odlin V, Zatterstrom C, et al. Abortion rate and contraceptive practices in immigrant and native women in Sweden. Scand J Public Health. 2003;31:405–10.

17. Rasch V, Gammeltoft T, Knudsen LB, Tobiassen C, Ginzel A, Kempf L. Induced abortion in Denmark: effect of socio-economic situation and country of birth. Eur J Pub Health. 2008;18:144–9.

18. Jones RK, Kost K. Underreporting of induced and Spontaneus abortion in the United States: analysis of the 2002 National Survey of family growth. Stud Fam Plan. 2007;38:187–97.

19. Catania J, Gibson D, Chitwood D, Coates T. Methodological problems in AIDS behavioural research: influences on measurement error and participation bias in studies of sexual behaviour. Psychol Bull. 1990;108:339–62.

20. Jagannathan R. Relying on surveys to understand abortion behavior: some cautionary evidence. Am J Public Health. 2001;91:1825–31.

21. Anderson BA, Katus K, Puur A, Silver BD. The validity of survey responses on abortion: evidence from Estonia. Demography. 1994;31:115–32.

22. Bumpass LL. The measurement of public opinion on abortion: the effects of survey design. Fam Plan Perspect. 1997;29:177–80.

23. Fu H, Darroch JE, Henshaw SK, Kolb E. Measuring the extent of abortion underreporting in the 1995 National Survey of family growth. Fam Plan Perspect 1998; 30:128–133 & 138.

24. Rossier C. Estimating induced abortion rates: a review. Stud Fam Plan. 2003; 34:87–102.

25. Udry JR, Gaughan M, Schwingl PJ, Van den Berg Bea J. A medical record linkage analysis of abortion underreporting. Fam Plan Perspect. 1996;28:228–31.

26. Smith LB, Adler NE, Tschann JM. Underreporting sensitive behaviors: the case of young women's willingness to report abortion. Health Psychol. 1999;18:37–43.

27. Castaneda A, Rask S, Koponen P, Mölsä M, Koskinen S. (eds.) Migrant Health and Wellbeing. A study on persons of Russian, Somali and Kurdish origin in Finland. Report 61/2012. Helsinki: National Institute for Health and Welfare (THL). (Report in Finnish with English Summary).

28. Lundqvist A, Mäki-Opas T. Health 2011 Survey – Methods. Report 8/2016. Helsinki: National Institute for Health and Welfare (THL).

29. The Medical Birth Register. https://thl.fi/en/web/thlfi-en/statistics/information-on-statistics/registerdescriptions/newborns. Accessed 23 May 2017.

30. Heino A, Niinimäki M, Mentula M, Gissler M. How reliable are health registers? Registration of induced abortions and sterilizations in Finland. Inform Health Soc Care. 2017; https://doi.org/10.1080/17538157.2017.129730.

31. Gissler M, Teperi J, Hemminki E, Meriläinen J. Data quality after restructuring a National Medical Registry. Scand J Public Health. 1995;23:75–80.

32. Robins J, Rotnitzky A, Zhao L. Estimation of regression coefficients when some regressors are not always observed. J Amer Statist Assoc. 1994;89: 846–66.

33. Lehtonen R, Pahkinen E. Practical methods for design and analysis of complex surveys. Revised. Chichester: John Wiley & Sons; 2004.

34. Graubard BI, Korn EL. Predictive margins with survey data. Biometrics. 1999;

35. Fleiss JL, Cohen J, Everitt BS. Large-sample standard errors of kappa and weighted kappa. Psychol Bull. 1969;72:323–7.

36. Rasch V, Wielandt H, Knudsen LB. Living conditions, contraceptive use and the choice of induced abortion among pregnant women in Denmark. Scand J of Public Health. 2002;30:293–9.

37. Regushevkaya R, Dubikaytis T, Laanpere M, Nikula M, Kuznetsova O, Haavio-Mannila E, Karro H, Hemminki E. Risk factors for induced abortions in St Petersburg, Estonia and Finland. Results from surveys among women of reproductive age. Eur J Contracept Reprod Health Care. 2009;14:176–86.

38. Degni F, Koivusilta L, Ojanlatva A. Attitudes towards and perceptions about contraceptive use among married refugee women of Somali descent living in Finland. Eur J Contracept Reprod Health Care. 2006;11:190–6.

39. Degni F, Mazengo C, Vaskilampi T, Essén B. Religious beliefs prevailing among Somali men living in Finland regarding the use of the condom by men and that of other forms of contraception by women. Eur J Contracept Reprod Health Care. 2008;13(3):298–303.

40. Westoff CF, Frejka T. Religiousness and fertility among European Muslims. Popul Dev Rev. 2007;33:785–809.

41. Merrill Ray M. Reproductive epidemiology: principles and methods. Brigham Young University Utah: Department of Health Science; 2010.

42. Kosunen EA, Vikat A, Gissler M, Rimpelä MK. Teenage pregnancies and abortions in Finland in the 1990s. Scand J Public Health. 2002;30:300–5.

43. Hennick M, Cooper P, Diamond I. Asian Women's use of family planning services. Br J Fam Plann. 1998;24:43–52.

44. Gure F, Yusuf M, Foster AM. Exploring Somali women's reproductive health knowledge and experiences: results from focus group discussions in Mogadishu. Reprod Health Matters. 2015;23:136–44.

45. Alvarez-Nieto C, Pastor-Moreno G, Grande-Gascón ML, Linares-Abad M. Sexual and reproductive health beliefs and practices of female immigrants in Spain: a qualitative study. Reprod Health. 2015; https://doi.org/10.1186/s12978-015-0071-2.

46. Tolonen H, Ahonen S, Jentoft S, Kuulasmaa K, Heldal J. Differences in participation rates and lessons learned about recruitment of participants-the European health examination survey pilot project. European Health Examination Pilot Project. Scand J Public Health. 2015;43:212–9.

47. Tolonen H, Koponen P, Borodulin K, Männistö S, Peltonen M, Vartiainen E. Language as a determinant of participation rates in Finnish health examination surveys. Scand J Public Health. 2018;46:240–3.

48. Ahlmark N, Holst Algren M, Holmberg T, Norredam ML, Smith Nielsen S, Blom AB, Bo A, Juel K. Survey nonresponse among ethnic minorities in a national health survey – a mixed-method study of participation, barriers. and potentials. Ethn Health. 2014;20:1–22.

19

Physical activity and depressive symptoms during pregnancy among Latina women

Kathleen Szegda[1,5,6*], Elizabeth R. Bertone-Johnson[1], Penelope Pekow[1], Sally Powers[2], Glenn Markenson[3], Nancy Dole[4] and Lisa Chasan-Taber[1]

Abstract

Background: Latina women are at increased risk for antenatal depressive disorders, which are common during pregnancy and are associated with elevated risk for poor maternal health and birth outcomes. Physical activity is a potential mechanism to reduce the likelihood of depressive symptoms. The purpose of the study was to assess whether total and domain-specific physical activity in early pregnancy reduced risk for elevated antenatal depressive symptoms in mid-late pregnancy in a population of Latina women at high-risk for depression.

Methods: Data from 820 Latina participants in the prospective cohort study Proyecto Buena Salud was examined using multivariable logistic regression. Total, moderate/vigorous, and domain-specific physical activity (household/caregiving, occupational, sports/exercise, transportation) were assessed using the Pregnancy Physical Activity Questionnaire. The Edinburgh Postnatal Depression Scale was used to assess depressive symptoms and identify women with elevated symptoms indicative of at least probable minor depression and probable major depression.

Results: A total of 25.9% of participants experienced at least probable minor depression and 19.1% probable major depression in mid-late pregnancy. After adjusting for important risk factors, no significant associations were observed between total physical activity (4th Quartile vs.1st Quartile OR = 1.02, 95% CI = 0.61, 1.71; p-trend = 0.62) or meeting exercise guidelines in pregnancy (OR = 0.96, 95% CI = 0.65, 1.41) and at least probable minor depression; similarly, associations were not observed between these measures and probable major depression. There was a suggestion of increased risk of probable major depression with high levels of household/caregiving activity (4th Quartile vs 1st Quartile OR = 1.51, 95% CI = 0.93, 2.46), but this was attenuated and remained not statistically significant after adjustment. When we repeated the analysis among women who did not have elevated depressive symptoms in early pregnancy ($n = 596$), findings were unchanged, though a nonsignificant protective effect was observed for sport/exercise activity and probable major depression in fully adjusted analysis (OR = 0.63, 95% CI = 0.30, 1.33).

Conclusion: Among Latina women at high-risk for antenatal depression, early pregnancy physical activity was not associated with elevated depressive symptoms in mid-to-late pregnancy.

Keywords: Physical activity, Antenatal depression, Antenatal depressive symptoms, Latina

* Correspondence: kszegda@schoolph.umass.edu
[1]Department of Biostatistics & Epidemiology, School of Public Health & Health Sciences, University of Massachusetts, 414 Arnold House, 715 North Pleasant Street, Amherst, MA 01003-9304, USA
[5]Baystate Medical Center, Springfield, MA, USA
Full list of author information is available at the end of the article

Background

Depressive disorders affect up to an estimated 18% of women during pregnancy [1]. Depression relapse rates are particularly high during pregnancy, with some studies finding relapse rates as high as 43% [2]. Latina women in the United States are at increased risk for antenatal depression with some studies finding almost double the prevalence among Latina women compared to non-Latina White women [3]. Factors that likely contribute to this disparity include economic, acculturation, and social challenges experienced by Latinas in the U.S. [4], which increases their likelihood of depression overall, and thus the likelihood of reoccurrence or initial onset of a depressive episode during pregnancy. Because depression during pregnancy has been associated with increased risk of poor maternal health outcomes during and following pregnancy (e.g., pre-eclampsia, post-partum depression) [5, 6], as well as poor birth outcomes (e.g., admission to neonatal nurseries, small-for-gestational age) [7, 8], it is important to identify ways to prevent antenatal depression and reduce depressive symptoms in this at-risk population.

Physical activity may prevent the onset of depression [9], which is particularly important in populations that experience a high prevalence of depression and are at high-risk for antenatal depression. Exercise and physical activity are believed to prevent depression and reduce depressive symptoms by altering neurotransmitter and hormone levels that are associated with depression. It is also believed that exercise may reduce depression by distracting from depressive symptoms and promoting self-efficacy [10, 11]. Among women with antenatal depression, physical activity is an alternative option to antidepressant medications and psychotherapy, which are current common depression treatment options that may be underutilized or contraindicated. Studies suggest some antidepressants may negatively impact the developing fetus [12], which may result in hesitancy among patients to take these medications. Psychotherapy can be inaccessible and unaffordable, particularly among disadvantaged populations that experience socioeconomic challenges [13, 14]. Among Latinos, mental health services such as psychotherapy may be particularly underutilized because of cultural beliefs and concerns about stigma and fatalism [15]. Though current U.S. Health and Human Services guidelines recommend that pregnant women engage in at least 150 min of moderate intensity aerobic activity per week [16], women often do not meet these guidelines.

Studies conducted among women in the general population have generally found that physical activity is inversely associated with depression [17], but research in pregnant populations has been limited. Among studies conducted with pregnant women, findings have varied with some finding an inverse association [18–21], and others finding no association [22–24]. Among studies finding an inverse association, a number have been limited by their cross-sectional examination of physical activity and depression [18, 21], making it difficult to ascertain whether physical activity affected depression status or whether depression status lead to decreased physical activity levels. In addition, the majority of prior studies focused on exercise or leisure time activity and did not examine other domains of physical activity (i.e., household/caregiving and occupational activity), which may be an important consideration in populations that have limited ability to participate in leisure time activity. In the one study to evaluate other domains of activity, Demissie et al. found that among 1220 well educated, predominantly White women in North Carolina, higher levels of activity perceived as moderate to vigorous were associated with a reduction in depressive symptoms. However, perceived moderate to vigorous levels of some forms of household/caregiving activity increased risk for depressive symptoms [20]. As some household/caregiving activities are included in the list of activities recommended by the U.S. Health and Human Services as a means to achieve physical activity guidelines, it is important to understand the association between different types of activities and depression.

In a recent meta-analysis conducted by Daley et al. that examined randomized clinical trials conducted to assess the effect of exercise on the prevention and treatment of antenatal depression [14], the meta-analysis found a reduction in depressive symptoms among the six studies examined (standardized mean difference = − 0.46, 95% CI = − 0.87, − 0.05), but the authors noted the limited number and quality of studies available. The authors called for additional research, citing the need for more studies to better understand subgroup effects, including the effects of physical activity among nondepressed women, as only one study examined the protective effects of physical activity among nondepressed women at baseline [14].

Our study aimed to extend prior work by prospectively examining associations between total physical activity and domain-specific physical activity on elevated depressive symptoms during pregnancy in a Latina population at high-risk for antenatal depression. In addition, we examined physical activity and elevated depressive symptoms among nondepressed women to better understand whether physical activity may be associated with the onset of depression among women at high-risk.

Methods

Data from Proyecto Buena Salud (PBS) was used to assess associations between physical activity and depressive symptoms. PBS was a prospective cohort study among Latina prenatal care patients conducted from 2006 to 2011 at Baystate Medical Center, a large tertiary care center in Western Massachusetts, which has approximately 4500 deliveries per year and serves an ethnically diverse population. Study design details have been published previously [25]. PBS was approved by the Institutional Review Boards at the University of Massachusetts, Amherst and Baystate Medical Center.

Women were recruited at prenatal care visits in early pregnancy (up to 20 weeks gestation). Participants were informed of study aims and procedures and asked to provide written informed consent. To reduce language and literacy barriers, interviews were conducted in English (73.7%) or Spanish by trained bilingual interviewers depending upon participant preference.

At the initial interview conducted at recruitment (mean = 12.4 weeks gestation), information was obtained on socio-demographic, acculturation, behavioral, physical activity, and depressive symptoms. Information on depressive symptoms was updated in mid-to-late pregnancy (mean = 25.7 weeks gestation). Information on medical history and clinical characteristics of the pregnancy were abstracted from the medical record after delivery.

Study population

Eligibility for PBS was restricted to Latina women of Puerto Rican or Dominican Republic descent who were either born on one of these islands, or had at least one parent or two grandparents born on these islands. Other exclusion criteria included: multiple gestation; history of diabetes, hypertension, heart or chronic renal disease; less than 16 or greater than 40 years of age; and current use of medications thought to adversely affect glucose tolerance.

A total of 1579 women were enrolled into PBS. Women were excluded if they had a miscarriage ($n = 68$). Among eligible participants, a total of 1040 women had information on early pregnancy physical activity information. Among these women, 820 had information on mid-to-late pregnancy depressive symptoms and were included in the final dataset for analysis.

Assessment of physical activity

Physical activity was assessed in early pregnancy using a modified version of the Pregnancy Physical Activity Questionnaire (PPAQ) [26]. The tool consists of a series of questions asking respondents to indicate intensity, frequency and time spent engaged in 35 activities from four domains: household/caregiving, occupational, sports/exercise, and transportation.

Average overall total early pregnancy physical activity weekly energy expenditure (metabolic equivalent [MET]-hrs/wk) was calculated by multiplying the amount of time spent on each activity by its intensity and then summing these values. Activity intensities were determined based on the Compendium of Physical Activities [27]; activities identified as having a different intensity

during pregnancy were assigned a modified intensity value [28]. Total energy expenditure by domain (household/caregiving, occupational, sports/exercise, transportation) and intensity (moderate, vigorous) were also calculated. Moderate and vigorous activity were combined into a single category because there were so few women who engaged in vigorous activity. Total physical activity levels as well as those for moderate/vigorous, household, and transportation activity were categorized into quartiles. Because a large percentage of women did not engage in sports/exercise activity during pregnancy, women were categorized into none, sport/exercise levels "at or below the median," and "above the median." For occupational physical activity levels, women were categorized as unemployed, "at or below the median" and "above the median."

Physical activity was also categorized as to whether participants met current U.S. Health and Human Services physical activity guidelines, which recommend that pregnant women engage in at least 150 min per week of moderate intensity aerobic physical activity [16]. Women were categorized as meeting the guidelines if they participated in > 7.5 MET-hrs per week of sports/exercise activities that were of moderate-intensity or greater (i.e., 30 min per day of activity at ≥ 3 METs multiplied by 5 days per week or 150 min). We focused on sports/exercise activity because studies suggest that household/caregiving or activities seen as burdensome may increase risk for depressive symptoms [29], whereas leisure time activity has most consistently found to reduce risk of depressive symptoms [17]. However, we also created a second variable for meeting guidelines that categorized women as meeting guidelines based on any domain of moderate or greater intensity activity.

The PPAQ has demonstrated good reliability and reasonable validity when compared to Actigraph accelerometer measures [26]. Intra-class correlations for two administrations of the PPAQ one week apart were 0.78, 0.82 and 0.81 for total, moderate and vigorous physical activity, and 0.83, 0.86 and 0.93 for sports/exercise, household/caregiving and occupational activity, respectively.

Assessment of depression

Depressive symptoms were assessed in early and mid-to-late pregnancy with the Edinburgh Postnatal Depression Scale (EPDS) [30], which has been validated as a depression screening tool in pregnant and postpartum women [31]. The EPDS is a 10-item scale that asks respondents to indicate how frequently they have felt various mood states within the past seven days. Examples of items on the EPDS include, "I have been so unhappy that I have been crying," and "Things have been getting on top of me." Total scores range from 0 to 30. Women were categorized as to whether or not they had elevated depressive symptoms indicative of at least probable minor depression (scores13 or higher) or probable major depression (scores 15 or higher) [32]. To be consistent with the prior literature, EPDS scores were imputed for participants missing fewer than 10% of EPDS scale items by replacing the missing value with the participant's average score of the nonmissing items [33].

The EPDS has been shown to have high sensitivity and specificity for major depression (sensitivity = 100%; specificity = 96%) and reasonable sensitivity and specificity for at least probable minor depression (sensitivity = 57%; specificity = 98%) using these cut-points in an English-speaking population [34]. The EPDS has also performed well as a depression screening tool in Spanish-speaking populations with good sensitivity and specificity for at least minor depression (sensitivity = 79%; specificity = 96%) and major depression (sensitivity = 83%; specificity = 97%) postnatally [35].

Covariates

Information on maternal age, education level, income, whether the participant was living with a partner, generation in the continental U.S., and overall acculturation (Psychological Acculturation Scale) [36] was obtained at the initial pregnancy interview. Smoking status and alcohol consumption were assessed at each pregnancy interview. Psychosocial stress was assessed by Cohen's Perceived Stress Scale [37] and anxiety was assessed via the State-Trait Anxiety Survey [38]. Pre-pregnancy weight, height, parity and presence of morning sickness during the pregnancy were obtained through the medical record. Body mass index (BMI) was calculated as weight (kg)/height (m^2).

Data analysis

Univariate statistics were used to describe the study population. Baseline characteristics were compared between women with each of the respective probable major depression measures and women who did not have elevated depressive symptom scores. Unadjusted and multivariable logistic regression analyses were used to assess associations between physical activity in early pregnancy and at least probable minor depression and probable major depression in mid-to-late pregnancy.

We examined associations between total physical activity, moderate/vigorous physical activity, domain-specific physical activity (household/caregiving, occupational, sports/exercise, transportation), and whether women met U.S. Health and Human Services (HHS) physical activity guidelines, and each of the elevated depressive symptom outcome measures in separate models. Maternal age, education, living with a partner/spouse and depression in early pregnancy (assessed at baseline via the EPDS) were included as a priori confounders in models because they have been identified as risk factors for depression, or

in the case of living with a partner/spouse, as a proxy for a strong protective factor (social support) [13, 39, 40]. Weeks between early and mid-to-late pregnancy interviews was also included in multivariable models in addition to any other potential confounders that changed the odds ratio for the depression measure by more than 10% with their inclusion in the model. Additional covariates identified for inclusion through this method included parity and generation in the U.S. For domain-specific multivariable models, we additionally adjusted for MET-hrs/wk. from all other domains of physical activity.

We chose not to include stress and anxiety in our multivariable models because they were both highly correlated with depression ($r = 0.61$–0.78) and we were interested in assessing associations for all cases of depression and their inclusion would have obscured associations when anxiety/stress and depression co-occurred. In a sensitivity analysis, we repeated analyses using U.S. HHS physical activity guidelines defined as moderate/vigorous physical activity from all domains of activity in early pregnancy and mid-to-late pregnancy.

Because the effects of physical activity on subsequent depression may vary by baseline depression status [41], we then repeated the above analyses among women who did not have elevated depressive symptoms in early pregnancy (i.e. did not have at least probable minor depression) ($n = 596$) [41]. Finally, we examined differences in characteristics between women with and without information on mid-to-late pregnancy depressive symptom to assess potential effects of missing data. All analyses were conducted using SAS version 9.2 (SAS Institute Inc., Cary, NC).

Results

Among study participants, 25.9% of women had elevated depressive symptoms indicative of at least probable minor depression and 19.1% had depressive symptoms indicative of probable major depression in mid-to-late pregnancy. The mean age was 21.6 years (SD = 4.9). Women were generally of low socioeconomic status with almost half (48.7%) reporting that they did not complete high school and only 6.1% of women reporting an annual household income of $30,000 or greater (Table 1). Almost half of participants (48.4%) were born in Puerto Rico or the Dominican Republic and over two thirds of the study population had low levels of acculturation (80.7%). Women who smoked during early pregnancy were more likely to have at least probable minor depression and probable major depression in mid-to-late pregnancy. In addition, women who were obese (BMI ≥ 30 kg/m^2) or who did not live with a partner/spouse were more likely to have at least probable minor depression in mid-to-late pregnancy; women who had higher levels of parity were more likely to have probable major depression in mid-to-late pregnancy.

Table 1 Participant Characteristics by Elevated Depressive Symptom Scores in Mid-to-Late Pregnancy: Proyecto Buena Salud, 2006–2011

	Total Population		At Least Probable Minor Depression (EPDS ≥13)			Probable Major Depression (EPDS ≥15)		
	n[a]	%	cases	%	p-value[b]	cases	%	p-value[b]
Maternal Age								
16–19	270	32.9	61	28.8	0.40	42	26.9	0.25
20–24	315	38.4	83	39.2		62	39.7	
25–29	144	17.6	40	18.9		30	19.2	
≥ 30	91	11.1	28	13.2		22	14.1	
Education								
Less than high school	396	48.8	111	52.9	0.37	87	56.1	0.09
High school graduate or GED	270	33.3	63	30.0		41	26.5	
Post high school	146	18.0	36	17.1		27	17.4	
Income								
less than $15,000	242	30.1	75	36.1	0.15	58	37.4	0.13
$15,000–$30,000	121	15.0	27	13.0		18	11.6	
$30,000 or greater	49	6.1	10	4.8		8	5.2	
Don't Know/Refused	393	48.8	96	46.2		71	45.8	
Acculturation								
Low	635	80.7	161	79.7	0.68	121	80.7	0.99
High	152	19.3	41	20.3		29	19.3	
Generation in U.S.								
Born in PR/DR	382	48.4	99	49.0	0.72	74	49.7	0.11
Parent born in PR/DR	363	46.0	94	46.5		72	48.3	
Grandparent born in PR/DR	44	5.6	9	4.5		3	2.0	
Live with partner/spouse								
no	405	50.3	117	56.0	0.05	82	52.9	0.46
yes	401	49.8	92	44.0		73	47.1	
Pre-Pregnancy BMI								
less than 18.5	43	5.3	11	5.3	< 0.01	7	4.6	0.22
18.5-< 25.0	395	48.8	109	52.4		78	51.3	
25.0-< 30.0	180	22.3	29	13.9		25	16.5	
30 or greater	191	23.6	59	28.4		42	27.6	
Parity								
0 live births	336	41.5	75	36.1	0.12	50	32.9	0.03
1 live birth	255	31.5	67	32.2		50	32.9	
2 or more live births	219	27.0	66	31.7		52	34.2	
Smoking (early pregnancy)								
no	672	86.6	162	79.0	< 0.01	117	77.0	< 0.01
yes	104	13.4	43	21.0		35	23.0	
Alcohol consumption (early pregnancy)								
no	756	97.4	197	26.1	0.06	147	19.4	0.24
yes	20	2.6	9	45.0		6	30.0	

[a]Numbers may not total to 820 due to missing data
[b]P-values were calculated using chi-square tests and are for comparisons between cases and noncases

On average, household/caregiving physical activity accounted for the largest average proportion of energy expenditure (56.0%) and sports/exercise activity the least (6.4%). Almost half of women did not engage in sports/ exercise activity in early pregnancy (46.5%) and 51.7% of women were not employed in early pregnancy.

We examined associations between total physical activity in early pregnancy and elevated depressive symptoms in mid-to-late pregnancy (Table 2). In unadjusted analyses, the odds ratio for at least probable minor depression for women with the highest level of total physical activity as compared to the lowest level was elevated, but not statistically significant (4th Quartile [Q_4] vs. 1st Quartile [Q_1] odds ratio [OR] = 1.28, 95% confidence interval [CI] = 0.83, 1.98; p-trend = 0.21). After adjustment for age, education, living situation, parity, generation in the U.S., at least probable minor depression in early pregnancy, and weeks between interviews, this odds ratio was attenuated to 1.02, (95% CI = 0.61, 1.71; p-trend = 0.62). Results were similar for probable major depression (unadjusted Q_4 vs. Q_1: OR = 1.28, 95% CI = 0.79, 2.05; p-trend = 0.27 vs. adjusted Q_4 vs. Q_1: OR = 0.96, 95% CI = 0.55, 1.70; p-trend = 0.83). Similarly, we did not observe significant associations between moderate/vigorous activity or meeting physical activity guidelines and mid-to-late pregnancy elevated depressive symptom outcomes. We also did not observe significant associations in a sensitivity analysis using U.S. HHS physical activity guidelines defined as moderate/vigorous physical activity from all domains of activity.

We then examined associations between domains of early pregnancy physical activity and mid-to-late pregnancy elevated depressive symptom outcomes (Table 2). Women with the highest level of household/caregiving activity had 1.51 times the odds of probable major depression compared to women with the lowest level (95% CI = 0.93, 2.46), but again this was not statistically significant and was further attenuated after adjustment for important risk factors (OR = 1.18, 95% CI = 0.63, 2.21). Point estimates for the other domains of physical activity (i.e., occupational, sports/exercise, and transportation) and odds ratios of at least probable minor depression or probable major depression were closer to 1.0 and also not statistically significant in both unadjusted and adjusted analyses (Table 2). In domain-specific analyses that included additional adjustment for MET-hrs/wk. from other domains of physical activity, we similarly observed no significant associations.

We then repeated the above analyses restricted to women who did not have elevated depressive symptoms (i.e. did not have at least probable minor depression) in early pregnancy (n = 596) (Table 3). Similar to our primary analysis, we did not observe significant associations between any of the physical activity measures and depressive symptom outcomes in unadjusted or adjusted

analyses. For example, for total activity the adjusted odds ratio for probable major depression when comparing Q_4 to Q_1 was 1.21 (95% CI = 0.56, 2.64; p-trend = 0.70) and for meeting exercise guidelines was 0.82 (95% CI = 0.43, 1.55) when compared to women who did not meet guidelines. Women with the highest levels of sports/exercise activity who did not have elevated depressive symptoms in early pregnancy appeared to have a lower odds of probable major depression (OR 0.63, 95% CI = 0.30, 1.33) after adjusting for important risk factors and other domains of activity, but this was not statistically significant.

Lastly, women who were missing mid-to-late pregnancy depressive symptom information did not differ from women with this information by early pregnancy probable depression status (at least probable minor depression or probable major depression) and also did not differ according to age, BMI, parity, generation in the U.S., whether they lived with a partner or spouse, or early pregnancy smoking status; however they had higher levels of education ($p < 0.01$), income ($p = 0.01$), and acculturation ($p = 0.02$) and were more likely to have had a preterm birth ($p < 0.001$).

Discussion

In our prospective cohort study of 820 Latina women, we did not observe statistically significant associations between total and domain-specific physical activity in early pregnancy and mid-to-late pregnancy elevated depressive symptoms. We similarly did not observe significant associations when restricting our analyses to women who did not have elevated depressive symptoms in early pregnancy.

Few studies have examined the association between total and domain specific physical activity and depression during pregnancy. Our findings that physical activity and sports/exercise activity were not associated with elevated depressive symptom outcomes are consistent with the findings of several other studies examining these associations [22–24]. Similar to our findings, Symons-Downs et al. did not find an independent association between exercise behavior and depressive symptoms in prospective analysis during pregnancy in their study of 230 predominantly White, highly educated women [22]. In the one study to evaluate other domains of activity, Demissie et al. similarly did not find significant associations between absolute levels (MET-hrs per week) of total (OR = 0.71, 95% CI = 0.42, 1.18) or domain-specific moderate to vigorous physical activity and elevated depressive symptoms among 1220 predominantly White women in North Carolina [20]. However, when the authors used participant perception of intensity to classify activities, they found that moderate levels of total moderate to vigorous activity was inversely associated with elevated depressive symptoms (OR = 0.56, 95% CI = 0.38, 0.83) and that moderate levels of moderate to vigorous household activity

Table 2 Odds ratios of mid-to-late pregnancy probable depression by various early pregnancy physical activity levels: Proyecto Buena Salud, 2006–2011

	At least Probable Minor Depression (EPDS≥13)								Probable Major Depression (EPDS≥15)							
	Cases		Unadjusted		Adjusted[b]		Adjusted[c]		Cases		Unadjusted		Adjusted[b]		Adjusted[c]	
	n	%	OR	95% CI	OR	95% CI	OR	95% CI	n	%	OR	95% CI	OR	95% CI	OR	95% CI
Total physical activity																
1st Quartile	53	27.9	referent		referent				40	21.1	referent		referent			
2nd Quartile	36	19.8	0.64	0.39, 1.03	0.52	0.30, 0.90	n/a		27	14.8	0.65	0.38, 1.12	0.55	0.30, 1.02	n/a	
3rd Quartile	44	22.1	0.73	0.46, 1.16	0.72	0.42, 1.23			32	16.1	0.72	0.43, 1.20	0.72	0.39, 1.31		
4th Quartile	64	32.5	1.28	0.83, 1.98	1.02	0.61, 1.71			49	25.4	1.28	0.79, 2.05	0.96	0.55, 1.70		
p-trend			0.21		0.62						0.27		0.83			
Met exercise guidelines[a]																
no	142	25.7	referent		referent				101	18.3	referent		referent			
yes	68	26.6	1.05	0.75, 1.46	0.96	0.65, 1.41	n/a		53	20.7	1.17	0.80, 1.69	1.12	0.73, 1.71	n/a	
Moderate/vigorous intensity																
1st Quartile	51	25.6	referent		referent				34	17.1	referent		referent			
2nd Quartile	44	21.8	0.81	0.51, 1.28	0.60	0.35, 1.03	n/a		36	17.8	1.05	0.63, 1.76	0.78	0.43, 1.43	n/a	
3rd Quartile	57	27.4	1.10	0.71, 1.70	0.73	0.44, 1.22			42	20.2	1.23	0.74, 2.03	0.86	0.48, 1.53		
4th Quartile	58	28.7	1.17	0.75, 1.82	0.89	0.53, 1.50			42	20.8	1.27	0.77, 2.10	0.94	0.52, 1.69		
p-trend			0.28		0.92						0.28		0.95			
Domain of Activity																
Household/ caregiving																
1st Quartile	49	26.6	referent		referent		referent		34	18.5	referent		referent		referent	
2nd Quartile	48	24.5	0.89	0.56, 1.42	1.11	0.64, 1.93	1.03	0.59, 1.81	39	19.9	1.10	0.66, 1.83	1.37	0.73, 2.55	1.26	0.67, 2.37
3rd Quartile	44	21.8	0.77	0.48, 1.22	0.67	0.38, 1.18	0.64	0.36, 1.13	27	13.4	0.68	0.39, 1.18	0.59	0.30, 1.14	0.56	0.29, 1.10
4th Quartile	60	30.0	1.18	0.76, 1.84	0.93	0.53, 1.64	0.85	0.48, 1.52	51	25.5	1.51	0.93, 2.46	1.18	0.63, 2.21	1.09	0.57, 2.08
p-trend			0.58		0.45		0.31				0.24		0.80		0.68	
Occupational																
unemployed	115	29.3	referent		referent		referent		86	21.9	referent		referent		referent	
at or below median	42	19.9	0.60	0.40, 0.90	0.74	0.47, 1.17	0.78	0.48, 1.26	31	14.7	0.62	0.39, 0.96	0.84	0.50, 1.42	0.96	0.56, 1.63
above median	52	25.7	0.84	0.57, 1.23	0.88	0.55, 1.39	0.85	0.53, 1.37	37	18.3	0.80	0.52, 1.23	0.85	0.51, 1.41	0.85	0.50, 1.44
Sports/Exercise																
none	94	25.0	referent		referent		referent		67	17.8	referent		referent		referent	
at or below median	59	27.8	1.16	0.79, 1.69	1.27	0.82, 1.97	1.1	0.70, 1.75	43	20.3	1.17	0.77, 1.80	1.33	0.81, 2.18	1.16	0.69, 1.94
above median	57	25.9	1.05	0.72, 1.54	0.98	0.63, 1.52	0.9	0.57, 1.44	44	20.0	1.15	0.76, 1.76	1.13	0.70, 1.83	0.98	0.59, 1.64
Transportation																
1st Quartile	61	26.2	referent		referent		referent		47	20.2	referent		referent		referent	
2nd Quartile	41	24.3	0.90	0.57, 1.43	0.82	0.48, 1.41	0.74	0.42, 1.30	26	15.4	0.72	0.43, 1.22	0.64	0.35, 1.19	0.55	0.29, 1.06
3rd Quartile	46	22.9	0.84	0.54, 1.30	0.99	0.60, 1.65	0.95	0.56, 1.62	34	16.9	0.81	0.49, 1.31	0.94	0.53, 1.65	0.82	0.45, 1.48
4th Quartile	62	30.1	1.21	0.80, 1.84	1.21	0.75, 1.97	1.22	0.72, 2.06	48	23.3	1.20	0.76, 1.90	1.10	0.65, 1.88	1.06	0.60, 1.90
p-trend			0.47		0.36		0.39				0.43		0.52		0.68	

[a]Met American College of Obstetricians and Gynecologists guidelines of > 7.5 MET-hrs/week in sports/exercise activities of moderate-intensity or greater
[b]Adjusted for age, education, live with partner or spouse, parity, generation in U.S., at least probable minor depression in early pregnancy and weeks between interviews
[c]Additionally adjusted for energy expenditure from other domains of physical activity

increased risk for elevated depressive symptoms, suggesting that perception of physical activity may impact the association.

Differences in findings may be due to differences in study populations, as well as, differential effects of different types of physical activity. For example, women in our study were predominantly of low socioeconomic status and had high levels of baseline depressive symptoms, which may impact associations as physical activity has been suggested to have different effects depending on levels of depression [41]. Importantly, the largest source of physical activity energy expenditure in our population was household/caregiving with almost half of women not participating in any sports/exercise activity. Studies suggest that type of physical activity has differential effects on depression in the general population, with exercise/leisure time activity generally having a positive effect on depression and household/caregiving physical activity either having no effect or increasing risk for depressive symptoms [17, 29]. Household/caregiving activity may be stressful for women, which could negate any positive effects of physical activity or increase risk for depressive symptoms. Indeed, a study by Molarius et al. found that the more burdensome study participants perceived domestic activities, the greater the risk for depressive symptoms [29].

A number of studies have examined associations between physical activity and antenatal depression among patients who were not diagnosed as clinically depressed at baseline [14, 42], however, antenatal depression is often undiagnosed [43] and no studies that we are aware of excluded women who had elevated depressive symptoms indicative of probable depression at baseline. In the recent meta-analysis by Daley et al., the authors identified one randomized controlled trial of an aerobic exercise program conducted among clinically nondepressed patients by Robledo-Colonia et al. which found an average four-point reduction in depressive symptom score among intervention group participants [14, 44]. However, some participants had baseline depressive symptom scores, as measured by the Center for Epidemiologic Studies - Depression Scale, which were higher than the widely used screening cut-point for significant depressive symptoms or depression [44, 45], suggesting that some women may have had undiagnosed depression at baseline. In our analysis, after excluding women with baseline depressive symptoms, sports/exercise may have had a protective impact on incident probable major depression, but this was not statistically significant.

Our study had several potential limitations. First, the EPDS is a tool that assesses depressive symptoms and is not a clinical measure of depression. However, the EPDS is widely used to indicate probable depressive disorder and has been demonstrated to have strong sensitivity and specificity for depression during pregnancy when validated compared to a structured clinical interview [34]. Though the validation studies for antenatal depression were conducted using the English version of the tool and the Spanish version has not been validated, we expect the Spanish version to have relatively comparable sensitivity and specificity because both the Spanish and English versions had good sensitivity and specificity for postnatal depression using the same cut-offs to define depression [34, 35]. If bias did occur as a result of misclassification of depression, results would have been biased towards the null. However, the EPDS minimizes

some other potential forms of bias because unlike other depression screening tools that have been used in many of the studies that have examined associations between physical activity and elevated depressive symptoms during pregnancy, the EPDS takes into account common somatic depressive symptoms that are also symptoms of pregnancy.

We had information on a number of important risk factors that may confound associations between physical activity and depression during pregnancy, however, we did not have information on history of pre-pregnancy depression, which is a risk factor for antenatal depression. Nonetheless, as depression relapse rates are high during pregnancy [2], we anticipate that many of these women would have a recurrence during pregnancy. By adjusting for early pregnancy depression, we were able to adjust for this confounding to some degree, though there are some women who may have had a recurrence later in pregnancy, which could lead to confounding if history of depression was associated with physical activity. In addition, we did not have information on diet, another potential confounder. Exercise behavior is positively associated with healthy eating [46] and studies suggest that nutrient deficiency (e.g. n-3 fatty acids, B vitamins, folate) and high energy intake (particularly that of unhealthy food) may be associated with depression [47, 48]. In addition, diet may be on the causal pathway between physical activity and depression because physical activity may suppress appetite and studies suggest caloric restriction may have an anti-depressant effect [49].

It is possible that women who were depressed in early pregnancy were less likely to complete the mid-to-late pregnancy interview on depression. We found that women missing mid-to-late pregnancy depressive symptom information did not differ by early pregnancy probable depression status or on the majority of sociodemographic, medical history, and behavioral factors than women not missing this information, although they had higher levels of education, income, and acculturation, and were more likely to have had a preterm birth. Socioeconomic status, which includes factors such as income and education, is positively associated with exercise activity [50, 51], and inversely associated with depression [52] with individuals of lower socioeconomic status experiencing higher rates of depression. Loss of women with higher incomes and levels of education during follow-up would have potentially biased a protective finding of sports/exercise activity towards the null. In addition, as a result of this loss to follow-up, we had lower power to detect effects than originally planned and the study needs replication in a larger sample. Finally, we used odds ratios as our estimates of effect. Though they are valid estimates of effect, caution should be taken in inferring risk as they may overestimate effects because the outcomes were not rare [53].

Table 3 Odds ratios of mid-to-late pregnancy probable depression by early pregnancy physical activity levels among nondepressed women in early pregnancy: Proyecto Buena Salud, 2006–2011

	At least Probable Minor Depression (EPDS ≥13)								Probable Major Depression (EPDS ≥15)							
	Cases		Unadjusted		Adjusted[b]		Adjusted[c]		Cases		Unadjusted		Adjusted[b]		Adjusted[c]	
	n	%	OR	95% CI	OR	95% CI	OR	95% CI	n	%	OR	95% CI	OR	95% CI	OR	95% CI
Total physical activity																
1st Quartile	24	17.1	referent		referent				16	11.4	referent		referent			
2nd Quartile	17	12.8	0.71	0.36, 1.39	0.66	0.33, 1.32	n/a		10	7.5	0.63	0.28, 1.44	0.57	0.24, 1.37	n/a	
3rd Quartile	19	12.6	0.70	0.36, 1.34	0.71	0.36, 1.43			12	8.0	0.67	0.31, 1.47	0.70	0.30, 1.62		
4th Quartile	22	17.3	1.01	0.54, 1.91	1.04	0.53, 2.03			16	12.6	1.12	0.53, 2.34	1.21	0.56, 2.64		
p-trend			0.96		0.94						0.79		0.70			
Met exercise guidelines[a]																
no	69	16.7	referent		referent		n/a		43	10.4	referent		referent		n/a	
yes	20	11.6	0.65	0.38, 1.11	0.69	0.40, 1.18			14	8.1	0.76	0.40, 1.42	0.82	0.43, 1.55		
Moderate/vigorous intensity																
1st Quartile	25	16.0	referent		referent		n/a		15	9.6	referent		referent		n/a	
2nd Quartile	23	15.2	0.94	0.51, 1.74	0.93	0.49, 1.77			16	10.6	1.11	0.53, 2.34	1.11	0.51, 2.41		
3rd Quartile	20	14.4	0.88	0.47, 1.67	0.92	0.47, 1.79			11	7.9	0.81	0.36, 1.82	0.90	0.39, 2.08		
4th Quartile	21	14.7	0.90	0.48, 1.70	0.90	0.46, 1.76			15	10.5	1.10	0.52, 2.34	1.14	0.51, 2.55		
p-trend			0.71		0.76						0.99		0.88			
Domain of Activity																
Household/ caregiving																
1st Quartile	25	18.3	referent		referent		referent		15	11.0	referent		referent		referent	
2nd Quartile	22	14.4	0.75	0.40, 1.41	0.94	0.48, 1.86	0.95	0.48, 1.91	16	10.5	0.95	0.45, 2.00	1.25	0.55, 2.85	1.20	0.52, 2.77
3rd Quartile	17	11.6	0.59	0.30, 1.15	0.67	0.32, 1.40	0.71	0.33, 1.50	8	5.5	0.47	0.19, 1.15	0.58	0.22, 1.56	0.57	0.21, 1.55
4th Quartile	21	15.9	0.85	0.45, 1.60	0.99	0.47, 2.06	0.98	0.46, 2.11	17	12.9	1.20	0.57, 2.52	1.60	0.67, 3.84	1.53	0.62, 3.78
p-trend			0.46		0.75		0.78				0.99		0.55		0.61	
Occupational																
unemployed	44	16.5	referent		referent		referent		28	10.5	referent		referent		referent	
at or below median	20	11.8	0.68	0.38, 1.20	0.58	0.32, 1.07	0.58	0.31, 1.09	13	7.7	0.71	0.36, 1.41	0.65	0.31, 1.37	0.68	0.32, 1.45
above median	23	15.5	0.93	0.54, 1.61	0.80	0.42, 1.53	0.72	0.37, 1.43	15	10.1	0.96	0.49, 1.86	0.77	0.35, 1.73	0.67	0.29, 1.56
Sports/Exercise																
none	45	16.0	referent		referent		referent		31	11.0	referent		referent		referent	
at or below median	26	16.7	1.05	0.62, 1.78	1.08	0.63, 1.87	0.93	0.52, 1.67	13	8.3	0.73	0.37, 1.45	0.80	0.40, 1.61	0.58	0.27, 1.24
above median	18	12.1	0.72	0.40, 1.30	0.76	0.41, 1.38	0.65	0.34, 1.42	13	8.7	0.77	0.39, 1.52	0.85	0.42, 1.71	0.63	0.30, 1.33
Transportation																
1st Quartile	27	15.7	referent		referent		referent		16	9.3	referent		referent		referent	
2nd Quartile	18	14.8	0.93	0.49, 1.78	0.87	0.44, 1.73	0.76	0.36, 1.57	12	9.8	1.06	0.48, 2.34	0.98	0.42, 2.26	0.88	0.37, 2.09
3rd Quartile	26	16.8	1.08	0.60, 1.95	1.11	0.59, 2.08	1.01	0.53, 1.95	18	11.6	1.28	0.63, 2.61	1.34	0.62, 2.86	1.05	0.47, 2.32
4th Quartile	18	13.0	0.80	0.42, 1.52	0.90	0.46, 1.75	0.76	0.36, 1.58	11	7.9	0.84	0.38, 1.87	0.94	0.41, 2.17	0.72	0.29, 1.80
p-trend			0.65		0.95		0.63				0.89		0.91		0.61	

[a]Met American College of Obstetricians and Gynecologists guidelines of > 7.5 MET-hrs/week in sports/exercise activities of moderate-intensity or greater
[b]Adjusted for age, education, live with partner or spouse, parity, generation in U.S., and weeks between interviews
[c]Additionally adjusted for energy expenditure from other domains of physical activity

Conclusion

Physical activity has been suggested as a potential mechanism to prevent the onset of antenatal depression and/or alleviate depressive symptoms. We found that total and domain-specific physical activity were not associated with elevated depressive symptom outcomes in mid- to late pregnancy in an at-risk population of Latina women with a high prevalence of elevated symptoms indicative of probable depression outcomes.

Abbreviations

95% CI: 95% confidence interval; BMI: Body mass index; EPDS: Edinburgh Postnatal Depression Scale; HHS: Health and human services; MET: Metabolic equivalent; OR: Odds ratio; PBS: Proyecto Buena Salud; PPAQ: Pregnancy physical activity questionnaire; Q1: 1st quartile; Q4: 4th quartile

Acknowledgements

The authors acknowledge the staff of Proyecto Buena Salud for their support on this study. We also express gratitude to the Proyecto Buena Salud study participants for their willingness to participate in this study.

Funding

This study was supported by NIH grant DK064902 from the National Institute of Diabetes and Digestive and Kidney Diseases.

Authors' contributions

KS, LCT, EBJ, SP, PP and GM provided substantial input into the study design, data analysis and interpretation. ND provided substantial input into study design and methods. KS conducted the literature review, analysis, and drafted the manuscript. All the authors reviewed and approved the final draft of the manuscript.

Competing interests

The authors declare that they have no competing interests.

Author details

[1]Department of Biostatistics & Epidemiology, School of Public Health & Health Sciences, University of Massachusetts, 414 Arnold House, 715 North Pleasant Street, Amherst, MA 01003-9304, USA. [2]Department of Psychological and Brain Sciences, University of Massachusetts, Amherst, MA, USA. [3]Baystate Medical Center, Springfield, MA, USA. [4]Carolina Population Center, University of North Carolina at Chapel Hill, Chapel Hill, NC, USA. [5]Baystate Medical Center, Springfield, MA, USA. [6]Public Health Institute of Western Massachusetts, Springfield, MA, USA.

References

1. Gavin N, Gaynes B, Lohr K, Meltzer-Brody S, Gartlehner G, Swinson T. Perinatal depression: a systematic review of prevalence and incidence. Obstet Gynecol. 2005;106(5):1071–83.
2. Cohen L, Altshuler L, Harlow B, Nonacs R, Newport DJ, Viguera A, Suri R, Burt V, Hendrick V, Reminick A, Loughead A, Vitonis A, Stowe Z. Relapse of major depression during pregnancy in women who maintain or discontinue antidepressant treatment. JAMA (Chicago, Ill). 2006; 295(5):499–507.
3. Gavin A, Melville J, Rue T, Guo Y, Dina K, Katon W. Racial differences in the prevalence of antenatal depression. Gen Hosp Psychiatry. 2011;33(2):87–93.
4. Mendelson T, Rehkopf D, Kubzansky L. Depression among Latinos in the United States: a meta-analytic review. J Consult Clin Psychol. 2008; 76(3):355–66.
5. Kurki T, Hiilesmaa V, Raitasalo R, Mattila H, Ylikorkala O. Depression and anxiety in early pregnancy and risk for preeclampsia. Obstet Gynecol. 2000; 95(4):487–90.
6. Josefsson A, Berg G, Nordin C, Sydsj G. Prevalence of depressive symptoms in late pregnancy and postpartum. Acta Obstet Gynecol Scand. 2001;80(3):251–5.
7. Grote N, Bridge J, Gavin A, Melville J, Iyengar S, Katon W. A meta-analysis of depression during pregnancy and the risk of preterm birth, low birth weight, and intrauterine growth restriction. Arch Gen Psychiatry. 2010; 67(10):1012–24.
8. Chung TK, Lau TK, Yip AS, Chiu HF, Lee DT. Antepartum depressive symptomatology is associated with adverse obstetric and neonatal outcomes. Psychosom Med. 2001;63(5):830–4.
9. Mammen G, Faulkner G. Physical activity and the prevention of depression: a systematic review of prospective studies. Am J Prev Med. 2013;45(5):649–57.
10. Paluska SA, Schwenk TL. Physical activity and mental health: current concepts. Sports Med. 2000;29(3):167–80.
11. Craft LL. Exercise and clinical depression: examining two psychological mechanisms. Psychol Sport Exerc. 2005;6(2):151–71.
12. Udechuku A, Nguyen T, Hill R, Szego K. Antidepressants in pregnancy: a systematic review. Aust N Z J Psychiatry. 2010;44(11):978–96.
13. O'Keane V, Marsh M. Depression during pregnancy. BMJ. 2007;334(7601):1003–5.
14. Daley AJ, Foster L, Long G, Palmer C, Robinson O, Walmsley H, Ward R. The effectiveness of exercise for the prevention and treatment of antenatal depression: systematic review with meta-analysis. BJOG. 2015;122(1):57–62.
15. Kouyoumdjian H, Zamboanga BL, Hansen DJ. Barriers to community mental health Services for Latinos: treatment considerations. Clin Psychol Sci Pract. 2003;10(4):394–422.
16. U.S. Health and Human Services Physical Activity Guidelines Advisory Committee. Chapter 7: additional considerations for some adults. In: Physical activity guidelines for Americans. U.S. Health and Human Services. 2008. http://www.health.gov/paguidelines/guidelines/chapter7.aspx. Accessed 16 June 2016.
17. Teychenne M, Ball K, Salmon J. Physical activity and likelihood of depression in adults: a review. Prev Med. 2008;46(5):397–411.
18. Orr S, James S, Garry J, Newton E. Exercise participation before and during pregnancy among low-income, urban, black women: the Baltimore preterm birth study. Ethnicity Disease. 2006;16(4):909–13.
19. Gjestland K, Bø K, Owe K, Eberhard-Gran M. Do pregnant women follow exercise guidelines? Prevalence data among 3482 women, and prediction of low-back pain, pelvic girdle pain and depression. Br J Sports Med. 2013; 47(8):515–20.
20. Demissie Z, Siega Riz A, Evenson K, Herring A, Dole N, Gaynes B. Physical activity and depressive symptoms among pregnant women: the PIN3 study. Arch Womens Ment Health. 2011;14(2):145–57.
21. Haas J, Jackson R, Fuentes Afflick E, Stewart A, Dean M, Brawarsky P, Escobar G. Changes in the health status of women during and after pregnancy. J Gen Intern Med. 2005;20(1):45–51.
22. Downs D, DiNallo J, Kirner T. Determinants of pregnancy and postpartum depression: prospective influences of depressive symptoms, body image satisfaction, and exercise behavior. Ann Behav Med. 2008; 36(1):54–63.
23. Goodwin A, Astbury J, McMeeken J. Body image and psychological well-being in pregnancy. A comparison of exercisers and non-exercisers. Aust N Z J Obstet Gynaecol. 2000;40(4):442–7.
24. Poudevigne M, O'Connor P. Physical activity and mood during pregnancy. Med Sci Sports Exerc. 2005;37(8):1374–80.
25. Chasan-Taber L, Fortner R, Gollenberg A, Buonnaccorsi J, Dole N, Markenson G. A prospective cohort study of modifiable risk factors for gestational diabetes among Hispanic women: design and baseline characteristics. J Women's Health. 2010;19(1):117–24.
26. Chasan-Taber L, Schmidt M, Roberts D, Hosmer D, Markenson G, Freedson P. Development and validation of a pregnancy physical activity questionnaire. Med Sci Sports Exerc. 2004;36(10):1750–60.
27. Ainsworth BE, Haskell WL, Whitt MC, Irwin ML, Swartz AM, Strath SJ, O'Brien WL, Bassett DR, Schmitz KH, Emplaincourt PO, Jacobs DR, Leon AS. Compendium of physical activities: an update of activity codes and MET intensities. Med Sci Sports Exerc. 2000;32(9 Suppl):S498–504.

28. Chasan-Taber L, Freedson P, Roberts D, Schmidt M, Fragala M. Energy expenditure of selected household activities during pregnancy. Res Q Exerc Sport. 2007;78(2):133–7.

29. Molarius A, Berglund K, Eriksson C, Eriksson H, Lindon-Bostram M, Nordstrom E, Persson C, Sahlqvist L, Starrin B, Ydreborg B. Mental health symptoms in relation to socio-economic conditions and lifestyle factors–a population-based study in Sweden. BMC Public Health. 2009;9:302.

30. Cox JL, Holden JM, Sagovsky R. Detection of postnatal depression. Development of the 10-item Edinburgh postnatal depression scale. British J Psychiatry. 1987;150:782–6.

31. Gibson J, McKenzie-McHarg K, Shakespeare J, Price J, Gray R. A systematic review of studies validating the Edinburgh postnatal depression scale in antepartum and postpartum women. Acta Psychiatr Scand. 2009;119(5):350–64.

32. Matthey S, Henshaw C, Elliott S, Barnett B. Variability in use of cut-off scores and formats on the Edinburgh postnatal depression scale: implications for clinical and research practice. Arch Womens Ment Health. 2006;9(6):309–15.

33. Dole N, Savitz DA, Hertz Picciotto I, Siega Riz AM, McMahon MJ, Buekens P. Maternal stress and preterm birth. Am J Epidemiol. 2003;157(1):14–24.

34. Murray DCJ. Screening for depression during pregnancy with the Edinburgh depression scale (EDDS). J Reprod Infant Psychol. 1990;8(2):99–107.

35. Garcia-Esteve L, Ascaso C, Ojuel J, Navarro P. Validation of the Edinburgh postnatal depression scale (EPDS) in Spanish mothers. J Affect Disord. 2003; 75(1):71–6.

36. Tropp L, Erkut S, Coll C, Alarcn O, Vzquez-Garca H. Psychological acculturation: development of a new measure for Puerto Ricans on the U.S. mainland. Educ Psychol Meas. 1999;59(2):351–67.

37. Cohen S, Williamson G. Perceived stress in a probability sample of the U.S. In: OS SS, editor. The social psychology of health: Claremont symposium on applied social psychology. Newbury Park: Sage; 1988.

38. Spielberger CD. Manual for the state-trait anxiety inventory. Palo Alto: Consulting Psychologists Press; 1983.

39. Ryan D, Milis L, Misri N. Depression during pregnancy. Can Fam Physician. 2005;51:1087–93.

40. Lusskin S, Pundiak T, Habib S. Perinatal depression: hiding in plain sight. Can J Psychiatr. 2007;52(8):479–88.

41. Carek P, Laibstain S, Carek S. Exercise for the treatment of depression and anxiety. Int J Psychiatry Med. 2011;41(1):15–28.

42. Shivakumar G, Brandon A, Snell P, Santiago-Muoz P, Johnson N, Trivedi M, Freeman M. Antenatal depression: a rationale for studying exercise. Depress Anxiety. 2011;28(3):234–42.

43. Marcus S, Flynn H, Blow F, Barry K. Depressive symptoms among pregnant women screened in obstetrics settings. J Women's Health. 2003;12(4):373–80.

44. Robledo-Colonia A, Sandoval-Restrepo N, Mosquera-Valderrama Y, Escobar-Hurtado C, Ramirez-Vlez R. Aerobic exercise training during pregnancy reduces depressive symptoms in nulliparous women: a randomised trial. J Physiother. 2012;58(1):9–15.

45. Radloff L. The CES-D scale: a self-report depression scale for research in the general population. Appl Psych Meas. 1977;1(3):385.

46. Johnson MF, Nichols JF, Sallis JF, Calfas KJ, Hovell MF. Interrelationships between physical activity and other health behaviors among university women and men. Prev Med. 1998;27(4):536–44.

47. Leung BMY, Kaplan B. Perinatal depression: prevalence, risks, and the nutrition link–a review of the literature. J Am Diet Assoc. 2009;109(9):1566–75.

48. Quirk S, Williams L, O'Neil A, Pasco J, Jacka F, Housden S, Berk M, Brennan S. The association between diet quality, dietary patterns and depression in adults: a systematic review. BMC Psychiatry. 2013;13:175.

49. Zhang Y, Liu C, Zhao Y, Zhang X, Li B, Cui R. The effects of calorie restriction in depression and potential mechanisms. Curr Neuropharmacol. 2015;13(4):536–42.

50. Giles Corti B, Donovan R. Socioeconomic status differences in recreational physical activity levels and real and perceived access to a supportive physical environment. Prev Med. 2002;35(6):601–11.

51. Sternfeld B, Ainsworth BE, Quesenberry CP. Physical activity patterns in a diverse population of women. Prev Med. 1999;28(3):313–23.

52. Everson S, Maty S, Lynch J, Kaplan G. Epidemiologic evidence for the relation between socioeconomic status and depression, obesity, and diabetes. J Psychosom Res. 2002;53(4):891–5.

53. Zhang J, Yu KF. What's the relative risk? A method of correcting the odds ratio in cohort studies of common outcomes. JAMA. 1998; 280(19):1690–1.

20

Mothers' reproductive and medical history misinformation practices as strategies against healthcare providers' domination and humiliation in maternal care decision-making interactions

Linda L. Yevoo[1,2]* (iD), Irene A. Agyepong[2], Trudie Gerrits[3] and Han van Dijk[1]

Abstract

Background: Pregnant women can misinform or withhold their reproductive and medical information from providers when they interact with them during care decision-making interactions, although, the information clients reveal or withhold while seeking care plays a critical role in the quality of care provided. This study explored 'how' and 'why' pregnant women in Ghana control their past obstetric and reproductive information as they interact with providers at their first antenatal visit, and how this influences providers' decision-making at the time and in subsequent care encounters.

Methods: This research was a case-study of two public hospitals in southern Ghana, using participant observation, conversations, interviews and focus group discussions with antenatal, delivery, and post-natal clients and providers over a 22-month period. The Ghana Health Service Ethical Review Committee gave ethical approval for the study (Ethical approval number: GHS-ERC: 03/01/12). Data analysis was conducted according to grounded theory.

Results: Many of the women in this study selectively controlled the reproductive, obstetric and social history information they shared with their provider at their first visit. They believed that telling a complete history might cause providers to verbally abuse them and they would be regarded in a negative light. Examples of the information controlled included concealing the actual number of children or self-induced abortions. The women adopted this behaviour as a resistance strategy to mitigate providers' disrespectful treatment through verbal abuses and questioning women's practices that contradicted providers' biomedical ideologies. Secondly, they utilised this strategy to evade public humiliation because of inadequate privacy in the hospitals. The withheld information affected quality of care decision-making and care provision processes and outcomes, since misinformed providers were unaware of particular women's risk profile.

(Continued on next page)

* Correspondence: Linda.Yevoo@wur.nl
[1]Sociology of Development and Change Group, Wageningen University, P. O. Box 8130, Hollandsweg 1, 6700 EW Wageningen, Netherlands
[2]Dodowa Health Research Centre, Research & Development Division, Ghana Health Service, P. O. Box DD 1, Dodowa-Accra, Ghana
Full list of author information is available at the end of the article

(Continued from previous page)

Conclusion: Many mothers in this study withhold or misinform providers about their obstetric, reproductive and social information as a way to avoid receiving disrespectful maternal care and protect their privacy. Improving provider client relationship skills, empowering clients and providing adequate infrastructure to ensure privacy and confidentiality in hospitals, are critical to the provision of respectful maternal care.

Keywords: Ghana, Care decision-making, Power, Empowerment, Ethnography, Pregnant women, Respectful maternal care

Background

Dufie, a high school graduate suddenly began to bleed 30 min after delivery of her baby. The healthcare provider re-examining the placenta, saying aloud as she checked over possible causes for the bleeding: *"There is no missing lobe, she had no tear [vagina], and her uterus is well contracted. What is making this woman bleed profusely?"* She massaged Dufie's lower abdomen gently and instructed the researcher to fetch an ampule of oxytocin injection.

Dufie's bleeding ceased about an hour later, after receiving nine more ampules of oxytocin injections.[1] Shortly thereafter, a gentleman came into the labour ward and said: *"My wife telephoned to inform me she had just delivered a baby girl and she is upset about it."*

The healthcare provider exploded with anger and asked him: *"Papa, are baby girls not human beings? She started bleeding suddenly because she disliked the baby's sex!"*

The gentleman replied: *"My wife insisted she wanted another male child although we have a son amongst our six children".* The healthcare provider became angrier at the revelation that a client who had told her she had had only three previous deliveries was actually a grand multiparous woman having her seventh delivery. She asked the gentleman: *"You mean your wife is a mother of seven instead of three? She nearly killed herself because she lied to us in her reproductive history. I would not have managed the bleeding the way I did, if I knew she was a mother of seven."*[2]

Reproductive care decision-making interactions: An encounter of domination and resistance

This labour ward scene is one of many observations made of pregnant women's with-holding vital medical, reproductive and social information from healthcare providers during field work. Withholding of information from healthcare providers by pregnant women (and clients) has also been reported in the literature from other healthcare settings [1–3]. Understanding why this happens in context, is critical for improving care decision-making and health outcomes. This is because the medical, obstetric, gynaecological and social history information pregnant women possess about themselves, is critical for healthcare providers' care decision-making. Healthcare providers combine clients' information with their expert knowledge and skills to arrive at what they hope is the appropriate

diagnosis and management plan that addresses the client's condition. Sometimes, with adequate information, healthcare providers may not require further physical examination or laboratory tests to determine the appropriate management clients require [4]. This article aims to provide insight as to why pregnant women in this study misinformed their healthcare providers or withheld specific information during antenatal care; and how this affected healthcare providers' care decisions and related clinical management and sometimes outcomes. This understanding is essential to inform interventions to improve maternal and newborn healthcare service and quality outcomes.

Researchers on provider-client care decision-making interactions have argued that asymmetrical relations of power between healthcare providers and clients, make healthcare providers dominate the care decision-making process [5]. For instance, healthcare providers may control the way clients -including pregnant women - should interact during the decision-making process, sometimes disregarding their complaints and concerns [6]. Other times, healthcare providers become angry, yell at, verbally abuse and make derogatory remarks about clients when they perceive they are not adopting the 'appropriate' medical practices and behaviours [5, 7–11]. In addition, healthcare providers sometimes conduct care interactions in environments that do not take into consideration confidentiality of information clients provide them and their privacy needs [2, 12]. These healthcare provider practices have been claimed to amount to human rights violations and denial of the right of pregnant women to receive respectful and dignified healthcare [13]. Despite this, empirical studies and qualitative synthesis suggest that the problem remains widespread globally, but more prevalent in low and middle-income countries including Ghana, the setting of the current study [8, 14–21]. Some consequences of disrespectful treatment of pregnant women include dissatisfaction, increased risk of experiencing obstetric complications and poor utilisation of reproductive and maternal healthcare services in subsequent pregnancies and deliveries [16, 22–25].

Other writers have suggested that healthcare providers' disrespectful treatment of mothers and practices of power, transforms clients from being independent decision-makers into passive actors during the care consultation [26].

On the contrary, some medical anthropologists and feminist scholars, argue that only analysing healthcare providers' enactment of (coercive) power during the care decision-making interaction is to overlook how clients respond to healthcare providers' attempts to dominate them [27–29]. These authors contend that clients including pregnant women do not remain passive. Rather they use whatever resources they possess – e.g., social knowledge about healthcare providers' attitudes, behaviours etc., – to develop strategies to maintain some control over their situation [30]. Foucault contends, where there is power, there is resistance ([31]: 95-96).

From this later perspective, empirical evidence from the medical literature shows that clients—including pregnant women—sometimes do not fully submit to healthcare providers' authority. They resist by concealing their medical information from healthcare providers during care decision-making interactions [1, 2]. A study among Latin American pregnant women found that pregnant women concealed some information about themselves from the healthcare providers because they were dissatisfied with the healthcare provider's relationship with them [32]. Similarly, Lazarus [29] observed that Puerto Rican pregnant women told healthcare providers what they wanted to hear as an expression of dissatisfaction with their healthcare providers behaviour towards them.

Some scholars have attributed similar client 'resistance' behaviours to gaps in their medical knowledge which prevent them from sharing vital health information even when given ample opportunity to do so [33].

In this article, we argue that clients' acts of resistance are directed towards healthcare providers' behaviours and healthcare delivery practices they perceive as unresponsive and humiliating to their personhood. We draw upon practice theory [34] and anthropological concepts of 'resistance', 'public transcript', 'front stage', 'hidden transcript' and 'back stage' from the work of James Scott [35, 36] to guide our analysis.

Practice theory

Practice theory highlights the puzzling and dialectical way(s) less powerful social actors behave in a relationship of domination. They respond by reproducing their own repression, acting in opposing ways or by resisting the submissive behaviour they have been socialised to use towards persons they consider as their superiors [34]. Some analysts contend that subordinated persons have consciousness and 'see' through the 'workings' of their domination [37] and hence, develop strategies to escape from being dominated [38]. Resistance - also defined as 'oppositional agency' [39] - is a strategy that less powerful persons may resort to in order to confront being dominated.

Resistance

James Scott [36] in his study 'The Weapons of the Weak: Everyday Forms of Peasant Resistance', conceptualizes resistance as act(s) that subordinated persons engage in with the intention to deny claims made on them by persons in a superordinate class. Scott argues that the relative powerlessness of subordinated persons, make them use covert resistance strategies (e.g. false compliance) as individualized self-help strategy to express dissent of their domination and confront superiors ([36]: 290). Feminists and scholars of subalterns argue that the strategies of these subordinated persons shed light on how they 'play with power' and express agency even under extreme domination ([40]: 12). In this article, we contend that because subordinates are not a homogeneous group, how they decide to act in power-laden relationships may vary depending on how they anticipate more powerful actors will (re)act towards them and on their interpretations of the dominator's behaviour.

'Public transcript', 'front stage', 'hidden transcript' and 'backstage'

'Public transcript' is a resistance strategy that subordinates use to evade domination and abuse of powerful persons' during public interactions [35]. 'Public transcript' consists of deliberately misrepresenting oneself by 'tilting' one's discourses (speech, emotions etc.) to conform to powerful persons' expectations on the 'front stage' [35]. The 'front stage', is a social space bounded by precepts of 'appropriate' conduct ([41]: 107), and a site where power relations are manifested and made visible. The 'front stage' is set to make subordinates act according to the 'rules' of conduct because subordinates' socialization tells them the way to behave on the 'front stage'; and to anticipate possible reactions of their superiors when they [subordinates] speak their mind or do not act according the 'rules' of the 'front stage' [35]. Therefore, on the 'front stage', subordinates' speak the lines of their superiors as a strategy to reassure their superiors they are in 'control' ([35]: xii). The accommodative attitude of the subordinates makes it difficult for their superiors to determine where subordinates' compliance ends and resistance begins ([36]: 289).

As a result, the way subordinates act in the presence of their superiors can diverge from their behaviours 'backstage'. Discovering what subordinates 'actually' feel, say and do, requires exploring their 'hidden transcript' [35]. 'Hidden transcript' to a large extent are discourses and practices that subordinates engage in whilst they are 'backstage' out of sight and earshot of superiors ([35]: 4). 'Backstage' is a 'social space' where subordinates interact with persons they 'trust' and take off the guises they put up whilst in the presence of their superiors [36]. These 'backstage' acts and 'hidden transcript', represent subordinates' agency. The 'front' and 'back stages' also include subordinates' behaviour surrounding concerns, anger, dissatisfaction and criticism of their superiors. In our work, uncovering pregnant women's 'hidden transcript' was essential to understanding their behaviour when interacting with healthcare providers in the antenatal care units and maternity wards in our study setting in southern Ghana.

Methods
Setting
Though Ghana's infant and maternal mortality have been falling over time, they remain unacceptably high. The maternal mortality ratio is estimated to have fallen from 634 per 100,000 livebirths in 1990 to 319 in 2015 [42] and neonatal mortality rates have declined from 41/1000 live births (1983–87) to 29/1000 live births (2010 to 2014) [43]. The Greater Accra Region where the study was conducted was one of the first sites in Ghana where institutionalisation of childbirth began [44, 45]. It currently holds the country's capital, the seat of government; and has relatively better roads and healthcare infrastructure than other regions in Ghana. These amenities make it a preferred region for healthcare professionals, contributing to the continuing geographical maldistribution of the country's critical healthcare professionals for maternal and newborn care [46]. Despite its relatively privileged status in the Ghanaian context, the region's institutional maternal mortality ratios were recorded to have worsened since 2011 [47, 48]. We conducted our study in two hospitals in this region which, for reasons of confidentiality we have named the Moon and Dawn hospitals. The Moon hospital was the smaller of the two study hospitals and the Dawn Hospital was relative better resourced in terms of healthcare infrastructure compared to the Moon Hospital. However, in absolute terms, both hospitals were resource and infrastructure constrained with severely limited operational working space and privacy for antenatal care and clinical consultations.[3,4]

Study design and data collection
This work was part of a larger ethnographic study undertaken in these two public hospitals to gain an in-depth understanding of care decision-making processes for mothers and newborn, and factors that influenced this process. The ultimate aim was to generate empirical evidence to inform design and implementation of interventions to accelerate improvements in maternal and new born health outcomes. The first author, henceforth, referred as the 'researcher', conducted ethnographic fieldwork to explore interactions between healthcare providers of maternal and newborn services and pregnant and delivering women in the antenatal, postnatal departments and labour wards in the two hospitals. The researcher spent a total of 22 months in the two hospitals in periods between a month and six months at a time between — February 2012 and July 2014— with participant observation used as the main approach to data collection.

Participant observation is the process whereby the researcher finds a credible role to facilitate the researcher's participation in the daily lives of research informants in their 'natural' setting [49]. This helps the researcher to participate, observe and create rapport between the researcher and the research informants [50]. In addition, it enables the researcher engage in conversations and seek clarification from informants about their behaviour and the meanings they attached to what they do. This process helps the researcher to understand what informants do within the context of their acts [51]. The in-depth interactions and observations are captured and written as field notes on daily basis. In the hospital settings the extent of the researcher's participation in informants' daily lives can sometimes be problematic for ethical and practical reasons like the researcher's personal identity and the subject of interest [49].

In this study, the researcher used her student researcher identity and the permission given by the hospital management, to participate in and observe care giving process and interactions between healthcare providers and pregnant women to answer the research questions. Using the student researcher identity enabled her to be present in the antenatal care units and the labour wards of the two hospitals. To prevent the researcher from being a nuisance to healthcare providers [52], and also play a meaningful role in the daily lives of healthcare providers and pregnant women, the researcher was 'informally' trained by healthcare providers to capture data about pregnant women. In the antenatal care unit she assisted the healthcare providers with recording data on mothers' socio-demographic and obstetric information, maternal weight and height. In the labour ward, she assisted with recording data such as date and time of delivery of the baby and placenta as well as the height and weight, chest and head circumferences of the baby. These are tasks healthcare providers also train female cleaners and student nurses to perform. During data capture in the antenatal care unit the researcher developed the habit of investing a little time to inform pregnant women about the importance of the accuracy of information for receiving quality care. She also took pregnant women a little away from the more public environment where the mother's histories were taken and invested time in answering women's questions repeatedly without showing signs of impatience and irritation. The practice she adopted made the history taking process longer but was possible because she had more time to spare as a student researcher. It also allowed her to gain the women's 'trust'. As this happened they started to tell her about their plans to limit the provision of some obstetric information and sometimes asked the researcher to correct information they had earlier misrepresented.[5,6,7,8]

This initial observation led to the researcher deciding to focus more time within her overall study on understanding what was happening in the area of histories provided by pregnant women at the antenatal clinic and why it was happening. She therefore focused on obtaining further insights from a sample of pregnant women on the range of information they withheld or misrepresented about themselves during history taking and observing care decision-making interactions between them and healthcare providers of over a longer period of time. In order to make these focused observations of the antenatal care history taking process, a total of 81 pregnant women who were within a gestational age of between 12 and 20 weeks were purposively selected and invited to participate in a longitudinal follow up.

The selected women were informed about the study's objective and data collection processes. Forty-two of these pregnant women - 24 in the Dawn and 18 in the Moon hospital - gave verbal consent to be followed-up when they reported on scheduled antenatal care appointments. Of the thirty-nine (39) women who refused to participate in the study, 15 of them needed spousal consent, 16 stated no reasons for their refusal and eight of them said they were considering the invitation but did not give a reply to the researcher, even though they subsequently often came into contact with the researcher. Given the context of 'mistrust' of healthcare providers, it is possible that the women who refused to participate were more inclined to keep their 'hidden transcript' hidden or were less trusting of the researcher's intent.

Upon acceptance, contact numbers were exchanged between the researcher and the pregnant women, and their socio-demographic information were documented. The exchange was to develop and facilitate long-term relationship and interactions between the researcher and the pregnant women. At pregnant women's antenatal care appointments, the researcher sat in the consultation process to observe the care interaction with healthcare providers, through several antenatal care appointments. Initially, the pregnant women seemed uncomfortable with the researcher's presence in the consultation process. Over time this changed, because at subsequent antenatal care appointments, pregnant women prompted her to come along when it was their turn to consult with healthcare providers. Brief field notes of interactions between healthcare provider and women were written and later expanded in the evenings in line with ethnographic standards and to aid analysis [53].

Subsequently, the researcher interviewed pregnant women to seek information they misrepresented about themselves or withheld from healthcare providers during history taking and in the care decision-making interactions and reasons that explained their actions. She used a semi-structured observation and interview guide (Additional file 1). At the end of the fieldwork period, the researcher had consistently observed all care decision-making interactions of 18 women at the Dawn Hospital from the first antenatal care registration until the postpartum period. For several practical reasons, the researcher was not able to consistently follow-up all the 24 women in the Moon hospital.[9]

To validate information generated from observation of the selected pregnant women in care decision-making interactions, and to verify whether the misinformation and withholding of information practices of pregnant women at the antenatal care was the norm rather than an exception, four focus group discussions were held with pregnant and postnatal women using a focus group discussion guide (Additional file 2). Three groups consisted of a mix of women with different levels of education and one consisted of women with a secondary education or higher. Two reasons accounted for the extra separate focus group discussion with the more highly educated pregnant women. First, women with a low level of education formed the majority of the hospitals' clientele and also made up the majority of pregnant women who participated in the study. Education and literacy can empower women and potentially reduce the power distance between healthcare providers and clients. It was therefore useful to find out practices and views between relatively highly educated (completed high school or more) and less highly educated women. The participants included women who had received prenatal, delivery and postnatal care from one of the two hospitals and women who attended antenatal care in other facilities (e.g., private or community clinics) but accessed skilled delivery care in the study hospitals because their prenatal clinics did not offer any skilled delivery services or they were high-risk cases referred for specialised obstetric care. Each focus group discussion was made up of between 7 and 10 women and was held with women 'backstage'. 'Backstage' [35] in this context was a rented premise located away from the hospital and healthcare providers. It provided the women with an environment to feel at ease and freely discuss their behaviours and experiences with the research team. Also, during the focus group discussions, women were asked not mention their names or the names of healthcare providers and to replace the names of their hospitals with the pseudonym 'my hospital' when making contributions. It was for anonymity reasons and to encourage them discuss issues freely.

A research assistant with experience in qualitative data collection including moderating focus group discussions was recruited as the facilitator for the discussions and the researcher took hand-written notes. The researcher paid the women's transportation costs to and from the venue and provided snacks during the discussions. The discussions lasted approximately 90 min each and were held in a local language (Twi) and audiotaped. Women's responses were transcribed verbatim by an independent research assistant for validity purposes; and were translated into English in the process.

Data analysis

Data collection and analysis was an iterative process according to the canons of grounded theory [54]. The data generated from the multiple sources were read line-by-line, and were sorted, integrated, organized and open-coded manually. The texts were categorised into themes and subthemes and given analytical labels. These categories were compared and contrasted between the various methods according to women's educational level and hospitals. The product of the process is presented as a 'thick description' [55] in the following sections.

Results

Managing obstetric and maternal information to resist healthcare providers' ideological 'domination' and humiliation

The researcher asked Dufie described in the vignette at the beginning of this paper, why she had not disclosed the number of children she had had during her history taking. She responded that her personal experiences with and observations of healthcare providers' relationships with multiparous pregnant women were often negative. She anticipated that the healthcare provider would have similar negative reaction towards her information about being a mother of six children and pregnant with a seventh. She said, the healthcare provider's likely comments to the 'right' information would be: "Why are you are having too many children? In contemporary Ghana with so much economic hardship; you are not practicing family planning." She went on to say:

"I make the decision to have ten children or less. Therefore, in my interactions with the healthcare provider, I expect her to talk to me nicely and explain why I should have fewer children rather than insulting me into submission. [...] you tell her what she wants to hear [...]. After all, they cannot follow me to my house to physically count the actual number of children I have." [10]

Dufie's position was confirmed by many of the pregnant and postpartum women who participated in the focus group discussions. The women interpreted healthcare providers' reactions as attempts to control them to think and act in ways that conformed to healthcare providers' reproductive ideologies and values. According to them, healthcare providers were ignoring the fact that they are autonomous individuals with the right to make their own fertility choices. [11,12]

Many of the women expressed concerns about healthcare providers' negative behaviour towards them such as making derogatory comments and criticising them when the obstetric information they gave did not conform to healthcare providers' reproductive ideologies. They explained in the focus group discussions and interviews that telling healthcare providers what they want to hear, prevented healthcare providers' verbal insults and also prevented them [women] from getting angry and starting arguments with the healthcare provider because of the insults. [11,12,13,14,15]

Pregnant women who sought antenatal care late in pregnancy - especially in the third trimester of pregnancy - sometimes reduced their gestational age to prevent healthcare providers from chastising them because they had failed to seek early antenatal care. Abigail a mother with no formal education attended her first antenatal care at a late gestational age. Though her ultrasound scan result indicated a higher gestational age, she told the attending healthcare provider a lower pregnancy gestational age. It was because she feared to be chastised by the healthcare provider if she told the truth of her real gestational age, which was too late for a first antenatal care visit. The healthcare provider found out her real gestational age through the ultrasound scan results and Abigail's fears of chastisement proved right. A part of the transcript of her interaction with the attendant healthcare provider shows below:

Healthcare provider: "Your scan result suggests you are almost due for delivery, but this is your first antenatal care visit. [...]. Pregnant women are stubborn. I am sure you are ill, the reason you are here today. Do you feel unwell?"

Abigail smiled at the healthcare provider and said: "I have leg pains and a headache". [16]

Despite being verbally abused, Abigail kept her fake smile. She told the researcher later: *"The healthcare provider's behaviour did not bother me because they always want to disgrace us."* [17]

Women in the focus group discussions confirmed that many pregnant women like Abigail gave a lower gestational age when they were registering for antenatal care in the third trimester because they feared healthcare providers would verbally assault and humiliate them. [11,12,13]

Rhoda, a highly educated mother criticised healthcare providers' for this behaviour during the group discussion. She said:

"If you start antenatal care around six months, these healthcare providers will get angry and treat you in

an inhuman way. They make sure to stand facing the crowd of pregnant women to criticize and insult you. If arriving for antenatal care later warrants such disgrace, when they [healthcare providers] ask you the pregnancy gestation, you reduce it by maybe three months. When the repercussions begin to manifest, we will both suffer because they would be running helter-skelter to save me." [12]

Women further explained that they often kept quiet when healthcare providers became angry, because engaging in open confrontation with them meant one may have to reluctantly terminate seeking care in the facility and move to another, located further away from your place of residence. Moving to another facility, the women said had negative consequences like incurring additional economic and social costs, such as increased transportation and time costs and social inconvenience. They also felt that healthcare providers were likely to neglect them for perceived act of insubordination if they openly confronted them. [12,13,17,18]

The women also indicated that some pregnant women - especially older women - sometimes altered information about their age to avoid being chastised and humiliated by the healthcare providers. Mothers revealed in the focus group discussions that they knew some older pregnant women – generally 40 years or older - who altered their age by at least ten years during history taking to prevent care provider reprimands. Susana, an uneducated mother observed that healthcare providers often berated these older women and made them feel like criminals for carrying a pregnancy at an older age. She stated:

"Many reasons account for women's decision to get pregnant at an older age. [...]. But these healthcare providers will humiliate her and associate the pregnancy with the refusal to adopt family planning. Generally, no one wants to be treated like a criminal when seeking care. [...] so under such situation you will reduce your age if asked." [19,20]

Comments made by some healthcare providers' in the study suggested that the women's concern about being chastised for "incorrect" behaviour was not misplaced. The healthcare providers also had motivations and pressures driving their behaviour. One healthcare provider stated in a conversation:

"Our less educated women do not understand that the simple use of family planning can reduce their risk of maternal morbidity and mortality. They think giving birth so many times is a reward." [21]

Another healthcare provider said a reason underlying their behaviour was the need to achieve the health sector's goals for mothers and babies. The healthcare provider stated:

"There is pressure on us to meet the country's health sector's goal of achieving zero maternal death and minimising neonatal mortalities. So you become frustrated that women cannot obey simple instructions or adopt practices that can save their lives and that of babies. That is why we get angry especially at the obstetric information" [22]

Managing medical information to evade stigmatisation and discrimination

A few of the women in the focus group discussions mentioned that they knew of pregnant women who had withheld vital medical information from healthcare providers because they feared stigmatisation and discrimination. Mandy, a highly educated pregnant woman said:

Many pregnant women who have HIV or a stigmatised disease like cancer would never disclose it to the doctors [healthcare providers] unless they test them. They do not provide them this information because if they [healthcare providers] get to know that one has HIV, they would pretend they care about her like any other woman. But some behaviour they put up when giving care, let you know that they are not treating her like a human being. For example, they would attend to her last and shout at her, not to touch them. [14]

Data from observations of skilled delivery care revealed that healthcare providers did indeed worry about being touched by pregnant women because of the healthcare providers' concerns and anxiety about occupational exposure to infections. This healthcare providers' behaviour created a sense that they visibly discriminated against some pregnant women because the adherence to standard infection prevention precautions were not consistently and routinely enforced in the same way for all pregnant women. For example, if a woman was known to be HIV positive, healthcare providers might wear extra pairs of examination gloves in addition to elbow length sterile gloves and any protective clothing they could lay their hands on. Also, they might caution colleagues who were unaware of the pregnant woman's HIV positive status to protect themselves by winking at them and mentioning a special HIV-positive code, while referencing the mother. [23,24,25,26]

Not all pregnant women responded to dominating and humiliating experiences by withholding information from healthcare providers. Women, who had had previous obstetric complications or had on-going complications particularly, used strategic perseverance as a counter-strategy against provider domination. An example was an uneducated mother, Samantha. She told the researcher that fear of the healthcare providers' wrath is a reason many expectant mothers withhold information from them during the care decision-making interaction. However, personally, she thought it was still necessary for pregnant women to provide accurate information to their healthcare providers to receive quality care. She explained how her decision to provide the healthcare providers with the required information, had helped her to overcome a threat to her pregnancy:

"I experienced complications at the early stages of this current pregnancy, so I told the doctors [healthcare providers] all information they required and it has helped me because they gave me the right management, now my condition has improved." [27]

In another example Patience, a high school graduate mother, recounted her experience in the focus group discussions:

"Not every one of them [healthcare providers] behaves towards us in a negative manner. In my previous pregnancy, the healthcare provider I met on my first care encounter in this hospital said one of the pregnant women had annoyed [her] so she refused to listen to [a] health complaint from the rest of us. I returned to the hospital again because I often encounter a lot of complications in my pregnancies. This time I met another healthcare provider, who was welcoming. I gave the healthcare provider all my past obstetric information. Immediately I was referred to see the appropriate healthcare provider for my health condition." [12]

Privacy and confidentiality

The environment in which pregnant women's reproductive history was taken did not offer privacy because of infrastructure and space constraints and related overcrowding. Healthcare providers took histories without a screen separating the other women waiting in both hospitals. [4,5]

The history-taking environment transformed a private interaction between client and healthcare provider into a 'public conversation' which others could listen to. Women considered providing certain histories such as induced abortions in such a 'public' history taking environment humiliating. Genevieve, a highly educated mother said:

"People call you a bad girl [promiscuous person] if you have had more than one self-induced abortion. However, as part of the information gathering, the healthcare provider will ask how many self-abortions

you have caused whilst other people listen. That is the reason pregnant women often reduce the figures in this context." [17,22,28,29]

At the Dawn Hospital, two doctors shared one consulting room and engaged in care decision interactions with pregnant women at the same time. [13,30,31]

Many of the mothers also expressed concerns about healthcare providers' inability to give them assurances about the protection of the confidentiality of the information they exchanged with them. [12,17,32,33] This prevented mothers from opening up completely because they were uncertain where their health and reproductive information could end up. The women felt that sharing confidential information could have negative repercussions on their relationship with family members, especially husbands. Ama, a high school graduate, complained:

"[The] healthcare providers are often unable to speak with clients [in an] undertone. While you give them information, they repeat it shouting because the hospital is noisy. As soon as this happens other patients' attention is drawn and then they start listening into the interaction. Thereafter, you hide the rest of the information." [34,35]

Discussion

Findings from this study corroborate the findings of some other studies [2, 19, 29, 56]. The unequal power relations between healthcare providers and women due in part to the biomedical knowledge healthcare providers have, which they consider as more 'authoritative' than that of pregnant women [7, 57]. Additionally, pregnant women desire to receive medical treatment and have access to medical resources like medications, which healthcare providers control [19, 29, 58]. Relatively lower educational and social status of many pregnant women [19, 21, 25, 59, 60] have also been stated as factors influencing pregnant women's decision to use covert 'resistance' strategies to confront healthcare providers, when dissatisfied with their – healthcare providers' - behaviours and practices of power.

While agreeing with these authors, we think that other practical and socio-cultural reasons may also account for the decision of pregnant women in this study to adopt these covert strategies to resist their domination. Some of the pregnant women in this study were secondary school graduates or even more highly educated than some of the healthcare providers. Despite this, they rarely openly confronted healthcare providers when they were upset with their dominating attitudes and practices of power. How can we understand these findings?

Firstly, it is possible that the general macro socio-cultural context of a fairly hierarchical society and a tendency towards unquestioned deference to authority and power-ful persons - whether based on age, social position and control of particular resources [61] - may be influencing the micro social context in the health care seeking and provision interactions. Socially, persons perceived as sub-ordinates would consider it unacceptable to either openly challenge their 'superiors' or question their authority, regardless of what they think. This social norm can make it possible for persons who find themselves in a super-ordinate position in any social, economic or bureaucratic organization to treat and relate to clients regarded as sub-ordinate with disrespect and perceive them as not having a voice to negotiate for services based on their prefer-ences. People, who find themselves in powerful positions, can frustrate less powerful persons who criticise them for perceived abuse of power, and may decide not to provide them with the required service. Some of the pregnant women expressed fears that they might be frustrated or 'punished' by the healthcare providers if they openly con-fronted them for perceived abuses of power. This concern could partially explain why they adopted 'public transcript' and 'front stage' behaviours. This finding would be keeping with McMahon et al's [19] study, which suggested that the fear of healthcare providers' neglect was a reason mothers in Tanzania resigned themselves to endure it, when they were verbally or physically abused by their healthcare provider during childbirth.

The pregnant women in our study - in their pragmatism [40] - evaded open conflict and resorted to more subtle strategies like 'public transcript' to respond to healthcare providers whose behaviour dominated, humiliated or stigmatised them.

Related to macro context factors is the general social pressure on individuals to be perceived as respectful [62] and good persons [63] rather than acquiring negative labels such as 'insolent' and 'trouble maker'. These socio-cul-tural values and pressures may also have prevented the preg-nant women in the study from speaking up about particular social interactions and relationships of domination. Adher-ence to these dominant social values can make women suppress their anger by adopting 'front stage' behav-iours like maintaining a false smile (as Abigail did). Ghanaian healthcare providers are embedded in the same socio-cultural context where these pregnant women operate, therefore, the way they act and interact with clients may be seen as a microcosm of what pertains in the Ghanaian socio-cultural context (cf. [64]), in relation to customer-patron relationship. Furthermore, healthcare providers often fail to acknowledge that pregnant women are part of a patriarchal system that compels them to have too many pregnancies and denies them the basic right to make their own reproductive decisions [65].

In this article our emphasis – based on a grounded analysis of the research findings – is on an analysis of

the reasons that make pregnant women withhold informa-tion from health care providers. However, the research also provided insight in the healthcare providers' behaviour. Some of the healthcare providers in this study mentioned that part of their behaviour is influenced by the pressures on them from their superordinates' in the healthcare system to reduce maternal and neonatal mortalities to the barest minimum and meet targets like the millennium and sustainable development goals in a resource constrained context. Another study from Ghana describes healthcare providers' physical abuse of mothers in labour as a strategy for gaining mothers' cooperation and compliance to improve neonatal outcomes [10].

Another explanation for some of our observations lies in street level bureaucracy theory. The study context is one of over stretched resources, overcrowding, heavy workloads and demand generally outstripping supply. Choices can also be limited, as clients like these pregnant women are "non-voluntary" ([66]: 54). They may not have ready access to private healthcare facilities in their local-ities and where they were available; the pregnant women may not be able to afford their relatively high costs. Also, clients cannot discipline healthcare providers and healthcare providers have little to lose, even when pregnant women would terminate their relations with their hospitals due to dissatisfaction with a healthcare provider's behaviour. Some research studies have documented healthcare providers putting quotas on the number of patients they can attend to in a day or sending clients away to minimise workload and reduce stress [9, 11, 67].

Healthcare providers behaviours may also be driven by motivational issues related to organizational conditions and processes such as poorly resourced healthcare facil-ities, overworked healthcare providers as well as superiors disrespectful treatment of subordinates by being quick to reproach them for mistakes committed while failing to provide equally swift commendation for good work done [24, 59, 67, 68]. Perceptions that employers and managers do not care or give adequate attention to their personal protection or healthcare needs in the face of the risk of injury in line of duty [67], could be part of the reasons for the described subtly stigmatisation and discrimination against HIV positive pregnant women.

As part of interventions to improve maternal and newborn care and outcomes, priority must be given to improving healthcare providers' client interactional skills by introducing and teaching it at both the basic and continuous learning levels. The skills acquisition may make healthcare providers more sensitive and aware of clients' aspirations and preferences during care interactions. The responsiveness may have positive effects on trust rela-tions between pregnant women and healthcare providers, and consequently minimise pregnant women's resistance acts against healthcare providers like withholding aspects of reproductive and medical information.

Healthcare providers' education should also include information on the importance of patients' autonomy, informed choices and shared-decision making.

Simultaneously, empowering pregnant women through education on interventions such as the patients' charter and patients' rights so that they are better able to speak up when dissatisfied with healthcare providers' attitude is important. Inventions like creating visible grievance centres in hospitals and a toll free customer hotlines to address clients concerns and prompt investigation to address them should be considered.

Facilitative supervision of healthcare providers to observe how they interact and relate to pregnant women during antenatal care history taking and care decision-making, can assist supervisors to identify peculiar challenges and concerns healthcare providers have other than interactional skills that promote disrespectful treatment of pregnant women. Addressing identified challenges and concerns, and correcting healthcare providers in a blame free manner, may minimise the negative behaviours towards pregnant women. Hospital managers should also recognise and reward staff who provide patient-centred care to minimise disrespectful care practices.

Healthcare administrators also need to pay attention to their responsiveness towards healthcare providers. This includes dealing with safety in the work place, adequate infrastructure and paying attention to work load and stress management. Ensuring the safety and healthcare needs of healthcare providers can improve health worker motivation and consequently may have positive influence on their relationship and attitudes towards clients. Finally, improving privacy and confidentiality in hospitals through provision of adequate infrastructure is critical, and should be seen as part of interventions for safe motherhood.

Limitations and strengths

The major limitation of the study is that it is focused on in-depth exploration and understanding of issues rather than statistical generalizability. It therefore cannot be assumed that the findings are generalizable beyond the two hospitals. The large number of invited women who refused to participate in the longitudinal observational study of their care interactions with providers means that it is possible that we missed some other unique perspectives peculiar to the pregnant women who refused to participate. There is the possibility that, in the same way that the pregnant woman withheld information from healthcare providers, they may have also hidden some information from the researcher. The use of focus group discussions with women away from the hospital to supplement the direct observational as well as triangulating the

responses and observations from focus group discussions, direct observations, interviews and conversations are all strategies that will reduce these possible errors in the data. The strength the methodology is that, it has provided valuable in-depth insights that could not have been uncovered by more statistically generalizable research methods like surveys.

Conclusion

In developing interventions to improve maternal and newborn health outcomes, much attention is paid to technical quality of care. Less attention has been paid to issues of responsiveness such as the quality of communication between healthcare providers and pregnant women during health care interactions and its implication for quality care provision. As our study shows, poor provider responsiveness can affect information provision by clients, which in turn can affect the quality of clinical decision-making and ultimately maternal and newborn health outcomes. The postpartum haemorrhage scene we described to start this article was in effect a near-miss influenced in part by the withholding of information from the healthcare provider.

Endnotes
[1]This insight also refers to the technical skills of the provider and organisational culture related issues. There is not the focus of this current article as they are addressed in another manuscript.
[2]Field notes observation
[3]Field notes observation
[4]Field notes observation
[6]Field notes observation
[7]The effect of the researcher's attitude and presence in the field on the data generated is discussed elsewhere
[8]Clients statements to the researcher such as: "You are different from what we know about most 'healthcare providers'. I had wanted to withhold some reproductive information to avoid the health care provider's scolding if I told the truth."
[9]In three cases the researcher was engaged in other school-related activities, three pregnant women had their babies closer to their parents; five did not attend their antenatal care appointment regularly. Another three of the women did not want the researcher's present at their baby's delivery. They cited embarrassments as reasons and five went into labour at times impossible for the researcher to be present
[10]Conversation
[11]FGD
[12]FGD
[13]FGD
[14]FGD
[15]Interview

[16]Field notes observation
[17]Conversation
[18]Conversation
[19]Conversation
[20]Conversation
[21]conversation
[22]Conversation
[23]Field notes observation
[24]Field notes observation
[25]Field notes observation
[26]Field notes observation
[27]Interview
[5]Conversation
[28]Field notes observation
[29]Field notes observation
[30]Interview
[31]Field notes observation
[32]Interview
[33]Field notes observation
[34]Conversation
[35]Interview

Additional files

Additional file 1: Semi-structured observation and conversation guide. Guide used to capture observations and interactions between pregnant women and healthcare providers during care provision. To also capture interactions between healthcare providers concerning mothers' care and interview with pregnant women.

Additional file 2: Focus Group Discussion Guide (FGD guide). A topic guide used to explore in-depth pregnant women reproductive and medical misinformation practices among pregnant women and postnatal mothers.

Abbreviations
ANC: Antenatal care; FGD: Focus group discussions; HIV: Human Immunodeficiency Virus; MDG: Millennium Development Goal

Acknowledgements
The authors are grateful to the Netherlands Organization for Scientific Research for funding this research. The researcher also thanks the pregnant women and lactating mothers who participated in the study and focus group discussions for their cooperation and insights on the subject of study. She also thanks Julia Challinor for her editorial comments, her research assistant for facilitating the group discussions and Dr. Kojo Arhinful for his useful comments on the ethnographic methods used in this study.

Funding
This study received financial support from the Netherlands Organization for Scientific Research (NWO/WOTRO) Global Health Policy and Health Systems Research grant for the project 'Accelerating progress towards attainment of MDG 4 and 5 in Ghana through basic health systems function strengthening' (grant number W 07.45.102.00). The Netherlands Organization for Scientific Research did not play any role in the study design, data collection, analysis and interpretations of data and writing of the manuscript.

Authors' contributions
LLY, HvD IAA and TG conceived and designed the study. LLY designed the study instruments and performed the investigation. LLY and HvD analysed the data. LLY wrote the first draft of the manuscript. HvD, IAA and TG reviewed and contributed to theoretical framework underpinning this article, read the first and subsequent drafts of the manuscript. HvD, IAA and TG also supported LLY in the finalisation of the final manuscript and agreed on the content of this article for publication. All authors read and approved the final manuscript.

Ethics approval and consent to participate
This research study obtained ethical approval, and verbal and written informed consent from management of the hospitals and research participants to participate in the study. The Ghana Health Service Ethical Review Committee granted ethical approval for the research (Ethical Review Number GHS-ERC: 03/01/12). Subsequently, the researcher obtained written approval and gained access into the two hospitals through an introductory letter from the Greater Accra Regional Director of Health Services to each of the District Director of Health Services who provides supervision and management support to the two hospitals. The District Directors also gave their written consent and forwarded their own approval letters, copies of the Regional Directors' letter and the researcher's ethical approval letter to the hospitals' managers for the study to be carried out in their hospitals. The hospitals' management in turn granted clearance for the study to be undertaken in their facilities with an approval letter to the researcher. Upon the approval, the hospital managers introduced the researcher to all members of staff and informed them about the research, its objectives, methodology and duration of the researcher's stay in the hospital.
In addition, the researcher obtained verbal consent from all pregnant women and healthcare providers involved in the study before observations and conversations were done.
Finally, the researcher obtained written informed consent from each mother in the longitudinal study and in the focus group discussions by providing them with consent information sheets. The information on the sheet was read in English and translated into a local language Twi by the researcher or the research assistant to the mothers, in the presence of an independent witness. The mothers were also informed that their participation was voluntary and could also withdraw from the study at any point if they were not comfortable. Mothers, who accepted to participate in the study, gave a written informed consent either by appending their signature or thumb printed on the informed consent sheets.

Competing interests
The authors declare that they have no competing interests.

Author details
[1]Sociology of Development and Change Group, Wageningen University, P. O. Box 8130, Hollandsweg 1, 6700 EW Wageningen, Netherlands. [2]Dodowa Health Research Centre, Research & Development Division, Ghana Health Service, P. O. Box DD 1, Dodowa-Accra, Ghana. [3]Graduate School of Social Sciences, Kloveiersburgwal 48 1012 CX Amsterdam, University of Amsterdam, Amsterdam, Netherlands.

References
1. Combs Thorsen V, Sundby J, Malata A. Piecing together the maternal death puzzle through narratives: the three delays model revisited. PLoS One. 2012; 7(12):e52090.
2. Yakong V, Rush K, Bassett-Smith J, Bottorff J, Robinson C. Women's experiences of seeking reproductive health care in rural Ghana: challenges for maternal health service utilization. J Adv Nurs. 2010;66(11):2431–41.
3. Senah K. Doctor-talk' and patient-talk'. Power and ethnocentrism in Ghana. In: van der Geest S, Reis R, editors. Ethnocentrism: Reflections on Medical Anthropology. Amsterdam: Aksant; 2002. p. 43–66.

4. Hampton J, Harrison M, Mitchell J, Prichard J, Seymour C. Relative contributions of history-taking, physical examination, and laboratory investigation to diagnosis and management of medical outpatients. Br Med J. 1975;2(5969):486.

5. Maternowksa M. A clinic in conflict: a political economy case study of family planning in Haiti. In: Russell A, Sobo E, Thompson M, editors. Contraception across cultures: technologies, choices, constraints. New York: Berg; 2000. p. 103–28.

6. Rogers M, Todd C. Information exchange in oncology outpatient clinics: source, valence and uncertainty. Psycho-Oncology. 2002;11(4):336–45.

7. Jewkes R, Abrahams N, Mvo Z. Why do nurses abuse patients? Reflections from south African obstetric services. Soc Sci Med. 1998;47(11):1781–95.

8. D'Ambruoso L, Abbey M, Hussein J. Please understand when I cry out in pain: women's accounts of maternity services during labour and delivery in Ghana. BMC Public Health. 2005;5(1):140.

9. Bohren M, Vogel J, Tunçalp Ö, Fawole B, Titiloye M, Olutayo A, Ogunlade M, Oyeniran A, Osunsan O, Metiboba L, et al. Mistreatment of women during childbirth in Abuja, Nigeria: a qualitative study on perceptions and experiences of women and healthcare providers. Reprod Health. 2017;14(1):9.

10. Rominski S, Lori J, Nakua E, Dzomeku V, Moyer C. When the baby remains there for a long time, it is going to die so you have to hit her small for the baby to come out: justification of disrespectful and abusive care during chidbirth among midwifery students in Ghana. Health Policy Plan. 2016; 32(2):215–24.

11. Mensah-Dapaah J. HIV/AIDS treatment in two Ghanaian hospitals: Experiences of patients, nurses and doctors, Monograph. Leiden: African Studies Centre; 2012.

12. Murira N, Lutzen K, Lindmark G, Christensson K. Communication patterns between health care providers and their clients at an antenatal clinic in Zimbabwe. Health Care Women Int. 2003;24(2):83–92.

13. World Health Organisation. WHO Statement: The prevention and elimination of disrespect and abuse during facility-based childbirth. Geneva: World Health Organisation; 2014.

14. Moyer C, Adongo P, Aborigo R, Hodgson A, Engmann C. 'They treat you like you are not a human being': maltreatment during labour and delivery in rural northern Ghana. Midwifery. 2014;30(2):262–8.

15. Miller S, Lalonde A. The global epidemic of abuse and disrespect during childbirth: hisotry, evidence, interventions and FIGO's mother-baby friendly birthing facilities initiative. Int J Gynaecol Obstet. 2015;131:S49–52.

16. Mannava P, Durrant K, Fisher J, Chersich M, Luchters S. Attitudes and behaviours of maternal health care providers in interactions with clients: a systematic review. Glob Health. 2015;11:36.

17. Kruk M, S K, Mbaruku G, K R, Moyo W, Freedman LP. Disrespectful and abusive treatment during facility delivery in Tanzania: a facility and community survey. Health Policy Planning. 2014;30(8):1–8.

18. Bohren M, Vogel J, Hunter E, Lutsiv O, Makh S, Souza J, Aguiar C, Coneglian F, Araújo Diniz A, Tunçalp Ö, et al. The mistreatment of women during childbirth in health facilities globally: a mixed-methods systematic review. PLoS Med. 2015;12(6):e1001847.

19. McMahon S, George A, Chebet J, Mosha I, Mpembeni R, Winch P. Experiences of and responses to disrespectful maternal care and abuse during childbirth; a qualitative study with women and men in Morogoro region, Tanzania. BMC Pregnancy Childbirth. 2014;14:268.

20. Engmann C, Crissman H, Engmann C, Adanu R, Nimako D, Crespo K, Moyer C. Shifting norms: pregnant women's perspectives on skilled birth attendance and facility based delivery in rural Ghana. Afr J Reprod Health. 2013;17(1):15–26.

21. 'th P, Dawson A, Homer C. Women's perspective of maternity care in Cambodia. Women Birth. 2013;26:71–5.

22. Bohren M, Hunter E, Munthe-Kaas M, Souza JP, Vogel J, Gülmezoglu A. Facilitators and barriers ti facility-based delivery in low and-income countries: a qualitative evidence synthesis. Reprod Health. 2014;11:71.

23. Roberts J, Sealy D, Marshak H, Manda TL, Gleason P, Mataya R. The patient-provider relationship and antenatal care uptake at two referral hospitals in Malawi: a qualitative study. Malawi Med J. 2015;27(4):145–50.

24. Asuquo E, Etuk S, Duke F. Staff attitude as barrier to the utilisation of university of Calabar Teaching Hospital for obstetric Care. Afr J Reprod Health. 2000;4(2):69–73.

25. Raj A, Dey A, Boyce S, Seth A, Bora S, Chandurkar D, Hay K, Singh K, Das A, Chakraverty A, et al. Associations between mistreatment by a provider during childbirth and maternal health complications in Uttar Pradesh, India. Matern Child Health J. 2017;21(9):1821–33.

26. Barry C, Bradley C, Britten N, Stevenson F, Barber N. Patients' unvoiced agendas in general practice consultations: qualitative study. Br Med J. 2000; 320(7244):1246–50.

27. Singer M. Cure, care and control: an Ectopic encounter with biomedical obstetrics. In: Baer H, editor. Encounters with biomedicine: case studies in medical anthropology, vol. 1. New York: Gordon and Breach Science Publishers; 1987. p. 249–93.

28. Martin E. The woman in the body: a cultural analysis of reproduction. 3rd ed. Boston: Beacon Press books; 2001.

29. Lazarus E. Theoretical considerations for the study of the doctor-patient relationship: implications of a perinatal study. Med Anthropol Q. 1988;2(1): 34–58.

30. Pappas G. Some implications for the study of the doctor-patient interaction: power, structure, and agency in the works of Howard Waitzkin and Arthur Kleinman. Soc Sci Med. 1990;30(2):199–204.

31. Foucault M: The history of sexuality, volume 1: an introduction London: Allan Lane; 1978.

32. Julliard K, Vivar J, Delgado C, Cruz E, Kabak J, Sabers H. What Latina patients don't tell their doctors: a qualitative study. Ann Fam Med. 2008;6(6):543–9.

33. Gott M, Hinchliff S. Barriers to seeking treatment for sexual problems in primary care: a qualitative study with older people. Fam Pract. 2003;20(6):690–5.

34. Ortner S. Anthropology and social theory: culture, power, and the acting subject. Durham: Duke University Press; 2006.

35. Scott J. Domination and the arts of resistance: hidden transcripts. New Haven: Yale University Press; 1990.

36. Scott J. Weapons of the weak: everyday forms of peasant resistance. New Haven: Yale University Press; 1985.

37. Giddens A. Central roblems in social theory: action, structure, and contradiction in social analysis. Berkeley: University of California Press; 1979.

38. Franz C, Stewart A. Introduction: women's lives and theories. In: Franz C, Stewart A, editors. Women Creating Lives: Identities, Resilience & Resistance, vol. 341. Oxford: Westview Press; 1994.

39. Ahearn L. Language and agency. Annu Rev Anthropol. 2001;30(1):109–37.

40. Lock M, Kaufert PA. Pragmatic women and body politics. Cambridge: Cambridge University Press; 1998.

41. Goffman E. The presentation of self in everyday life. New York: Anchor Books; 1959.

42. Trends in maternal mortality: 1990 to 2015. Estimates by WHO, UNICEF, UNFPA, World Bank Group and the United Nations Population Division. http://www.who.int/gho/maternal_health/countries/gha.pdf. Accessed 17 July 2017.

43. Ghana Statisical Service, Ghana Health Service, ICF I. Ghana demographic and health survey 2014. Maryland: Rockville; 2015.

44. Ofosu-Amaah S. The maternal and childbirth cervices in Ghana. J Trop Med Hyg. 1981;84(6):265–9.

45. Amponsah NA. Colonizing the womb: women, midwifery, and the state in colonial Ghana, Monograph. Texas: University of Texas; 2011.

46. Ghana health workforce observatory: Human resources for health country profile. http://www.moh.gov.gh/wp-content/uploads/2016/02/Ghana-hrh-country-profile.pdf. Accessed 20 Apr 2017.

47. Ghana Health Service: 2014 Family health report. Accra. Ghana Health Service; 2014. p. 119.

48. Ghana Health Service. 2016 Annual Report. Accra: Ghana Health Service; 2017. p. 125.

49. van der Geest S, Finkler K. Hospital ethnography: introduction. Soc Sci Med. 2004;59(10):1995–2001.

50. Hammersley M, Atkinson P. Ethnography: principles in practice. 7th ed. London: Routledge; 1993.

51. Spradley J. Participant observation. New York: Wadsworth Cengage Learning; 1980.

52. Wind G. Negotiated interactive observation: doing fieldwork in hospital settings. Anthropol Med. 2008;15(2):79–89.

53. Emerson R, Fretz R, Shaw L. Writing Ethnographic Field notes. 2nd ed. Chicago: The Universtity of Chicago Press; 2011.

54. Strauss A, Corbin J. Grounded theory methodology. In: Denzin N, Lincoln Y, editors. Handbook of Qualitative Research. 1st ed. Thousand Oaks: Sage Publications; 1994. p. 273–85.

55. Geertz C. Thick description: Toward an interpretive theory of culture. New York: Basic Books Inc. Publishers; 1973.

56. Bloor M, McIntosh J. Surveillance and concealment: a comparison of

techniques of client resistance in therapeutic communities and health
visiting. In: Cunninigham-Burley S, McKeganey N, editors. Readings in
Medical Sociology. London: Routledge; 1990. p. 159–81.

57. Irwin S, Jordan B. Knowledge, practice, and power: court-ordered cesarean
sections. Med Anthropol Q. 1987;1(3):319–34.

58. Mulemi B. Coping with cancer and adversity: hospital ethnography in
Kenya, Doctoral Thesis. Leiden: University of Amsterdam; 2010.

59. Rahmani Z, Brekke M. Antenatal and obstetric care in Afghanistan – a
qualitative study among health care receivers and health care providers.
BMC Health Serv Res. 2013;13(1):166.

60. Afsana K, Rashid S. The challenges of meeting rural Bangladeshi women's
needs in delivery care. Reprod Health Matters. 2001;9(18):79–89.

61. Assimeng M. Social structure of Ghana: A study in persistence and change.
2nd ed. Tema: Ghana Publishing Corporation; 1999.

62. van der Geest S. Between respect and reciprocity: managing old age in
rural Ghana. Southern African J Gerontol. 1997;6(2):20–5.

63. Adinkrah M. Better dead than dishonored: masculinity and male suicide
behavior in contemporary Ghana. Soc Sci Med. 2012;74(2012):474–81.

64. Zaman S. Broken limbs, broken lives: ethnography of a hospital ward in
Bangladesh, Ph.D. Thesis. Amsterdam: University of Amsterdam; 2005.

65. Adongo P, Phillips J, Kajihara B, Fayorsey C, Debpuur C, Binka F. Cultural
factors constraining the introduction of family planning among the
Kassena-Nankana of Northern Ghana. Soc Sci Med. 1997;45(12):1789–804.

66. Lipsky M. Street-level bureaucracy: dilemmas of the individual in public
services. New York: Russell Sage Foundation; 1980.

67. Aberese-Ako M, van Dijk H, Gerrits T, Arhinful DK, Agyepong IA. 'Your health
our concern, our health whose concern?': Perceptions of injustice in
organizational relationships and processes and frontline health worker
motivation in Ghana. Health Policy Plan. 2014;29(suppl 2):ii15–28.

68. Agyepong IA, Anafi P, Asiamah E, Ansah E, Ashon D, Narh-Dometey C.
Health worker (internal customer) satisfaction and motivation in the public
sector in Ghana. Int J Health Plann Manag. 2004;19:319–36.

21

Prevalence, risk factors and associated adverse pregnancy outcomes of anaemia in Chinese pregnant women

Li Lin[1], Yumei Wei[1], Weiwei Zhu[2], Chen Wang[1], Rina Su[1], Hui Feng[1], Huixia Yang[1]* and on behalf of the Gestational diabetes mellitus Prevalence Survey (GPS) study Group

Abstract

Background: Anaemia in pregnant women is a public health problem, especially in developing countries. The aim of this study was to assess the prevalence and related risk factors of anaemia during pregnancy in a large multicentre retrospective study ($n = 44{,}002$) and to determine the adverse pregnancy outcomes in women with or without anaemia.

Methods: The study is a secondary data analysis of a retrospective study named "Gestational diabetes mellitus Prevalence Survey (GPS) study in China". Structured questionnaires were used to collect socio-demographic characteristics, haemoglobin levels and pregnancy outcomes from all the participants. Anaemia in pregnancy is defined as haemoglobin < 110 g/L. We used SPSS software to assess the predictors of anaemia and associated adverse pregnancy outcomes.

Results: The overall prevalence of anaemia was 23.5%. Maternal anaemia was significantly associated with maternal age ≥ 35 years (AOR = 1.386), family per capita monthly income< 1000 CNY (AOR = 1.671), rural residence (AOR = 1.308) and pre-pregnancy BMI < 18.5 kg/m² (AOR = 1.237). Adverse pregnancy outcomes, including GDM, polyhydramnios, preterm birth, low birth weight (< 2500 g), neonatal complications and NICU admission, increased significantly ($P < 0.001$) in those with anaemia than those without.

Conclusions: The results indicated that anaemia continues to be a severe health problem among pregnant women in China. Anaemia is associated with adverse pregnancy outcomes. Pregnant women should receive routine antenatal care and be given selective iron supplementation when appropriate.

Keywords: Anaemia, Pregnant women, Associated factors, Pregnancy outcomes, China

Background

Anaemia is defined as a condition in which haemoglobin (Hb) level in the body is lower than normal, which results in a decreased oxygen-carrying capacity of red blood cells to tissues [1]. It affects all age groups, but pregnant women and children are more vulnerable. Stevens et al. [2] reported that the global prevalence of anaemia in non-pregnant women, pregnant women and children is 29, 38 and 43%, respectively.

According to the WHO guidelines, anaemia in pregnancy is defined as a haemoglobin level < 110 g/L [3, 4]. The prevalence of anaemia is an important health indicator. A study in 2013 showed that anaemia is more prevalent in developing countries (43%) than developed countries (9%) [5]. Previous studies have reported that the prevalence of anaemia in pregnancy varies in women with different socio-economic conditions, lifestyles, or health-seeking behaviours across different cultures [6, 7].

* Correspondence: yanghuixia@bjmu.edu.cn
[1]Department of Obstetrics and Gynaecology, Peking University First Hospital, Xi'anmen Street No.1, Xicheng District, Beijing 100034, China

Anaemia is one of the most prevalent complications during pregnancy. It is commonly considered a risk factor for poor pregnancy outcomes and can result in complications that threaten the life of both mother and foetus, such as preterm birth [8], low birth weight [9], foetal impairment, and maternal and foetal deaths [10].

Physiologically, plasma volume expands by 25–80% of pre-pregnancy volumes between the second trimester and the middle of the third trimester of pregnancy [11, 12]. This induces a modest decrease in Hb levels during pregnancy. Previous studies show that the best time to investigate any risk factors associated with anaemia may be up until 20 weeks of gestation [13]. Thus, in this study, we took the haemoglobin level estimated before the 14th week of gestation to determine factors associated with anaemia in pregnant women. Considering the physiological changes in plasma volume, we used the third trimester's Hb level to assess the pregnancy outcomes of anaemia.

In the present study, associated factors, including socio-demographic factors, body mass index, parity and age were analysed, and we evaluated the maternal and foetal outcomes among anaemic and non-anaemic women.

Methods
Data sources
We conducted a large retrospective study entitled "Gestational diabetes mellitus Prevalence Survey in China (the GPS study)" in 21 hospitals, including 15 centres in Beijing, 5 centres in Guangzhou and 1 centre in Chengdu. Medical records of 44,002 pregnant women who delivered between June 2013 and May 2015 were collected. We designed a structured questionnaire to collect the socio-demographic, obstetric and medical history of pregnant women [14]. An additional file shows the questionnaire in more details (see Additional file 1). The GPS study aimed to investigate the prevalence of pregnancy diseases and the factors associated with the determined diseases.

Study design and population
The present analysis was based on data from the GPS study. We recorded the haemoglobin level of pregnant women in three trimesters. Excluding 599 cases that lacked haemoglobin values in either trimester, 43,403 pregnancies were included in the study. We demonstrated the current status of anaemia during pregnancy in China from three aspects, including the prevalence of anaemia, related risk factors and the relationship between anaemia and pregnancy outcomes.

Prevalence of anaemia
Since three trimesters' haemoglobin levels of pregnant women were recorded, we found that the diagnosis of

anaemia should be made when the haemoglobin value in any trimester was lower than 110 g/L. Thus, 43,403 participants were included.

Related risk factors
To analyse the factors associated with anaemia, we selected the Hb value of the early trimesters as a subgroup, which included 26,924 pregnant women. Women with pre-pregnancy diabetes mellitus (PGDM), chronic hypertension and chronic renal disease were excluded.

Anaemia and adverse pregnancy outcomes
To evaluate the risk of adverse pregnancy outcomes in women with and without anaemia, we used the Hb value in the 3rd trimester, which included 41,569 women. Women with PGDM, twin or multiple pregnancies, chronic hypertension, or other foetal factors (foetal malformations, foetal death) were excluded. We analysed the maternal outcomes, including caesarean section, GDM, hypertension, premature rupture of membranes (PROM), foetal distress, placenta abruption, polyhydramnios, and oligohydramnios; and infant complications, such as preterm labour, low birth weight, neonatal complications and NICU admission.

Definitions
Based on WHO criteria, we defined anaemia in pregnancy as Hb < 110 g/L. Mild, moderate and severe anaemia were defined as Hb measurements between 100 and 109 g/L, 70-79 g/L and less than 70 g/L, respectively [3].

Gestational age was based on the number of days between the first day of an expectant mother's last menstrual period (LMP) and date of delivery and was expressed in the week after the LMP. The 1st, 2nd and 3rd trimester were defined as a gestational age less than 14 weeks, 14–27.9 weeks and 28–42 weeks, respectively. Body mass index (BMI) was divided into four groups based on WHO recommendations for Asian populations: underweight: BMI < 18.5 kg/m^2, normal: 18.5-23.9 kg/m^2, overweight: 24-27.9 kg/m^2, and obesity: ≥28 kg/m^2 [15].

Definition of maternal and neonatal outcomes: macrosomia was defined as new-born birth weight ≥ 4000 g, while new-born birth weight < 2500 g represented low birth weight. Preterm birth is defined as the time of delivery between the 28 and 36^{+6} gestational weeks. GDM was diagnosed according to the Chinese MOH 2011 criteria [16], which recommend that the diagnosis should be made when any one of the following values is met or exceeded in the 75 g oral glucose tolerance test (75 g OGTT) at 24-28 weeks: 0 h (fasting), 5.1 mmol/L; 1 h, 10.0 mmol/L; and 2 h, 8.5 mmol/L. Hypertensive disorders include preeclampsia, eclampsia, pregnancy-induced hypertension and haemolysis, elevated liver enzymes and low platelet syndrome (HELLP).

Statistical analysis

Data were entered into EPI data version 3.1 and cleaned. Finally, data were analysed using SPSS software version 22.0 for Mac (Chicago, IL, USA). Data were summarized in tables and figures. Continuous variables were presented as the mean ± standard deviations (SDs). Bivariate and multivariate logistic regression analyses were performed to adjust for potential confounding factors. Variables with P-value≤0.25 by the bivariate analysis were candidates for the multiple logistic regression model. The results of group comparisons of risk factors and pregnancy outcomes were expressed as ORs (95% CIs) for categorical variables. The P-value was set at < 0.05 for statistical significance.

Results

Prevalence of anaemia among pregnant women

We included 43,403 pregnant women in our study. The number of participants in the anaemia and non-anaemia groups was 10,199 and 33,204, respectively. The prevalence of anaemia in total was 23.5% (10,199/43,043). The maternal demographic characteristics are shown in Table 1. Sorted by city, we found that the prevalence of anaemia in Beijing, Guangzhou and Chengdu was 19.3%, 38.8% and 23.9%, respectively (Fig. 1).

In this study, we collected the Hb value of three trimesters, and there were 26,924, 33,879 and 41,569 effective Hb values in the 1st, 2nd and 3rd trimester, respectively. We found that the mean Hb values in the three trimesters were 129.89 ± 9.90 g/L, 118.99 ± 9.78 g/L and 121.21 ± 12.62 g/L, respectively (Table 2). The prevalence of anaemia was higher in the 2nd trimester (14.7%) and 3rd trimester (16.6%) than in the 1st trimester (2.7%) (Table 3). The severity of anaemia in pregnancy is shown in Table 3. Few pregnant women suffered from severe anaemia, while most of the participants had mild and moderate anaemia.

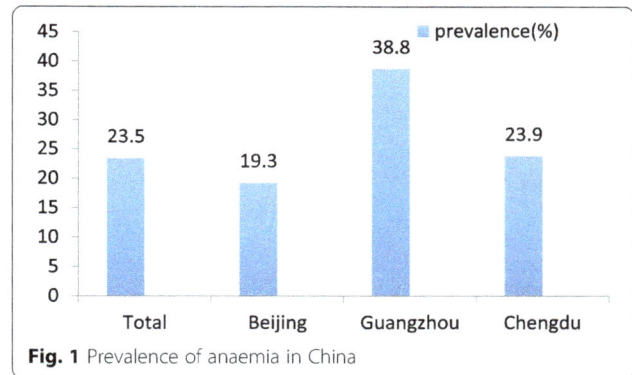

Fig. 1 Prevalence of anaemia in China

Factors associated with anaemia

A total of 26,255 women were included to evaluate the associated risk factors. Table 4 shows the maternal characteristics of the anaemia group versus the non-anaemia group. We found that the differences in maternal age, educational status, city, family monthly income, residence, pre-pregnancy BMI and parity were significant between anaemic and non-anaemic women (Table 5).

A binary logistic regression model was performed to identify the factors affecting maternal anaemia. After adjusted by other variables, maternal age ≥ 35 years (AOR = 1.386, 95%CI:1.103-1.742), women from Guangzhou (AOR = 7.293, 95%CI:5.455-9.751) or Chengdu (AOR = 2.147, 95%CI:2.174-3.777), family per capita monthly income < 1000 CNY (AOR = 1.671, 95%CI:1.291-2.162), rural residence (AOR = 1.308, 95%CI:1.095-1.563) and pre-pregnancy BMI < 18.5 kg/m^2 (AOR = 1.237, 95%CI:1.021-1.498) were the predictors of anaemia among the pregnant women (Table 6).

The risk of adverse pregnancy outcomes

We enrolled 39,439 women with singleton pregnancies. Table 7 shows the maternal characteristics of the anaemia group and the non-anaemia group. We found that the prevalence of polyhydramnios, preterm birth, low birth weight (< 2500 g), neonatal complications and NICU admission increased in the women with anaemia, while GDM, foetal distress and oligohydramnios increased in non-anaemic women (Table 8).

Table 1 Maternal demographic characteristics. Data are expressed as the means ± SDs or n (%)

Variables	Anaemic	Non-anaemic	Total
Pregnant women	10,199 (23.5%)	33,204 (76.5%)	43,403 (100.0%)
Maternal age (years)	29.50 ± 4.46	29.80 ± 4.19	29.73 ± 4.25
Gravidity	1.94 ± 1.20	1.85 ± 1.13	1.87 ± 1.15
Parity	0.78 ± 0.73	0.59 ± 0.67	0.64 ± 0.69
Pre-pregnancy BMI (kg/m^2)	20.57 ± 4.39	21.31 ± 4.41	21.13 ± 4.42
Pre-pregnancy height (cm)	54.00 ± 8.38	56.42 ± 9.18	55.85 ± 9.06
Pre-pregnancy weight (kg)	160.48 ± 4.96	161.56 ± 4.92	161.30 ± 4.95

Table 2 Hb level of three trimesters in pregnancy

	Number	Percent	Hb (g/L)	Testing time (week)
1st trimester	26,924	61.2	129.89 ± 9.90	10.65 ± 2.72
2nd trimester	33,879	77.0	118.99 ± 9.78	23.17 ± 3.39
3rd trimester	41,569	94.5	121.21 ± 12.62	37.24 ± 2.71

Table 3 Anaemia and its severity in three trimesters in pregnancy

	Total	Anaemia		Severity of anaemia					
				Mild		Moderate		Severe	
	N	N	%	N	%	N	%	N	%
1st trimester	26,924	732	2.7	567	77.5	165	22.5	0	–
2nd trimester	33,879	4996	14.7	4144	82.9	848	17.0	4	0.1
3rd trimester	41,569	6888	16.6	5073	73.6	1800	26.1	15	0.2

Discussion

Anaemia is one of the most common complications during pregnancy and could cause adverse pregnancy outcomes. It is a public health problem not only in developing but also in industrialized countries. In the present study, the overall prevalence of anaemia is 23.5%. According to the WHO classification of the public health importance of anaemia [3], it was a moderate public health problem among the pregnant women in our study. However, compared to the prevalence of anaemia in developed countries [5], it remains a severe health problem in China.

To our knowledge, this study is the first to compare the prevalence of anaemia in three big cities, which may partially represent the Western, Northern and Southern China. We found that the prevalence of anaemia in Guangzhou (38.8%) and Chengdu (23.9%) was significantly higher than the total, while it was lower in Beijing (19.3%). This prevalence was comparable to a study conducted in rural Western China (45.7%) [17]. The results may have been due to the different levels of local economic development, lifestyle, and diet, and may also be related to the altitude of the area.

Our study showed that the prevalence of anaemia increased with the progress of pregnancy. We found that the anaemia prevalence gradually increased from early pregnancy (2.7%) to middle pregnancy (14.7%), then became the highest in late pregnancy (16.6%). The change

Table 4 Maternal characteristics of the selected population. Data expressed as the means ± SDs or n (%)

Variables	Anaemic	Non-anaemic	Total
Haemoglobin (g/L)	103.31 ± 5.88	130.55 ± 8.89	129.80 ± 9.88
Gestation week (weeks)	11.32 ± 2.38	10.63 ± 2.73	10.65 ± 2.72
Maternal age (years)	29.91 ± 4.43	30.02 ± 3.93	30.01 ± 3.94
Gravidity	1.96 ± 1.21	1.77 ± 1.09	1.78 ± 1.10
Parity	0.83 ± 0.72	0.51 ± 0.63	0.52 ± 0.63
Pre-pregnancy BMI (kg/m²)	20.34 ± 3.88	21.23 ± 4.13	21.20 ± 4.13
Pre-pregnancy height (cm)	160.45 ± 4.67	161.77 ± 4.91	161.74 ± 4.91
Pre-pregnancy weight (kg)	53.00 ± 7.64	56.13 ± 8.76	56.05 ± 8.75

Table 5 Clinical variables in association with anaemia among pregnant women [N (%)]

Variables	Anaemic	Non-anaemic	χ^2	P-value
Pregnant women	719 (23.5%)	25,536 (76.5%)		
Maternal age				
< 20y	5 (8.2%)	56 (91.8%)	15.424	< 0.001*
20-35	616 (2.6%)	22,850 (97.4%)		
≥ 35	98 (3.6%)	2630 (96.4%)		
Educational status				
College and above	485 (2.3%)	20,168 (97.7%)	69.346	< 0.001*
Junior or senior	224 (4.5)	4748 (95.5%)		
Primary or illiteracy	3 (3.3%)	88 (96.7%)		
Cities				
Beijing	296 (1.6%)	17,951 (98.4%)	477.503	< 0.001*
Guangzhou	164 (10.5%)	1400 (89.5%)		
Chengdu	259 (4.0%)	6185 (96.0%)		
Family per capita monthly income (CNY)				
< 1000	140 (2.2%)	6170 (97.8%)	9.256	0.010*
1000-4999	262 (2.9%)	8667 (97.1%)		
≥ 5000	308 (2.9%)	10,141 (97.1%)		
Residence				
Urban	487 (2.4%)	19,671 (97.6%)	36.801	< 0.001*
Rural	226 (3.9%)	5580 (96.1%)		
Pre-pregnancy BMI (kg/m²)				
< 18.5	152 (3.6%)	4046 (96.4%)	35.163	< 0.001*
18.5-23.99	483 (2.8%)	17,737 (97.2%)		
24-27.99	62 (1.7%)	3589 (98.3%)		
≥ 28	13 (1.3%)	980 (98.7%)		
Parity				
0	246 (1.7%)	14,316 (98.3%)	148.303	< 0.001*
1-3	463 (4.0%)	11,101 (96.0%)		
≥ 4	8 (11.0%)	65 (89.0%)		

The results are reported as the frequency (percentage) and *P-value< 0.05 was statistically significant

in the haemoglobin level during the second trimester may be related to physiological changes during pregnancy, which is due to plasma dilution. In the third trimester, physiologically, the increased plasma volume velocity slows down and women may undergo routine antenatal care and iron supplementation, which will elevate the Hb level [18]. However, we found an increased prevalence in the third trimester, which may have been due to inadequate iron supplementation.

Considering the degree of anaemia, Desalegn et al. [19] reported that of 66 anaemic pregnant women, 40. 92% had mild, 54.54% had moderate, and 4.54% had severe anaemia. Another study showed that among 224 pregnant women, 37% women had anaemia (26% mild

Table 6 Predictors of anaemia among pregnant women

Variables	COR	95%CI	P-value	AOR	95%CI	P-value
Maternal age						
< 20y	3.312	1.322-8.297	0.011*	2.489	0.958-6.467	0.061
20-35	1			1		
≥ 35	1.382	1.113-1.717	0.003*	1.386	1.103-1.742	0.005*
Educational status						
College and above	1			–		
Junior or senior	0.705	0.222-2.237	0.553	–		
Primary or illiteracy	1.384	0.434-4.408	0.583	–		
Cities						
Beijing	1			1		
Guangzhou	7.104	5.826-8.663	< 0.001*	7.293	5.455-9.751	< 0.001*
Chengdu	2.540	2.144-3.008	< 0.001*	2.847	2.147-3.777	< 0.001*
Family per capita monthly income (RMB, CYN)						
< 1000	0.747	0.610-0.915	0.005*	1.671	1.291-2.162	< 0.001*
1000-4999	0.995	0.842-1.176	0.956	1.157	0.968-1.382	0.109
≥ 5000	1			1		
Residence						
Urban	1			1		
Rural	1.636	1.393-1.921	< 0.001*	1.308	1.095-1.563	0.003*
Pre-pregnancy BMI (kg/m^2)						
< 18.5	1.302	1.081-1.567	0.005	1.237	1.021-1.498	0.030*
18.5-23.99	1			1		
24-27.99	0.599	0.458-0.782	< 0.001*	0.662	0.506-0.867	0.003*
≥ 28	0.460	0.264-0.800	0.006*	0.506	0.283-0.906	0.022*
Parity						
0	1			1		
1-3	2.427	2.075-2.839	< 0.001*	1.071	0.842-1.363	0.576
≥ 4	7.162	3.400-15.089	< 0.001*	2.130	0.920-4.932	0.078

COR Crude Odds Ratio, AOR Adjusted Odds Ratio, CI Confidence interval
*P-value< 0.05 was statistically significant

Table 7 Maternal characteristics of the selected population. Data expressed as the means ± SDs or n (%)

Variables	Anaemic	Non-anaemic	Total
Pregnant women	6476 (16.4%)	32,963 (83.6%)	39,439 (100%)
Haemoglobin (g/L)	102.16 ± 6.64	125.09 ± 9.64	121.32 ± 12.53
Gestation week	22.65 ± 3.61	23.25 ± 3.36	23.17 ± 3.40
Maternal age (years)	29.21 ± 4.48	29.74 ± 4.18	29.66 ± 4.23
Gravidity	1.99 ± 1.21	1.83 ± 1.13	1.86 ± 1.14
Parity	0.86 ± 0.74	0.59 ± 0.67	0.63 ± 0.69
Pre-pregnancy BMI (kg/m^2)	20.48 ± 4.51	21.14 ± 4.33	21.04 ± 4.36
Pre-pregnancy height (cm)	160.39 ± 4.92	161.48 ± 4.92	161.30 ± 4.93
Pre-pregnancy weight (kg)	53.96 ± 8.30	55.93 ± 8.89	55.61 ± 8.83

Table 8 Adverse pregnancy outcomes in anaemic and non-anaemic women. [N (%)]

Variables	Anaemic	Non-anaemic	χ^2	P
Caesarean section	2986(46.1%)	15,031(45.6%)	0.565	0.452
GDM	1031(15.9%)	6575(19.9%)	56.368	< 0.001*
Hypertensive disorder	165 (2.5%)	863 (2.6%)	0.105	0.746
PROM	1319(20.4%)	7021 (21.3%)	2.820	0.093
Foetal distress	611(9.4%)	4119(12.5%)	48.049	< 0.001*
Placenta abruption	28 (0.40)	147(0.4%)	0.23	0.880
Polyhydramnios	125 (1.95)	386 (1.2%)	24.394	< 0.001*
Oligohydramnios	168 (2.6%)	1202 (3.6%)	17.876	< 0.001*
Preterm labour	529 (8.2%)	1600 (4.9%)	116.45	< 0.001*
Low birth weight (< 2500 g)	319 (4.9%)	1108(3.4%)	37.991	< 0.001*
Neonatal complications	687 (10.6%)	2501 (7.6%)	66.489	< 0.001*
NICU admission	631 (9.7%)	2000 (6.1%)	117.492	< 0.001*

*$P < 0.05$ is statistically significant

and 11% moderate). Our results showed findings similar to those studies.

The results of our study showed that pregnant women with lower family per capita income were more anaemic than the higher one. The higher prevalence of anaemia was also found among pregnant women from rural areas. The results of a study in Pakistan showed that patients with low income comprised a higher portion of patients with anaemia compared to those with a high income [20]. This is likely related to the lack of information about adequate nutrition during pregnancy, economic factors and the inaccessibility of health care centres. Interestingly, our study also indicated that pre-pregnancy BMI < 18.5 kg/m^2 was a predictor of anaemia, which may be due to the inadequate nutrition during pregnancy. Previous studies have shown an association of anaemia with low education status [5, 21] and multiparity [22]. However, we did not find this association in our study. This might have been due to variations in the methods and study subjects involved. These predictors of anaemia (including age, income, area, pre-pregnancy BMI) may provide clinical guidance. Women with these risk factors should appropriately increase their nutrition during pregnancy, and pregnant women diagnosed with anaemia should take iron supplements.

It has been suggested that anaemia in pregnancy is associated with an increased risk of adverse pregnancy outcomes, such as preterm birth, hypertensive disorders, and low birth weight [13, 23, 24]. Preterm labour and low birth weight have been reported to be suboptimal pregnancy outcomes of anaemia in previous studies [8, 25, 26]. These results were in accordance with our findings. We also found that an increase of NICU admission in anaemic women. This may be due to the higher prevalence of preterm birth and low

birth weight in anaemic women than non-anaemic women.

The association between GDM and anaemia has not been well reported. In our study, we observed that anaemia reduced the prevalence of GDM. Lao et al. [27] reported that the prevalence of GDM is reduced in iron deficiency anaemia. These results indicate that haemoglobin level is positively associated with the prevalence of GDM. Our study also first reported that anaemia is associated with polyhydramnios, which may occur in parallel with the GDM outcome.

Although the sample size and the study sites included 21 centres in China, there may be bias in our results, as the data were collected in a retrospective manner. Studies reported that the inter pregnancy interval [22] and history of parasitic infection [7, 28] were associated with the prevalence of anemia, which could not be estimated in this study due to the lake of the factors. Recent studies noted that both low and high iron intake was associated with mortality among women [29] and elevated iron level may increase the risk of GDM [30]. However, the present study did not record the iron supplementation of the participants, which may have impacted the results of adverse pregnancy outcomes of anaemia.

Conclusion

This study showed that anaemia in pregnancy continues to be a health problem in China, and economic factors may contribute to the situation. Therefore, we should vigorously promote early prenatal care for these at-risk pregnant women. This would allow for iron and folic acid supplementation during pregnancy, which would potentially reduce the prevalence of anaemia.

Abbreviations

75 g OGTT: 75 g oral glucose tolerance test; AOR: Adjusted odds ratio; BMI: Body mass index; CI: Confidence interval; CNY: China Yuan; COR: Crude odds ratio; GDM: Gestational diabetes mellitus; GPS study: Gestational diabetes mellitus Prevalence Survey study; Hb: Haemoglobin; HELLP syndrome: Haemolysis, elevated liver enzymes and low platelet syndrome; LMP: Last menstrual period; NICU: Neonatal Intensive Care Unit; OR: Odds ratio; PGDM: Pre-pregnancy diabetes mellitus; PROM: Premature rupture of membranes; SD: Standard deviation

Acknowledgements

We appreciate all the investigators' efforts in data collection. We acknowledge and thank the GPS study group for providing medical records from the 21 hospitals.

Funding

The study was supported by the World Diabetes Foundation (Grant no. WDF10-517) and (Grant no. WDF14-908), Beijing Municipal Science and Technology Project (Z151100001615051) and National Key Technology Research and Development Program of China (2015BAI13B06). These funding bodies accepted the study as proposed and played roles in protocol development, data collection, analysis and manuscript writing.

Authors' contributions

LL collected the data, conducted the data analysis and prepared the manuscript; HY, YW and WZ contributed to the design and analysis of the study; and CW, RS and HF were involved in the collection of the data. All authors have read and approved the final version of the manuscript.

Competing interests

The authors declare that they have no competing interests.

Author details

[1]Department of Obstetrics and Gynaecology, Peking University First Hospital, Xi'anmen Street No.1, Xicheng District, Beijing 100034, China. [2]National Institute of Hospital Administration, Beijing 100191, China.

References

1. Grewal A. Anaemia and pregnancy: Anaesthetic implications. Indian J Anaesth. 2010;54(5):380–6.
2. Stevens GA, Finucane MM, De-Regil LM, Paciorek CJ, Flaxman SR, Branca F, et al. Global, regional, and national trends in haemoglobin concentration and prevalence of total and severe anaemia in children and pregnant and non-pregnant women for 1995-2011: a systematic analysis of population-representative data. Lancet Glob Health. 2013;1(1):e16–25.
3. WHO. Haemoglobin concentrations for the diagnosis of anaemia and assessment of severity. Edited by World Health Organization. 2011 Available online from: http://apps.who.int/iris/bitstream/10665/85839/3/WHO_NMH_NHD_MNM_11.1_eng.pdf.
4. World Health Organization. Worldwide prevalence of anaemia 1993–2005: WHO global database on anaemia. Edited by Bruno de Benoist, Erin McLean, Ines Egli and Mary Cogswell. 2008 Available online from: http://apps.who.int/iris/bitstream/10665/43894/1/9789241596657_eng.pdf.
5. Balarajan Y, Ramakrishnan U, Ozaltin E, Shankar AH, Subramanian SV. Anaemia in low-income and middle-income countries. Lancet. 2011; 378(9809):2123–35.
6. Gebre A, Mulugeta A. Prevalence of anemia and associated factors among pregnant women in north western zone of Tigray, Northern Ethiopia: a cross-sectional study. J Nutr Metab. 2015;2015:165430.
7. Kefiyalew F, Zemene E, Asres Y, Gedefaw L. Anemia among pregnant women in Southeast Ethiopia: prevalence, severity and associated risk factors. BMC Res Notes. 2014;7:771.
8. Levy A, Fraser D, Katz M, Mazor M, Sheiner E. Maternal anemia during pregnancy is an independent risk factor for low birthweight and preterm delivery. Eur J Obstet Gynecol Reprod Biol. 2005;122(2):182–6.
9. Banhidy F, Acs N, Puho EH, Czeizel AE. Iron deficiency anemia: pregnancy outcomes with or without iron supplementation. Nutrition. 2011;27(1):65–72.
10. Haas JD, Brownlie T. Iron deficiency and reduced work capacity: a critical review of the research to determine a causal relationship. J Nutr. 2001; 131(2S-2):676S–88S. discussion 688S-690S
11. Chesley LC. Plasma and red cell volumes during pregnancy. Am J Obstet Gynecol. 1972;112(3):440–50.
12. Goodlin RC. Maternal plasma volume and disorders of pregnancy. Br Med J (Clin Res Ed). 1984;288(6428):1454–5.
13. Haider BA, Olofin I, Wang M, Spiegelman D, Ezzati M, Fawzi WW. Anaemia, prenatal iron use, and risk of adverse pregnancy outcomes: systematic review and meta-analysis. BMJ. 2013;f3443:346.
14. Wang C, Zhu W, Wei Y, Su R, Feng H, Lin L, et al. The predictive effects of early pregnancy lipid profiles and fasting glucose on the risk of gestational diabetes mellitus stratified by body mass index. J Diabetes Res. 2016;2016: 3013567.
15. WHO Expert Consultation. Appropriate body-mass index for Asian populations and its implications for policy and intervention strategies. Lancet. 2004;363(9403):157–63.
16. Yang HX. Diagnostic criteria for gestational diabetes mellitus (WS 331-2011). Chin Med J. 2012;125(7):1212–3.
17. Pei L, Ren L, Wang D, Yan H. Assessment of maternal anemia in rural Western China between 2001 and 2005: a two-level logistic regression approach. BMC Public Health. 2013;13:366.
18. Scholl TO. Iron status during pregnancy: setting the stage for mother and infant. Am J Clin Nutr. 2005;81(5):1218s–22s.
19. Desalegn S. Prevalence of anaemia in pregnancy in Jima town, southwestern Ethiopia. Ethio Med J. 1993;31(4):251–8.
20. Ayub R, Tariq N, Adil MM, Iqbal M, Jaferry T, Rais SR. Low haemoglobin levels, its determinants and associated features among pregnant women in Islamabad and surrounding region. J Pak Med Assoc. 2009;59(2):86–9.
21. Chowdhury HA, Ahmed KR, Jebunessa F, Akter J, Hossain S, Shahjahan M. Factors associated with maternal anaemia among pregnant women in Dhaka city. BMC Womens Health. 2015;15:77.
22. Obse N, Mossie A, Gobena T. Magnitude of anemia and associated risk factors among pregnant women attending antenatal care in Shalla Woreda, West Arsi Zone, Oromia Region, Ethiopia. Ethio J Health Sci. 2013;23(2):165–73.
23. Xiong X, Buekens P, Alexander S, Demianczuk N, Wollast E. Anemia during pregnancy and birth outcome: a meta-analysis. Am J Perinatol. 2000;17(3):137–46.
24. Pena-Rosas JP, De-Regil LM, Garcia-Casal MN, Dowswell T. Daily oral iron supplementation during pregnancy. Cochrane Database Syst Rev. 2015;7: CD004736.
25. Malhotra M, Sharma JB, Batra S, Sharma S, Murthy NS, Arora R. Maternal and perinatal outcome in varying degrees of anemia. Int J Gynaecol Obstet. 2002;79(2):93–100.
26. Scholl TO, Hediger ML, Fischer RL, Shearer JW. Anemia vs iron deficiency: increased risk of preterm delivery in a prospective study. Am J Clin Nutr. 1992;55(5):985–8.
27. Lao TT, Ho LF. Impact of iron deficiency anemia on prevalence of gestational diabetes mellitus. Diabetes Care. 2004;27(3):650–6.
28. Getachew M, Yewhalaw D, Tafess K, Getachew Y, Zeynudin A. Anaemia and associated risk factors among pregnant women in Gilgel Gibe dam area, Southwest Ethiopia. Parasit Vectors. 2012;5:296.
29. Shi Z, Zhen S, Zhou Y, Taylor AW. Hb level, iron intake and mortality in Chinese adults: a 10-year follow-up study. Br J Nutr. 2017;117(4):572–81.
30. Rawal S, Hinkle SN, Bao W, Zhu Y, Grewal J, Albert PS, et al. A longitudinal study of iron status during pregnancy and the risk of gestational diabetes: findings from a prospective, multiracial cohort. Diabetologia. 2017;60(2):249–57.

Permissions

All chapters in this book were first published in P&C, by BioMed Central; hereby published with permission under the Creative Commons Attribution License or equivalent. Every chapter published in this book has been scrutinized by our experts. Their significance has been extensively debated. The topics covered herein carry significant findings which will fuel the growth of the discipline. They may even be implemented as practical applications or may be referred to as a beginning point for another development.

The contributors of this book come from diverse backgrounds, making this book a truly international effort. This book will bring forth new frontiers with its revolutionizing research information and detailed analysis of the nascent developments around the world.

We would like to thank all the contributing authors for lending their expertise to make the book truly unique. They have played a crucial role in the development of this book. Without their invaluable contributions this book wouldn't have been possible. They have made vital efforts to compile up to date information on the varied aspects of this subject to make this book a valuable addition to the collection of many professionals and students.

This book was conceptualized with the vision of imparting up-to-date information and advanced data in this field. To ensure the same, a matchless editorial board was set up. Every individual on the board went through rigorous rounds of assessment to prove their worth. After which they invested a large part of their time researching and compiling the most relevant data for our readers.

The editorial board has been involved in producing this book since its inception. They have spent rigorous hours researching and exploring the diverse topics which have resulted in the successful publishing of this book. They have passed on their knowledge of decades through this book. To expedite this challenging task, the publisher supported the team at every step. A small team of assistant editors was also appointed to further simplify the editing procedure and attain best results for the readers.

Apart from the editorial board, the designing team has also invested a significant amount of their time in understanding the subject and creating the most relevant covers. They scrutinized every image to scout for the most suitable representation of the subject and create an appropriate cover for the book.

The publishing team has been an ardent support to the editorial, designing and production team. Their endless efforts to recruit the best for this project, has resulted in the accomplishment of this book. They are a veteran in the field of academics and their pool of knowledge is as vast as their experience in printing. Their expertise and guidance has proved useful at every step. Their uncompromising quality standards have made this book an exceptional effort. Their encouragement from time to time has been an inspiration for everyone.

The publisher and the editorial board hope that this book will prove to be a valuable piece of knowledge for researchers, students, practitioners and scholars across the globe.

List of Contributors

Gordon Abekah-Nkrumah
Department of Public Administration and Health Services Management, University of Ghana Business School, Legon, Accra, Ghana

Lilian Mselle
Muhimbili University of Health and Allied Sciences, School of Nursing, Dar es salaam, Tanzania

Gorrette Nalwadda
Department of Nursing, Makerere University, Kampala, Uganda

Mike Kagawa
Department of Obstetrics and Gynecology, Makerere University, Kampala, Uganda

Khadija Malima
Tanzania Commission for Science and Technology, Dar es Salaam, Tanzania

Shigeko Horiuchi
St. Luke's International University, 10-1 Akashi-cho, Chuo-ku, Tokyo 104-0044, Japan

Putu Duff
British Columbia Centre for Excellence in HIV/AIDS, St. Paul's Hospital, 608-1081 Burrard Street, Vancouver, BC, Canada
Department of Medicine, University of British Columbia, St. Paul's Hospital, 608-1081 Burrard Street, Vancouver, BC, Canada
Kirby Institute for Infection and Immunity (formerly the National Centre in HIV Epidemiology and Clinical Research), UNSW Australia I, Wallace Wurth Building, Sydney, NSW 2052, Australia

Jennifer L. Evans and Ellen S. Stein
Institute for Global Health, Department of Epidemiology, University of California-San Francisco, San Francisco, California, USA

Lisa Maher
Kirby Institute for Infection and Immunity (formerly the National Centre in HIV Epidemiology and Clinical Research), UNSW Australia I, Wallace Wurth Building, Sydney, NSW 2052, Australia

Kimberly Page
Institute for Global Health, Department of Epidemiology, University of California-San Francisco, San Francisco, California, USA
Division of Epidemiology, Biostatistics and Preventive Medicine, Department of Internal Medicine, University of New Mexico Health Sciences Center, Albuquerque, NM, USA

Jerry Ictho, Jean Nyamwiza, Emmanuel Lako Ernesto Loro, John Mukisa, Angella Musewa, Annet Nalutaaya, Ronald Ssenyonga, Ismael Kawooya and Benjamin Temper
Clinical Epidemiology Unit, Makerere University College of Health Sciences, Kampala, Uganda

Sam Ali
Clinical Epidemiology Unit, Makerere University College of Health Sciences, Kampala, Uganda
Department of Radiology, UMC Victoria Hospital Bukoto, Kampala, Uganda

Rosemary Kusaba Byanyima
Department of Radiology, Mulago Hospital Complex, Kampala, Uganda

Sam Ononge
Department of Obstetrics and Gynaecology, Makerere University College of Health Sciences, Kampala, Uganda

Achilles Katamba
Clinical Epidemiology Unit, Makerere University College of Health Sciences, Kampala, Uganda
Department of Medicine, Makerere University College of Health Sciences, Kampala, Uganda

Joan Kalyango
Clinical Epidemiology Unit, Makerere University College of Health Sciences, Kampala, Uganda
Department of Pharmacy, Makerere University College of Health Sciences, Kampala, Uganda

Charles Karamagi
Clinical Epidemiology Unit, Makerere University College of Health Sciences, Kampala, Uganda
Department of Pediatrics and Child Health, Makerere University College of Health Sciences, Kampala, Uganda

Beatrice Mwilike
Muhimbili University of Health and Allied Sciences, School of Nursing, Dar es salaam, Tanzania
St. Luke's International University, 10-1 Akashi-cho, Chuo-ku, Tokyo 104-0044, Japan

Kathryn L. Andersen and Valerie Acre
Ipas, 300 Market Street, Suite 200, Chapel Hill, NC 27516, USA

Mary Fjerstad
San Diego, CA, USA

Indira Basnett and Sharad Sharma
Kathmandu, Nepal

Shailes Neupane
Valley Research Group (VaRG), Lalitpur, Nepal

Emily Jackson
Los Angeles, CA, USA

Deirdre O'Malley
Health Research Board, Research Fellow, School of Nursing and Midwifery, Trinity College Dublin, Dublin, Ireland

Agnes Higgins, Deirdre Daly and Valerie Smith
School of Nursing and Midwifery, Trinity College Dublin, Dublin, Ireland

Cecily Begley
School of Nursing and Midwifery, Trinity College Dublin, Dublin, Ireland
Institute of Health and Care Sciences, The Sahlgrenska Academy, University of Gothenburg, Gothenburg, Sweden

Elizabeth R. Bertone-Johnson, Penelope Pekow and Lisa Chasan-Taber
Department of Biostatistics & Epidemiology, School of Public Health & Health Sciences, University of Massachusetts, 414 Arnold House, 715 North Pleasant Street, Amherst, MA 01003-9304, USA

Sally Powers
Department of Psychological and Brain Sciences, University of Massachusetts, Amherst, MA, USA

Glenn Markenson
Baystate Medical Center, Springfield, MA, USA

Nancy Dole
Carolina Population Center, University of North Carolina at Chapel Hill, Chapel Hill, NC, USA

Kathleen Szegda
Department of Biostatistics & Epidemiology, School of Public Health & Health Sciences, University of Massachusetts, 414 Arnold House, 715 North Pleasant Street, Amherst, MA 01003-9304, USA
Baystate Medical Center, Springfield, MA, USA
Public Health Institute of Western Massachusetts, Springfield, MA, USA

Han van Dijk
Sociology of Development and Change Group, Wageningen University, Hollandsweg 1, 6700 EW Wageningen, Netherlands

Irene A. Agyepong
Dodowa Health Research Centre, Research & Development Division, Ghana Health Service, Dodowa-Accra, Ghana

Linda L. Yevoo
Sociology of Development and Change Group, Wageningen University, Hollandsweg 1, 6700 EW Wageningen, Netherlands Dodowa Health Research Centre, Research & Development Division, Ghana Health Service, Dodowa-Accra, Ghana

Trudie Gerrits
Graduate School of Social Sciences, Kloveiersburgwal 48 1012 CX Amsterdam, University of Amsterdam, Amsterdam, Netherlands

Satu Jokela, Eero Lilja and Anu E. Castaneda
Department of Welfare, National Institute for Health and Welfare, Mannerheimintie 166, 00271 Helsinki, PL 30, Finland

Tarja I. Kinnunen
Faculty of Social Sciences, University of Tampere, PL 100, Arvo Ylpön katu 34, Tampere 33520, Finland

Mika Gissler
Department of Information Services, National Institute for Health and Welfare, PL 30, Mannerheimintie 166, Helsinki 00271, Finland
Department of Neurobiology, Care Sciences and Society, Division of Family Medicine, Karolinska Institute, Stockholm, Sweden

Päivikki Koponen
Department of Public Health Solutions, National Institute for Health and Welfare, Mannerheimintie 166, 00271 Helsinki, PL 30, Finland

Dagne Addisu
Department of midwifery, College of medicine and health science, Debre Tabor University, Debre Tabor, Ethiopia

Azezu Asres and Simegnew Asmer
Department of midwifery, College of medicine and health science, Bahir Dar University, Bahir Dar, Ethiopia

Getnet Gedefaw
Department of midwifery, College of medicine and health science, Wolidia University, Wolidia, Ethiopia

Itzel N. Alvarado-Maldonado
Division of Reproductive Medicine, Instituto Nacional de Perinatología Isidro Espinosa de los Reyes, Mexico City, Mexico

Alfredo Castillo-Mora, Carlos Ortega-González, Nayeli Martínez-Cruz, Lidia Arce-Sánchez and Mabel Ramos-Valencia
Department of Endocrinology, Instituto Nacional de Perinatología Isidro Espinosa de los Reyes, Mexico City, Mexico

Anayansi Molina-Hernández
Departament of Physiology and Cellular Development, Instituto Nacional de Perinatología Isidro Espinosa de los Reyes, Mexico City, Mexico

Guadalupe Estrada-Gutierrez
Direction of Research, Instituto Nacional de Perinatología Isidro Espinosa de los Reyes, Mexico City, Mexico

Salvador Espino Y. Sosa
Division of Clinical Research, Instituto Nacional de Perinatología Isidro Espinosa de los Reyes, Mexico City, Mexico

Enrique Reyes-Muñoz
Division of Obstetrics and Gynecology, Hospital Regional Universitario de Colima, Colima, Mexico

Ruth Hernández-Sánchez
Department of Gynecological and Perinatal Endocrinology, Instituto Nacional de Perinatología Isidro Espinosa de los Reyes, Montes Urales 800, Lomas Virreyes, Miguel Hidalgo, CP 11000 Mexico City, DF, Mexico

Cristina M. Sánchez-González and Yesenia Recio-López
Division of Reproductive Medicine, Instituto Nacional de Perinatología Isidro Espinosa de los Reyes, Mexico City, Mexico
Programa de Maestría en Ciencias Médicas de la Universidad Anáhuac Norte, Mexico City, Mexico

Sucheta Mehra, Lee Shu-Fune Wu, Alain B. Labrique, Rolf D. W. Klemm, Keith P. West Jr and Parul Christian
Center for Human Nutrition, Department of International Health, Johns Hopkins Bloomberg School of Public Health, 615 North Wolfe St., Room E2519, Baltimore, MD 21205-2179, USA

Donna M. Strobino
Department of Population, Family and Reproductive Health, Johns Hopkins Bloomberg School of Public Health, Baltimore, MD 21205-2179, USA

Pamela J. Surkan
Center for Human Nutrition, Department of International Health, Johns Hopkins Bloomberg School of Public Health, 615 North Wolfe St., Room E2519, Baltimore, MD 21205-2179, USA
Department of Population, Family and Reproductive Health, Johns Hopkins Bloomberg School of Public Health, Baltimore, MD 21205-2179, USA

Abu Ahmed Shamim, Mahbubur Rashid, Hasmot Ali and Barkat Ullah
The JiVitA Project, Johns Hopkins University in Bangladesh, Gaibandha, Bangladesh

Nang Thu Thu Kyaw and Myo Minn Oo
Department of Operational Research, International Union Against Tuberculosis and Lung Disease (The Union), Mandalay, Myanmar

Srinath Satyanarayana
Center for Operational Research, International Union Against Tuberculosis and Lung disease (The Union), Paris, France

Khaing Hnin Phyo, Aye Aye Mon and Thet Ko Aung
HIV unit, International Union Against Tuberculosis and Lung Disease (The Union), Mandalay, Myanmar

Than Than Lwin, Zaw Zaw Aung, Nang Seng Noon Kham and Htun Nyunt Oo
National AIDS Programme, Department of Public Health, Ministry of Health and Sports, Nay Pyi Taw, Myanmar

Thurain Htun
Monitoring, Evaluation, Accountability and Learning Unit, HIV, International Union Against Tuberculosis and Lung Disease (The Union), Mandalay, Myanmar

Theingi Mya
Department of Obstetrics and Gynecology, Central Women Hospital, Mandalay, Myanmar

Ajay M. V. Kumar
Center for Operational Research, International Union Against Tuberculosis and Lung disease (The Union), Paris, France
Department of Operational Research, International Union Against Tuberculosis and Lung Disease (The Union), Delhi, India

Khine Wut Yee Kyaw
Department of Operational Research, International Union Against Tuberculosis and Lung Disease (The Union), Mandalay, Myanmar

Oluwasegun Jko Ogundele and Milena Pavlova
Department of Health Services Research, CAPHRI, Maastricht University Medical Center, Faculty of Health, Medicine and Life Sciences, Maastricht University, 6200MD Maastricht, The Netherlands

Wim Groot
Department of Health Services Research, CAPHRI, Maastricht University Medical Center, Faculty of Health, Medicine and Life Sciences, Maastricht University, 6200MD Maastricht, The Netherlands
Top Institute Evidence-Based Education Research (TIER), Maastricht University, Maastricht, The Netherlands

Ola Jahanpour
Institute of Public Health, Department of Epidemiology and Biostatistics, Kilimanjaro Christian Medical University College (KCMUCo), Moshi, Tanzania

Sia E. Msuya
Institute of Public Health, Department of Epidemiology and Biostatistics, Kilimanjaro Christian Medical University College (KCMUCo), Moshi, Tanzania
Department of Community Medicine, Kilimanjaro Christian Medical Centre (KCMC), Moshi, Tanzania
Better Health for African Mother and Child (BHAMC), Moshi, Tanzania

Jim Todd
Institute of Public Health, Department of Epidemiology and Biostatistics, Kilimanjaro Christian Medical University College (KCMUCo), Moshi, Tanzania
London School of Hygiene and Tropical Medicine, bloomsbury, UK

Babill Stray-Pedersen
Division of Women, Oslo University Hospital, University of Oslo, Oslo, Norway
Institute of Clinical Medicine, University of Oslo, Oslo, Norway

Melina Mgongo
Institute of Public Health, Department of Epidemiology and Biostatistics, Kilimanjaro Christian Medical University College (KCMUCo), Moshi, Tanzania
Better Health for African Mother and Child (BHAMC), Moshi, Tanzania
Institute of Clinical Medicine, University of Oslo, Oslo, Norway

Elizabeth A. Claydon, Danielle M. Davidov and Keith J. Zullig
Department of Social & Behavioral Sciences, West Virginia University School of Public Health, Robert C. Byrd Health Sciences Center, West Virginia University, One Medical Center Drive, Morgantown, WV 26506-9190, USA

Christa L. Lilly
Department of Biostatistics, West Virginia University School of Public Health, Morgantown, WV, USA

Lesley Cottrell
Department of Social & Behavioral Sciences, West Virginia University School of Public Health, Robert C. Byrd Health Sciences Center, West Virginia University, One Medical Center Drive, Morgantown, WV 26506-9190, USA Department of Pediatrics, West Virginia University School of Medicine, Morgantown, WV, USA

Stephanie C. Zerwas
Department of Biostatistics, West Virginia University School of Public Health, Morgantown, WV, USA Department of Psychiatry, UNC School of Medicine, Chapel Hill, NC, USA

Rajan Paudel
Department of Community Medicine and Public Health, Maharajgunj Medical Campus, Institute of Medicine, Tribhuvan University, Kathmandu, Nepal

Kwan Lee and Seok-Ju Yoo
Department of Preventive Medicine, College of Medicine, Dongguk University, 123 Dongdae-ro, Gyeongju-si 38066, Republic of Korea

Jitendra Kumar Singh
Department of Community Medicine and Public Health, Janaki Medical College, Tribhuvan University, Janakpur, Nepal

Rajendra Kadel
Personal Social Services Research Unit, London School of Economics and Political Science, London, UK

Samaj Adhikari
Maharajgunj Medical Campus, Institute of Medicine, Tribhuvan University, Kathmandu, Nepal

Mohan Paudel
Southgate Institute for Health, Society and Equity, Flinders University, Adelaide, Australia

Narayan Mahotra
Department of Physiology, Maharajgunj Medical Campus, Institute of Medicine, Tribhuvan University, Kathmandu, Nepal

Dilaram Acharya
Department of Preventive Medicine, College of Medicine, Dongguk University, 123 Dongdae-ro, Gyeongju-si 38066, Republic of Korea Department of Community Medicine, Kathmandu University, Devdaha Medical College and Research Institute, Rupandehi, Nepal

Virginie Scotet, Marianne Uguen and Carine L'Hostis
UMR1078 "Génétique, Génomique Fonctionnelle et Biotechnologies", Inserm, EFS, Université de Brest, ISBAM, 22 avenue Camille Desmoulins, 29200 Brest, France

Philippe Saliou
UMR1078 "Génétique, Génomique Fonctionnelle et Biotechnologies", Inserm, EFS, Université de Brest, ISBAM, 22 avenue Camille Desmoulins, 29200 Brest, France Laboratoire d'Hygiene et de Sante Publique, Hopital Morvan, Brest, France

Marie-Christine Merour, Céline Triponey and Brigitte Chanu
Etablissement Français du Sang – Bretagne, Site de Brest, Brest, France

Jean-Baptiste Nousbaum
UMR1078 "Génétique, Génomique Fonctionnelle et Biotechnologies", Inserm, EFS, Université de Brest, ISBAM, 22 avenue Camille Desmoulins, 29200 Brest, France Service d'Hepato-Gastroenterologie, Hopital La Cavale Blanche, Brest, France

Gerald Le Gac
UMR1078 "Génétique, Génomique Fonctionnelle et Biotechnologies", Inserm, EFS, Université de Brest, ISBAM, 22 avenue Camille Desmoulins, 29200 Brest, France Laboratoire de Genetique Moleculaire et d'Histocompatibilite, Hopital Morvan, Brest, France

Claude Ferec
UMR1078 "Génétique, Génomique Fonctionnelle et Biotechnologies", Inserm, EFS, Université de Brest, ISBAM, 22 avenue Camille Desmoulins, 29200 Brest, France Etablissement Français du Sang – Bretagne, Site de Brest, Brest, France Laboratoire de Genetique Moleculaire et d'Histocompatibilite, Hopital Morvan, Brest, France

Maxine Johnson, Barbara Whelan, Clare Relton, Kate Thomas, Mark Strong and Elaine Scott
School of Health and Related Research (ScHARR), University of Sheffield, Sheffield, UK

Mary J. Renfrew
Mother and Infant Research Unit, School of Nursing and Health Sciences, University of Dundee, Dundee, UK

Ingvil Krarup Sørbye and Lise C. Gaudernack
Department of Obstetrics, Oslo University Hospital Rikshospitalet, Nydalen, 0424 Oslo, Norway

Mirjam Lukasse
Oslo and Akershus University College, Faculty of Health Sciences, Department of Nursing and Health Promotion, 0130 Oslo, Norway

Kjersti Engen Marsdal
Department of Obstetrics, Oslo University Hospital Rikshospitalet, Nydalen, 0424 Oslo, Norway
Oslo and Akershus University College, Faculty of Health Sciences, Department of Nursing and Health Promotion, 0130 Oslo, Norway

Li Lin, Yumei Wei, Chen Wang, Rina Su, Hui Feng and Huixia Yang
Department of Obstetrics and Gynaecology, Peking University First Hospital, Xi'anmen Street No.1, Xicheng District, Beijing 100034, China

Weiwei Zhu
National Institute of Hospital Administration, Beijing 100191, China

Index

www.ingramcontent.com/pod-product-compliance
Lightning Source LLC
Chambersburg PA
CBHW082037190326
41458CB00010B/3388